KEYGUIDE TO INFORMATION SOURCES IN

Dentistry

KEYGUIDE TO INFORMATION SOURCES IN

Dentistry

Margaret A. Clennett

MANSELL PUBLISHING LIMITED
London and New York

First published 1985 by Mansell Publishing Limited
(A subsidiary of The H. W. Wilson Company)
6 All Saints Street, London N1 9RL, England
950 University Avenue, Bronx, New York 10452, U.S.A.

British Library Cataloguing in Publication Data

Clennett, Margaret A.
Keyguide to information sources in
dentistry.—(Keyguides)
1. Dentistry—Bibliography 2. Dentistry—Information services
I. Title II. Series
617.6'007 Z6668

ISBN 0-7201-1747-X

Library of Congress Cataloging in Publication Data

Clennett, Margaret A.
Keyguide to information sources in dentistry.

Includes index.
1. Dentistry—Bibliography. 2. Dentistry—Abstracts.
3. Dentistry—Directories. 4. Dentistry—Information
services. I. Title. [DNLM: 1. Dentistry—abstracts.
2. Dentistry—directories. 3. Information Services.
ZWU 100 C627k]
Z6668.C55 1985 [RK51] 016.6176. 85-21373

ISBN 0-7201-1747-X

Typeset by Latimer Trend & Company Ltd, Plymouth
Printed in Great Britain by Whitstable Litho Ltd., Whitstable, Kent

For CMC, DNC and PS

Contents

Introduction

When I was appointed Librarian of the Institute of Dental Surgery in 1973, I was at first bemused by the range of material available, and mystified by the terminology. In many ways, therefore, this *Keyguide* is the sort of book I would have liked to have had on the shelf at that time, and I trust that librarians today who are not familiar with dentistry will find that it answers many of their questions. It is intended to offer the information worker or non-dental researcher an overview of the major sources in the field as a whole, and in specialized subject areas. The dentist beginning research, or one who is interested in a speciality other than his own, will find the subject sections of particular interest.

Part I comprises a narrative description of the kinds of information sources available, such as indexing services, journals and directories. Chapter 1, on the history and scope of dentistry, will be of particular interest to the non-dentist, while research workers will find in Chapter 4 a critique on the *Index to dental literature*, dentistry's principal indexing tool.

Part II contains annotated entries for sources relating to dentistry in general, and its component specialities. Core journals and major specialist serials, in a range of languages, are included. For monographs and textbooks the emphasis is, however, on English-language titles, and these lists are not intended to be comprehensive. Titles which are listed are regarded as important contributions to the field, or have already demonstrated their value or usefulness to the reader.

Part III is an address directory, with listings for national associations, dental schools, and selected libraries, associations and publishers. Although it was correct at the time of going to press, secretaries of societies regularly change and some addresses may therefore be out of date.

Acknowledgements

I am indebted to the many people who have given advice and assistance during the preparation of this book, notably the former and present staff of the Institute of Dental Surgery, Eastman Dental Hospital, who have provided valuable assistance with the subject sections in Part II. I am particularly grateful in this respect for the comments and advice given by Dr. R. D. Holt, Mr. R. J. Ibbetson and Miss S. M. Wright. Dr. S. Gelbier gave support with the historical sections. Finally, thanks are due to Mr. G. Bolas, who spent considerable time on scrutiny and suggestions with respect to Chapter 1.

PART I

Survey of dentistry and its literature

1 The History and Scope of Dentistry

1.1 Historical Introduction

A precise date when dental disease was first described and treated cannot be identified, but as early as 4000 BC the ancient Egyptians were using an assortment of remedies to treat afflictions of the mouth. The Chinese, around 2000 BC, described toothache and gum diseases, and the Etruscans, around 800 BC, have left specimens of restorative dentistry. Around 400 BC Hippocrates wrote about dental treatment in the Greek civilization. In the period of the Roman Empire in the first century AD Celsus described tooth extraction and Martial reported on the wearing of artificial teeth.

Later, in Western Europe the clergy undertook medicinal work, until in 1163 the Pope prohibited priests from performing any operation that drew blood. As a result, extractions became a function of the barbers, and by the fourteenth century guilds of barber-surgeons had evolved with rules governing the conduct of their members, in keeping with the general movement towards organized trade guilds. As there were insufficient numbers of barbers, extractions were also undertaken by itinerant tooth drawers, who appeared, garishly dressed, at fairs and markets throughout Europe. It is during this period of history that documentary evidence of dental practice becomes more plentiful, with contemporary paintings, drawings and cartoons depicting the scene; *Figure 1.1* is an example.

It was common for the teeth to be discussed in medical texts before the sixteenth century, but the first book devoted entirely to dentistry was a text intended for the general public, the *Artzney Buchlein*, published in Leipzig in 1530. Eustachius produced his *Libellus de dentibus* in 1563, and gave the first accurate

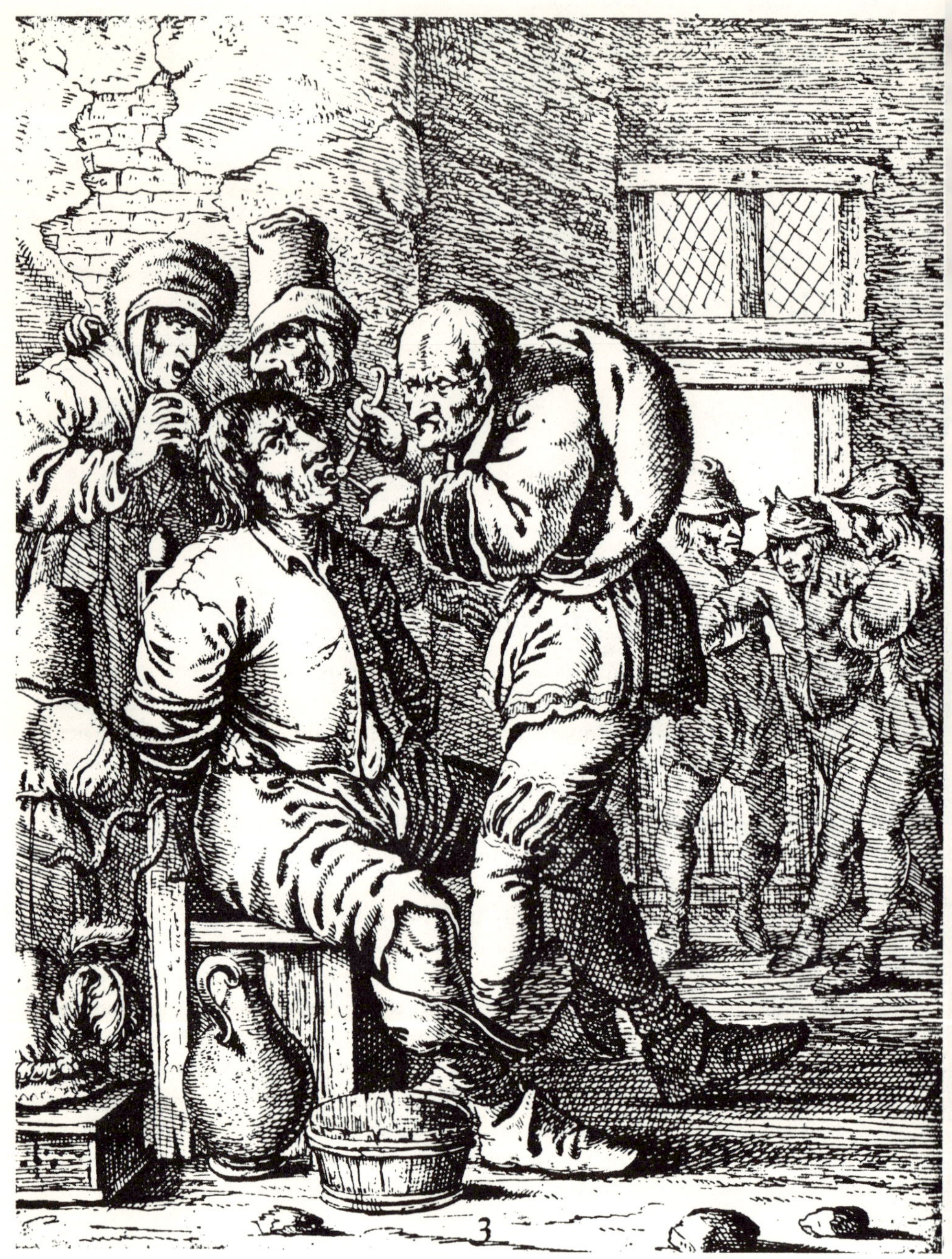

Figure 1.1 'Das Gefühl' by Adriaen Brouwer (1606–1638).

acccount of the anatomy of the teeth. The first book on dentistry to be written in English was Charles Allen's *Operator for the teeth*, published in York in 1685.

Pierre Fauchard is acknowledged as the father of modern dentistry, mainly because of the techniques expounded in his book *Le chirurgien dentiste*, published in 1728. He stressed the importance of sound teeth and described appliances to straighten crooked ones, and the manufacture of dentures. Later in the eighteenth century John Hunter, the Scottish anatomist and surgeon, celebrated for his research work, turned his attention to the mouth, and in 1771 published his classic work on anatomy and physiology, *Natural history of the human teeth*. Hunter recommended that surgeon-dentists should receive lectures on dentistry, and these were started by William Rae in 1782. On a more formal basis, Joseph Fox became the first of many eminent teachers to give regular lectures at Guy's Hospital, commencing in 1798.

The first dental school to be formally constituted, however, was in the United States, the Baltimore College of Dental Surgery founded in Maryland in 1839. In the same year the first periodical, the *American journal of dental science*, was published.

It was not until the 1850s that reform came to Britain and opposition to dentistry from the influential Royal College of Surgeons of England was overcome. In 1856 the Odontological Society was founded, and in 1858 the Society opened the Dental Hospital of London followed, in 1859, by the first British dental school, the London School of Dental Surgery. These were later to become the Royal Dental Hospital and School. The College of Dentists, also formed in 1856, opened the Metropolitan School of Dental Science in 1859, and the associated National Dental Hospital two years later; these are now part of University College. An amendment to the 1858 Medical Act empowered the Royal College of Surgeons of England to examine for, and award, the LDS diploma, and the first licences were awarded in 1860.

The first woman to qualify as a dentist in Britain was Lilian Lindsay (née Murray), who received her LDS from Edinburgh in 1895. She then had a distinguished career, being at various points a general practitioner, sub-editor of the *British dental journal*, honorary librarian at the British Dental Association, and its only woman president to date, holding that office in 1946. Her published output was prolific, and included many historical papers, a book entitled *Short history of dentistry* [374]* and a translation of Fauchard's *Le chirurgien dentiste*.

Education in other countries took longer to develop. The first school in Canada was not established until 1875, although Canada was in fact the first country to pass an act restricting the practice of dentistry to authorized persons—in 1868, ten years before Britain. Schools were set up in Switzerland and Denmark in 1881, Germany in 1884, Russia in 1891 and France in 1892.

The British parliament passed its first Dentists Act in 1878, thereby establishing a register of those entitled to practise dentistry and restricting the titles of

*Numbers in square brackets refer to entries in the bibliography (Part II).

'dentist' and 'dental practitioner' to such persons. A significant loophole remained nevertheless, enabling the unqualified to continue as before by using descriptions such as 'dental consulting rooms'. The British Dental Association was established in 1880 to uphold and promote the interests and ethical standards of the profession, and was instrumental in the passing of the 1921 Dentists Act, which succeeded in making dentistry a closed profession.

Advances in dental science itself were few and far between until the nineteenth century. Hunter initiated a fashion for transplanting teeth as substitutes for those extracted, his experiments in this field resulting from his dissatisfaction with denture materials. Ivory or bone was traditionally used for false teeth during the eighteenth century, but tended to discolour and deteriorate. A notable step forward in prosthetic dentistry came when the Frenchman Nicolas Dubois de Chemant invented 'mineral paste', now known as porcelain, in 1789.

Dental caries was for centuries believed to be caused by worms in the teeth, a theory still not rejected when Anton Van Leeuwenhoek identified oral bacteria through a microscope in 1683. William Robertson and Emile Magitot, in the mid-nineteenth century, studied the causative factors of caries, notably the effects of food and saliva, but it was Willoughby Dayton Miller who demonstrated that acids formed by bacteria in the mouth were responsible for tooth decay. His 'chemico-parasitic' theory was published in his *Microorganisms of the human mouth* in 1882, and is still broadly accepted today.

Improvements in techniques and materials have meant that teeth are being treated instead of extracted, pain can be alleviated, and procedures can be undertaken more speedily. Amalgam, still today the most commonly used filling material, was first introduced in 1834 but was regarded with suspicion until Greene Vardiman Black's experimental work in the 1890s demonstrated that it was an acceptable material. Improvements to the composition and properties of amalgam are still being made. A mid-twentieth-century development has been the use of polymers and cements which have better adhesive properties and which are tooth-coloured. The acid etch and bonding techniques used in conjunction with polymeric materials, pioneered by Michael G. Buonocore in 1955, require a lesser amount of healthy tooth substance to be removed for the purposes of retaining the filling. The new materials are tooth-coloured, and therefore have significant aesthetic advantages.

Dentures, too, are more sophisticated. Vulcanized rubber (vulcanite) was introduced as a denture base in the 1850s, shortly after dental applications for Goodyear's invention had been appreciated, and because of its low cost and ease of production, dentures became affordable by the lower classes. A common procedure was, in fact, to have all one's natural teeth extracted early on in life, and false ones fitted, in order to avoid potential toothache and expensive treatment. Plastics, the denture-base materials in use nowadays, started to replace vulcanite in the 1930s.

Progress in the field of anaesthesia has made dental treatment a less daunting prospect for both patient and operator. Horace Wells became aware of the anaesthetic properties of nitrous oxide when he attended one of the then fashionable 'laughing gas' entertainments in Hartford, Connecticut, in 1844, and two years later William Morton, a fellow American, discovered that ether too could be used to anaesthetize patients. It was soon realized that there were disadvantages in the administration of these general anaesthetics, and following experimentation, cocaine was introduced as the first reliable local anaesthetic in 1884. Further developments, especially in intravenous techniques, came after the Second World War.

Excavating cavities in pre-anaesthetic days would not only have been a painful, but an extremely laborious operation. In 1871 the Morrison foot engine was marketed, but the notable advance of our own time was the development of the high-speed drill in the 1950s, making cavity preparation a faster and less traumatic procedure.

The first chair for dental patients which had an adjustable back was devised by James Snell in 1831, and designs have undergone numerous modifications since then. Important features were a headrest and footrest, until the 1970s when the supine position became popular, so that now patients lie down for their treatment.

Preventive dentistry is a twentieth-century phenomenon, although the caries-inhibiting properties of fluoride were described in the late nineteenth century. Fluoridation of water supplies is still a controversial subject, despite the surveys which show that people drinking water with appropriate levels of fluoride, either naturally occurring or artificially added, have fewer cavities. Fluoride toothpastes were introduced in Britain in 1959, and currently comprise over 95 percent of UK toothpaste sales. Dental health information is now reaching children and adults not only from dentists, but from the oral hygiene industry, educational organizations and the popular press. There is, therefore, a greater public awareness of the importance of oral health, and people are expecting to keep, and are in fact keeping, their natural teeth until later in life. This situation was demonstrated in the British survey *Adult dental health, 1978* [645] conducted by the Office of Population, Censuses and Surveys (published 1980), which showed an overall improvement in oral health since the previous survey conducted ten years earlier. In consequence, restorative treatment is more complex. The introduction of the British National Health Service in 1948 made dental treatment available to large numbers of patients who could not have afforded fees.

The adage taught to dental students twenty years ago, that it was not necessary to fit dentures to patients over the age of sixty, has been put aside, because the potential life span of the geriatric patient has now increased from the former 'three score years and ten' to eighty years and more. As general health improves, so too does the number of elderly patients, and hence the demand for prosthetic work.

This brief review is intended only to highlight the more important events and trends in the history of dentistry. The subject is a speciality in its own right, and is treated as such in Part II, where appropriate texts are listed which describe the growth and advance of the profession in considerable detail.

An excellent general overview, also useful for the non-specialist, is given by J. M. Campbell (1970), while the 'Centenary review', a series of papers in the *British dental journal* (1980), discusses the progress of various disciplines during the last hundred years.

1.2 The Scope of Dentistry Today

Dentistry may be defined as the branch of medicine concerned with diseases of the mouth and teeth, and their prevention and treatment, and with oral prostheses. Stomatology is often used as a synonym, although, strictly speaking, it is the medical speciality concerned with the mouth and its diseases, rather than the teeth.

Dentistry includes a range of specialities; although dental students receive a grounding in all aspects of the subject, some practising dentists have now chosen to specialize in one aspect, for instance orthodontics or periodontology.

1.2.1 Dental Specialities and Their Relationships

The brief definitions that follow are for the guidance of the reader who is not familiar with clinical dentistry. The scope of different specialities can vary from one country to another, and dictionaries or glossaries should be consulted if more precision is required.

Conservative dentistry is undertaken by most general dental practitioners, and comprises the replacement of diseased or injured tooth tissue by fillings, crowns (caps) and bridges (appliances attached permanently to natural teeth to replace missing teeth). The term *operative dentistry* is often used for this kind of treatment, but strictly speaking refers only to cavity preparation and fillings. *Prosthetic dentistry*, sometimes called prosthodontics, concerns the design, construction and fitting of prostheses to replace missing teeth; these are normally full or partial dentures, which can be removed by the patient at will. Crown and bridgework may be regarded as a form of prosthetic rather than conservative dentistry and the American terminology does in fact use the phrase 'fixed prosthodontics'. *Periodontology* is the study of diseases of the supporting tissues of the teeth, that is to say, the gingivae (gums) and supporting bone. These three aspects of dental treatment together make up *restorative dentistry*.

Children's dentistry, *paedodontics*, is regarded as a separate speciality although the same kind of treatment may be carried out as on adults. There may be particular problems with management, however, such as uncooperative behaviour perhaps through fear. Another factor to be taken into account when treating children is the potential changes, as the child grows, to the teeth and jaws, which are still in the course of development.

Orthodontics deals with the causes, prevention and treatment of irregularities of shape of the jaws, and position of the teeth. Most but not all orthodontic patients are children, and paedodontics and orthodontics are often linked, particularly in hospitals and dental schools. Adults are increasingly being accepted for treatment, however, especially in North America.

Relationships between the specialities are becoming closer, because the effects of different treatments are interrelated. For example, a crown with poorly shaped margins at gum level may cause gingival problems, involving the conservative dentist and his periodontal colleague. An oral surgeon may be required to remodel an area of bone in order that the prosthetic specialist can provide dentures capable of being retained effectively in the mouth of an elderly patient. Children fitted with orthodontic appliances must take special care in maintaining a high standard of oral hygiene, to prevent decay developing in parts of the mouth that may be difficult to keep clean on account of the wires fixed to their teeth. The links between various specialities are shown in *Figure 1.2*.

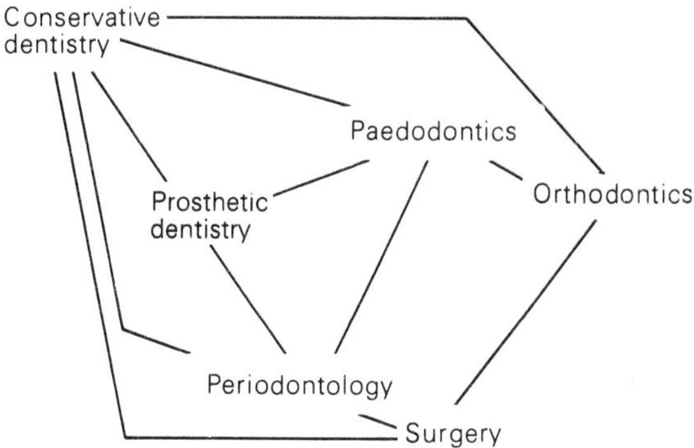

Figure 1.2 Relationship between dental specialities.

1.2.2 Relationships with Other Disciplines

An understanding of the biological sciences—the anatomy, physiology and biochemistry of the body as whole—is a necessary basis for the study of these mechanisms in relation to oral tissues, and fundamental for subsequent research on oral diseases. Thus the British Royal Colleges' postgraduate Fellowship in Dental Surgery examinations require a wide knowledge of basic biological science.

It must not be forgotten that dentistry is a profession related to medicine, and that the dentist is treating not a single tooth, but a human patient. Systemic disease may present symptoms in the mouth or affect treatment given by the dentist. For example, a haemophiliac may need a tooth extracted; a patient who is allergic to nickel, which is used in amalgam (the most commonly used filling material), may need a tooth filled. The dentist in these cases must obviously take into account the medical problems involved and modify his treatment accordingly. The importance of the relationship of clinical medicine to dentistry cannot be overemphasized.

Oral surgery made major advances following developments in plastic surgery during the Second World War, and there is still a close link between plastic surgery and dentistry for treatment of facial injuries. Orthodontists are increasingly cooperating with surgeons to operate on the jaws to correct gross deformities or improve facial aesthetics for cosmetic purposes.

Public health is a broad field in which workers in the community dental service, discussed below, play an important role. This area of health care involves planning and implementing the provision of dental facilities for populations or special categories of patients, such as handicapped persons, rather than individuals. Hence there will be liaison with public health bodies and officials locally and nationally. Public health dentists need to have a knowledge of the demand for and provision of social services in general, and be familiar with epidemiological methods.

Dentists running their own practices will need to be aware of business methods and appropriate legislation. The latter will cover such general topics as health and safety regulations, laws on dismissal of staff and sick pay. Managerial skills as well as clinical expertise are therefore necessary to administer a successful practice.

Science and technology, although they affect the clinical dentist as regards the adoption of new materials and techniques in general practice, impinge primarily on the research aspect of the profession. Researchers developing new materials may not necessarily be qualified dentists, but can be metallurgists or chemists. New materials and procedures are extensively tested *in vitro*, in the laboratory, before trials involving humans are undertaken, and there is therefore a need for specialists with the appropriate advanced knowledge.

Figure 1.3 illustrates the relationship of dentistry to other subjects.

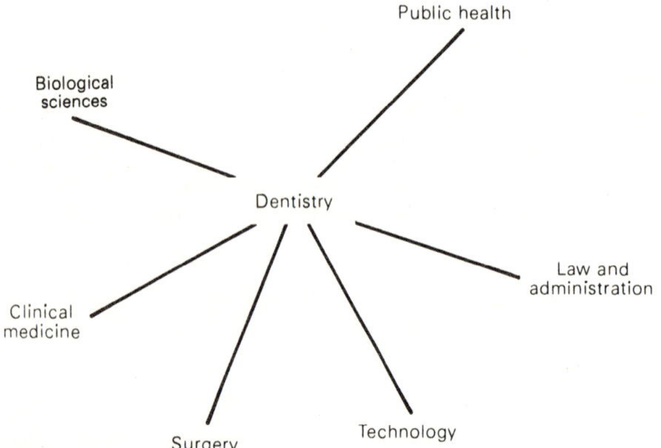

Figure 1.3 Relationship of dentistry to other disciplines.

1.3 Organization of the Subject Field

1.3.1 Varieties of Dental Practice

Clinical dentistry is predominantly undertaken by dentists in general practice, either under some control from the state or independently. The degree of state control varies from country to country.

In Britain approximately eighty percent of dentists are independent contractors within the National Health Service, and are paid on a fee per item basis from government funds via the Dental Estimates Board. Many of these dentists in the General Dental Service (GDS) offer some treatment—for instance, crowns—outside the NHS on a private basis, but only a small number of dentists operate entirely in private practice. In many other countries (for instance Australia, France, West Germany and the United States), general dental practitioners are predominantly in private practice, their charges being met either by the patients directly or by their insurance agencies.

Specialists work mainly in private practice, or in dental hospitals. Britain has no official list of specialists in private practice; any dentist wishing to treat patients privately or restrict his practice to a particular branch of dentistry is free to do so. In the hospital service, the specialities of oral surgery, orthodontics and restorative dentistry are recognized. The United States recognizes more: endodontics, oral pathology, oral and maxillofacial surgery, orthodontics, paedodontics, periodontology, prosthodontics and public health dentistry, and has speciality boards for each which hold examinations for accreditation. European countries vary in the number of specialities that are formally recognized.

The hospital dental service has two aspects, the dental department of a general hospital, which may encompass oral surgery or orthodontic units, and the specialized dental hospitals. Dental schools are linked to dental hospitals or to general hospitals with large dental departments. Most hospital patients are referred from general dental practitioners and tend to need complex treatment or the ready availability to hand of back-up medical facilities because of an existing medical condition; other patients present as emergency cases.

Dentists working in the field of public health dentistry are salaried employees of local or central government, who organize and implement treatment for specific groups of people within the community. Traditionally the dental care of schoolchildren has been of particular importance; today dental care for the handicapped, housebound patients and elderly people is a significant aspect of the work of the community dentist.

Academic dentistry is concerned with the education of dental students. The full-time teaching staff in dental schools are salaried employees of their university, and have an established career structure from (in Britain) lecturer to professor. Because the dental schools are attached to dental hospitals or departments, there are close links with the hospital service. Many university staffs have honorary hospital appointments, and vice versa.

Less common areas of dental practice include the armed forces and industrial dentistry. Provision of dental care to the services and to employees of commercial organizations requires only limited manpower, so the number of dentists in these fields is small.

The Council for Postgraduate Medical Education in England and Wales (1980) has issued a useful booklet entitled *Careers in dentistry*, of particular interest to newly qualified dentists or final-year students, but also useful for anyone wishing to know more about the variety of dental practice. It describes the scope of each branch of dentistry, and the kind of further training required.

1.3.2 Ancillary Personnel

Dental surgery assistants (DSAs), often called nurses, help the dentist in his clinical work, for instance by passing instruments and mixing fillings, but they do not undertake actual treatment. DSAs are usually trained by the dentist, but may attend a full-time or part-time course to sit for a national certificate. The Association of British Dental Surgery Assistants is a typical national body, and publishes a journal entitled *British dental surgery assistant.*

Hygienists are often qualified DSAs who have taken a further examination, and they are qualified to perform a defined range of procedures in the patient's mouth. Typically hygienists work in large practices or hospitals, or with periodontologists, and a large part of their time is spent scaling and polishing teeth, and providing dental health education. Examples of professional organizations are the British Dental Hygienists' Association, which publishes *Dental health*, and the American Dental Hygienists' Association, issuing the journal *Dental hygiene.*

The small number of school dental nurses/dental therapists (an occupation pioneered in New Zealand) are employed in school or hospital dental services. They are trained to undertake simple treatment for children, including fillings, and extraction of deciduous teeth.

Technicians make dentures, crowns and other prosthetic appliances according to a dentist's specifications. They are not allowed by British law to have dealings directly with patients regarding the provision of new dentures, although they can legally advertise their services as menders of appliances.

Denturists are an expanding group, now legally permitted in some countries and certain American states, but generally the subject of controversy. Where so entitled by law, denturists provide dentures for patients without the prior involvement of a dentist.

1.4 Statutory and Professional Bodies

There is a pattern, not unique to medicine, in which three distinct kinds of authority have separate but overlapping interests in the organization and development of the profession. These comprise the academic institutions to be discussed in section 1.5, the statutory bodies, vested with authority from government, and the voluntary societies, namely the professional organizations whether international, national, local or speciality. The interrelationship between them is discussed with special reference to South Africa by Van Reenen (1981), but the principles he expounds are widely applicable. The statutory body has the regulatory and controlling power, but the voluntary body is the voice of the profession, while the universities provide the manpower.

1.4.1 Statutory Bodies and Legislation

Although there are variations from country to country, the practice of dentistry is generally regulated by national or regional government laws, which are administered by a statutory body appointed by the government concerned. The newly qualified dentist, therefore, having gained his degree or diploma, must register with the appropriate authority before he is entitled to provide treatment. This arrangement is intended to maintain high standards of education and professional conduct, and protect the interests of the patient.

In Britain, for example, the Dentists Act of 1984 is implemented by the General Dental Council. This body has some of its members nominated by the government health departments and by the universities, and others elected by the profession. The GDC deals with disciplinary matters and ethics, and is under statutory obligation to publish the *Dentists register* [193] annually. It is mandatory for dentists who wish to practise in Britain to remit an annual retention fee to the GDC, and thereby be listed in the *Register* each year.

An important function of the GDC is the assessment of educational standards, which involves liaison with the universities and Royal Colleges, as discussed in sections 1.5 and 1.6. The acceptability of foreign qualifications for eligibility to practise in Britain is included in this remit. Hindley-Smith (1970) provides a more detailed review of the history and functions of the GDC.

Following extensive negotiation, the European Economic Community dental directives were issued in 1978, coming into force in 1980. They were published in the *British dental journal* (1978) and were followed by a commentary (1978) explaining the directives in plain, non-legal terms. Any dentist who is a national of an EEC member country, with an approved qualification and legally entitled to practise in the country granting it, may now also practise in any other EEC member country (except Italy) on the same terms as that country's own practitioners. Working parties are studying the implications of the various educational systems of member countries, and the recognition of specialities, with a long-term view towards achieving compatibility in training, career structure and identification of specialities between the member countries. At present, language barriers remain for many dentists a practical obstacle to working abroad.

In Australia, dentists have to register with the state in which they practise, and each state government printer publishes its own list of practitioners.

Each state in the USA has its own licensing board, which issues its own regulations, and a dentist licensed to practise in one state will have to obtain a new licence to practise in another. Although national written examinations, monitored by the American Dental Association, have superseded locally held ones, most states still hold individual examinations to assess clinical competence, which aspiring incomers, regardless of age, experience or qualifications, must pass. Binder (1981) provides a useful review of the function and work of the state boards. According to a report issued by the ADA (1978), foreign dental graduates wishing to practise in the United States encounter considerable problems in securing licensure; they are subject initially to the provisions of the Immigration and Nationality Act, and are constrained by the licensure requirements themselves and by the lack of reciprocity between states. A booklet on education and registration was issued for the guidance of foreign dentists by the ADA in 1981.

Brief details on legislation and registration for over one hundred countries together with addresses for further information are supplied in the Fédération Dentaire Internationale publications *Basic fact sheets* (1981) [217] and *Handbook of regulations of dental practice* (1976) [587].

1.4.2 International Organizations

Dentistry is practised worldwide, and cooperation among practitioners, academics and policy-makers is regarded as essential for the advancement of the profession. Special-interest groups have national, intercontinental and international organizations to bring together people working in the same field. Usually such bodies issue newsletters or journals, as will be seen in Part II of this book. The diversity of specialist organizations can be seen in the directory of organizations which forms Part III.

The need for liaison and cooperation on a general as opposed to special-subject basis has long been recognized. Although there are a number of international organizations, the two bodies held in greatest esteem, and having a considerable influence on policy and practice throughout the world, are the Fédération Dentaire Internationale and the International Association for Dental Research.

International Association for Dental Research

The International Association for Dental Research (IADR) was founded in 1920 as a result of the efforts of William J. Gies, an American biochemist who was also a successful researcher in the dental field. Its objectives are to promote the advancement of research in all branches of dental science, and to encourage and facilitate cooperation between investigators. Annual meetings are conducted, and the Association acts as a national and international force for the support of research.

The IADR has regional subgroups called geographical divisions, which are important in their own right, having independent officers and holding their own annual meetings. Inevitably, the North American one, entitled the American Association for Dental Research, is the largest, and has evolved from the original membership; other divisions were established in due course: British division, 1953 (from 1983 entitled the British Society for Dental Research); Japanese, 1954; Continental European, 1964; South African, 1966; Australian, 1968 (to become Australia and New Zealand the following year); and Scandinavian NOF (linked to the Scandinavian Dental Federation), 1969. Within divisions there may be local sections; these are an important feature in North America.

The IADR has three subject groups: craniofacial biology; dental materials; and periodontology research group.

The important *Journal of dental research* [77] was acquired by the IADR in 1934, and its monthly issues promote and communicate research. The *Program and abstracts of papers* of the annual general session, commonly known as the *IADR abstracts*, are published as a special issue of the *Journal of dental research* each year together with the *AADR abstracts*, while divisional abstracts are included in a conventional monthly part or published as a separate issue. The *Journal* also publishes conference reports from time to time, usually as special issues.

A detailed history of this important organization has been written by Orland (1973).

Fédération Dentaire Internationale

The Fédération Dentaire Internationale (FDI) was established in 1900 at the instigation of the Frenchman Charles Godon. Its objectives are 'to represent the profession of dentistry on a voluntary non-governmental international basis, to sponsor an annual world congress, and to establish and encourage international programmes which will advance the science and art of dentistry and the state of the profession'. In 1979 membership comprised seventy-eight member associations, that is, national dental associations, and 13,784 supporting members who are individual dentists. Its headquarters are in London.

An important function of the FDI is its annual congress, held in a different location each year. Papers presented are generally published in the *International dental journal* [72], the FDI's official organ, which was established in 1949 and is issued quarterly.

Four commissions undertake scientific work: Oral Health, Research and Epidemiology; Dental Education and Practice; Dental Products; and Defence Forces Dental Services. Their findings are published in the *International dental journal* and in the FDI Technical Report series. Issued monthly is the *FDI newsletter*, with items of topical interest. The FDI has a unique asset in the support of the national associations, and is thereby able to issue useful guides to manpower figures, legislation and oral conditions for its member countries. These data are available in the publications *Basic fact sheets* [217] and *Handbook of regulations of dental practice* [587]. Other publications are listed in appropriate sections of this *Keyguide*. Ennis (1967) wrote the official comprehensive history of the FDI, while Leatherman (1981) produced a smaller publication to mark its eightieth anniversary in which he described highlights of the earlier years, with personal recollections and details of important events from 1952 to 1980.

World Health Organization

Although it does not fit into any of the categories already discussed, the World Health Organization (WHO) is an international body of considerable importance, particularly in the field of public health dentistry. Its Oral Health Unit, based at WHO headquarters in Geneva, has been responsible for the development and adoption of standard methods to facilitate the collection of dental data on a global basis, and has published a number of reports on epidemiological techniques and methodology for oral health surveys, as well as reports on dental health in various regions. Barmes and Infirri (1977) discuss this aspect of the work of WHO, and also describe its Global Epidemiology Data Bank. This data bank includes information on surveys undertaken to examine oral conditions throughout the world. In 1977 data were available on caries for ninety-five countries, and on periodontal diseases for fifty countries. Also included are details of the sample population studied, and the type of survey such as national, quasi-national or pilot study. Access to this type of information is particularly important for planners of oral health services, but requests are accepted from governmental and non-governmental bodies, research organizations and individuals.

WHO is also concerned with dental manpower and training, but has produced fewer published reports on this topic.

Individual WHO publications are discussed in appropriate subject chapters of this *Keyguide* so will not be discussed here. Their physical format is varied. Some of the most useful are booklets published in the WHO Technical Report series, others are reproduced from typescript and are part of the WHO Offset series. Publications dealing with particular geographical areas may be issued by the regional office concerned, such as the WHO Regional Office for Europe in Copenhagen. It is usual for English and French versions to be produced of any document; other languages used when appropriate include Spanish, Russian and Arabic.

Close collaboration is maintained between WHO and the FDI, since there are many areas of common concern.

1.4.3 National Associations

Most countries have their own professional dental society to promote the interests of their members, liaise and negotiate with other bodies on dental matters, and offer assistance to members at a personal level. The dental society is therefore the voice of the national profession, representing its view to the public, government, educational and other relevant institutions. Some countries, including Belgium, have more than one national association, but such a situation is the exception rather than the norm. Whereas registration with the appropriate statutory body is mandatory, membership of the national professional society is not; nevertheless, support is generally good. By definition, a national association caters for all dentists: general dental practitioner or specialist, student, academic or clinician. Often the society will produce a journal and/or newsletter, with papers of general interest and topical information; these may be available to nonmembers on subscription. The appropriate national dental association is a useful source of information on dentistry in that country, particularly for details not widely available elsewhere.

Two representative national bodies are described below; a complete list is given in Part III.

American Dental Association

The American Dental Association (ADA) is the largest of all the associations, numerically and in published output. Founded in 1859, it now has over 135,000 members. Much of the work of the ADA is carried out under the aegis of specialized subdivisions: councils, bureaux, and commissions whose reports are frequently published in the monthly *Journal of the American Dental Association* (*JADA*) [74] and are highly regarded in the profession.

There are sixteen councils, whose interests range from clinical matters, such as the Council on Materials, Instruments and Equipment, to specialized practice, with the Council on Hospital and Industrial Dental Services. Other councils include those for Dental Education, Dental Research and Dental Journalism. ADA commissions oversee the interests of continuing dental education/dental accreditation; national dental examinations; and relief and disaster fund activities. The bureaux comprise eight departments, one of which, the Bureau of Library Services, is discussed in more detail in Chapter 2, Section 2.5.2. Other bureaux include those for communications, economic and behavioural research, and health education and audiovisual services. A complete list of councils and bureaux is given in each issue of *JADA*. Also part of the organization are the ADA Health Foundation and the American Dental Political Action Committee. ADA publications range through reference books for the dentist, dental health education for the patient, and audiovisual material, and are listed under appropriate sections of this book. The history of the ADA is described by R. W. McCluggage (1959).

British Dental Association

The British Dental Association (BDA) was established in 1880 to be a scientific society and ensure the effective operation of the 1878 Dentists Act, though its purpose has been modified with time. Today one of its prime functions is to maintain the honour and interests of its members, especially in negotiating with government health departments the terms and conditions of service under which dental services are provided to the public. The membership comprises some 16,000 dentists, and local activity is through the twenty-one regional branches and 120 sections, which are local subdivisions of the branches. Most British dentists work in general practice, but three BDA groups—hospitals, community dental services, and university dental teachers and research workers—serve the special interests of members in these sections of the profession. As in the ADA, although the nomenclature is slightly different, there are committees monitoring various spheres of practice, such as ethics, dental health and science, and ancillary personnel. The scale of operation is, however, considerably smaller, and therefore more typical of other national organizations. The official organ is the *British dental journal* [62] published twice a month; *BDA news* is a monthly topical newsletter available only to BDA members. A centenary history of the Association was published in 1979.

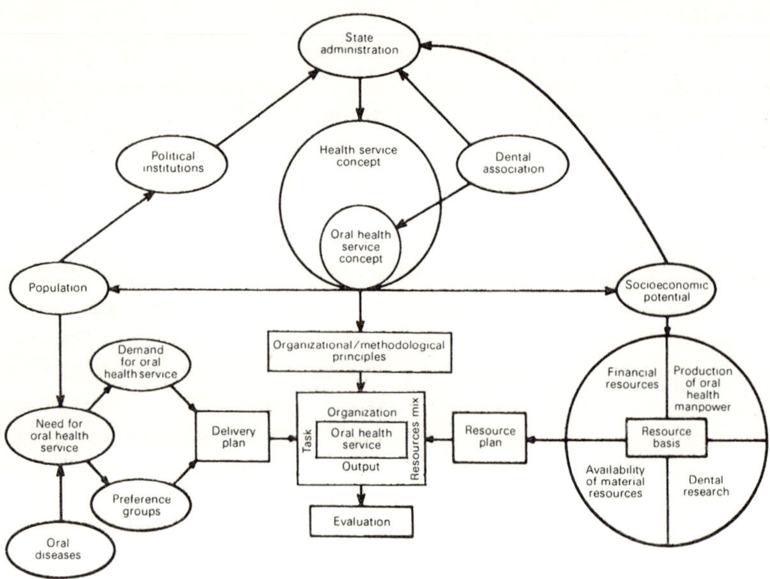

Figure 1.4 The oral health service system and its national and community setting.

(Reproduced by courtesy of the World Health Organization from Kostlan, J. *Oral health services in Europe*. Copenhagen: WHO, 1979).

1.4.4 Other Associations

Countries which occupy large geographical areas have networks of regional organizations. In the USA, each state has its own association; France too has regional societies. Their purpose, as with the BDA branches and sections, is to meet the needs of dentists in a particular area, and provide a forum for local meetings and ideas. Details of American state societies are given in the *American dental directory* [198]; for other countries the national association is a useful source of information.

An important British medical society to which dentists may belong is the Royal Society of Medicine, which assumed its present name in 1907 when the Medical and Chirurgical Society, founded in 1805, amalgamated with a number of other medical societies. These bodies voluntarily surrendered their independence, and were incorporated to form a single society that would present a stronger professional voice. One such association which ceased to exist in its own right was the influential Odontological Society; this became the Section of Odontology, one of the speciality sections of which the RSM is composed.

The Society is a prestigious body in medicine today, being particularly influential in the areas of policy-making and research. Membership is primarily for the professionally qualified, and is on a subscription basis; benefits to members include the monthly *Journal of the Royal Society of Medicine* (*JRSM*) [94], which is highly regarded, and use of the library facilities. Since the RSM has one of the most extensive postgraduate medical collections in Europe and is rich in historical material, it is of particular value to academics, authors and research workers.

Each section holds regular meetings, papers from which may be published in the *JRSM*.

1.5 Education

In order to practise dentistry, an appropriate qualification must be obtained. In Britain and most Commonwealth countries this is usually the university degree of Bachelor in Dental Surgery (BDS); the United States and many other countries award a Doctorate in Dental Surgery (DDS). Undergraduate training is of four to six years' duration, depending on the institution attended, and is provided by schools of dentistry, which are normally part of the medical faculty of an established university, as is the case in all of the British schools. In the USA about 92 percent of the schools, of which there are over sixty, have this arrangement.

Preclinical sciences, for instance anatomy and physiology, are studied in relation to the whole body, usually before the detailed curriculum on the oral structures. Practical procedures on patients are undertaken in the final year or years of the course, and follow extensive sessions using phantom heads (life-sized replicas).

The USA operates a system of accreditation and licensure. The ADA is responsible for accrediting dental schools by regular evaluation to ensure that high educational standards are maintained, and it is necessary for students to have attended an accredited school to be eligible to sit speciality certification exams or obtain state licensure.

After qualification, a dentist is generally eligible to pursue his career with no further training, but in Britain vocational training schemes for the newly qualified are being introduced. These are part-time courses of one or two years' duration, organized on a regional basis for new recruits to the general dental service (GDS) and the community dental service (CDS). Trainees attend lectures for approximately one day per week and receive more detailed tuition on their chosen field of practice than was feasible to fit into a standard undergraduate curriculum. GDS trainees, for example, benefit from sessions on the business side of practice, which may have been only briefly discussed in a predominantly clinically-orientated undergraduate course. Vocational trainees may undertake a research project.

Higher degrees are awarded by the universities and the medical dental societies. Students for a British Master of Science (MSc) degree attend a taught course of one to two years' duration at a dental school and study a particular speciality, for instance children's dentistry or periodontology. The examination comprises written papers, clinical and practical work, and the submission of a dissertation. Students attend not only from Britain, but also from a variety of overseas countries, and the MSc degree is highly regarded.

The universities are also responsible for the research-orientated higher degrees, such as Doctor of Philosophy (PhD). For this type of award there are no taught lectures, but applicants undertake a specialized research project on which is based a substantial thesis. To achieve high academic rank in Britain, possession of a research degree is an important factor.

Professional bodies too offer higher diplomas which are much sought after, particularly by those wishing to start climbing the academic ladder. The Royal Colleges of Surgeons of England, Edinburgh and Glasgow each award the Fellowship in Dental Surgery (FDS). This is a two-part, broadly based qualification, awarded to candidates successful in the written, clinical and viva voce parts of the examination. A similar qualification, the Fellowship of the Faculty of Dentistry (FFD), is offered by the Royal College of Surgeons in Ireland.

A higher diploma tailored for general practitioners awarded by the Royal Colleges of England, Edinburgh, and Glasgow is the Membership in General Dental Surgery (MGDS). An important element of this examination is the casebook aspect, in which courses of treatment for a specified number of patients are recorded in detail; models and photographs are submitted as appropriate, and the patients themselves are available for inspection by the examiners. Other diplomas awarded by the Royal Colleges are described in section 1.6.

Continuing education is available for those who wish to attend short courses, either arranged by independent organizations on a profit-making basis, or at regional level by postgraduate tutors under the aegis of the National Health Service. Many of these are approved under the NHS Act as 'Section 63' courses for which participants can claim travelling and other appropriate expenses.

In the United States not only do the universities award higher degrees, but the eight speciality boards hold examinations for dentists wishing to acquire a recognized higher qualification in a particular branch of the profession. Continuing education is growing in importance in the USA, and is in fact mandatory in some states.

Dental manpower, together with its educational implications, is a topic of current concern to the governing and professional bodies in both the USA and Britain. The American Association of Dental Schools (1980), in its report on advanced dental education, recommended that the number of places on speciality courses be reduced, while in Britain an independent report by the Nuffield Foundation (1980), with a wider remit, made recommendations relating to the undergraduate and postgraduate curriculum, staffing and finance of schools and the provision of general dental care. The extent to which the recommendations made by these impartial organizations will be implemented by the appropriate authorities remains to be seen although the total intake of students to British dental schools has been reduced by ten percent.

Finding the addresses of dental schools throughout the world can be a lengthy process, there being no regularly updated, published list. For this reason a worldwide list of schools is given in Part III. The *World directory of dental schools, 1963* was issued by the World Health Organization in 1967, but unfortunately has never been revised. While it can still be useful for some background information, such as licensure, or the year in which schools were established, it is otherwise too out of date to be regarded as reliable nowadays. National directories may list schools in the country concerned; for example, those in North America are listed in the annual *American dental directory* [198].

For information on individual courses it is advisable to contact the schools of interest or scan appropriate journals for advertisements. For the United States, the American Association of Dental Schools produces an annual directory entitled *Admission requirements of US and Canadian dental schools*. Every two or three years the *British dental journal* publishes in a September issue an *Educational directory*, also available as a separate pamphlet. This gives brief descriptions of entry requirements and undergraduate courses at dental schools in Britain. Also provided are outline details on postgraduate education and organizations of interest to potential students. An independent survey of British undergraduate courses is provided by the *Dentistry degree course guide*, edited biennially by the Careers Research and Advisory Centre, and showing the variation in content and structure between the courses available.

Lists of approved training posts for prospective candidates for the Fellowship in Dental Surgery (FDS) or Diploma in Orthodontics (DOrth) awarded by the Royal College of Surgeons of England (RCS), or for newcomers to the United Kingdom hospital dental service, have been published. For the latter, the British Dental Students' Association issues annually a *Directory of dental house officer appointments in Great Britain and Northern Ireland*, a booklet arranged by town, and listing the number and length of appointments at each hospital, with details of accommodation, scope of the post, and names of consultants. Recognized hospital appointments for RCS purposes are listed in appendices to the regulations, available from the RCS, for the FDS and DOrth examinations.

The Council for Postgraduate Medical Education (1983) has issued a second edition of *Guide to postgraduate degrees, diplomas and courses in dentistry*, which gives more information than the *British dental journal*'s *Educational directory*, and is a valuable guide to the locations and length of courses for prospective postgraduate students in Britain.

Short courses, primarily for continuing education or updating clinical knowledge or techniques, are advertised in the national dental press. For the United States, the *Journal of the American Dental Association* publishes a comprehensive list in its June and December issues, for the following six months. The list is arranged by broad subject groups, and by region within each group. Individual entries give the name of the course, location, date, type of participant (e.g. specialist, technician) and educational method. Some courses outside the USA are listed, most of which are in Canada.

The British Postgraduate Medical Federation (BPMF) is the central organizing body for vocational and short courses in London and the surrounding counties, and issues an *Annual list of courses in the four Thames regions*, which covers an academic year. Of particular interest are the BPMF vocational training schemes for the newly qualified, and the wide range of short courses for keeping the general practitioner and specialist up to date.

Of value to administrators and teachers is the *Journal of dental education*, first published in 1936 and issued monthly by the American Association of Dental Schools. Although primarily aimed at North American educationalists, it also publishes papers on teaching methods, curricula and sociological aspects which are of broader appeal. Also included are book reviews, and advertisements for teaching positions in North America.

Other papers related to education are scattered throughout the periodical literature. Policy matters or national surveys tend to appear in journals published by the national associations, while teaching models or techniques, for instance, may be described in the appropriate speciality publications.

1.6 Royal Colleges

The four British Royal Colleges occupy a significant place in education and research. To give their full titles, they are the Royal College of Surgeons of England (RCS England), Royal College of Surgeons of Edinburgh (RCS Edin.), Royal College of Physicians and Surgeons of Glasgow (RCS Glas.) and Royal College of Surgeons in Ireland (RCS Irel.).

During the first half of the nineteenth century, the RCS England was vigorously opposed to the concept of dentistry's being a profession of equal standing to medicine. Following reform in the dental profession, and greater cohesion brought about by the formation of the Odontological Society in 1856, it changed its view and in 1859 established the diploma of Licenciate in Dental Surgery (LDS). This was to remain the only British dental qualification obtainable until the University of Birmingham awarded the first degree in dentistry in 1900. With the expansion in university education, few students now sit for the LDS alone; exemptions are permitted for all examinations except for the final LDS to candidates who have passed the comparable university exams. Many dentists consider it a privilege to become a Licenciate, however, and therefore sit the final LDS in addition to the final BDS, their university degree.

The RCS England established a separate Faculty of Dental Surgery in 1947, in appreciation of the special administrative aspects of the field.

All the Royal Colleges today play an important role in postgraduate education. As mentioned earlier, the Fellowship in Dental Surgery (FDS) requires extensive knowledge in basic medical and dental science. It is a sought-after qualification, particularly for those wishing to pursue an academic career, not only in Britain, where senior teaching staff are expected to have the FDS, but in other countries too. There is reciprocity between Edinburgh, Glasgow and England, so that a candidate who has part I from one college can sit part II at another. The RCS Irel. diploma, the Fellowship in the Faculty of Dentistry (FFD), is granted either in the practice of dentistry, or in a special subject: oral surgery, orthodontics, prosthetics, public health dentistry or restorative dentistry.

For general practitioners, the recently instituted Membership in General Dental Surgery (MGDS) is offered to successful candidates by the London and Scottish Colleges. The RCS Edin. also awards a higher diploma covering conservative dentistry, periodontology and prosthetics, which is entitled the Diploma in Restorative Dentistry (DRD) and, in orthodontics, the Diploma in Dental Orthopaedics. Available from the RCS England are other specialist awards, the Diploma in Orthodontics (DOrth) and the Diploma in Dental Public Health (DDPH).

Liaison with other bodies is an important function of the Royal Colleges, notably in relation to education and training. Close links are therefore retained with the General Dental Council and the universities.

Research has traditionally occupied an important role at RCS England. The Institute of Basic Medical Sciences, founded in 1951 and, from 1961, jointly administered by the College and the University of London, has been responsible for significant advances in a wide range of medical fields, including dentistry. The College also has its own dental research sections, the central London unit investigating oral soft-tissue diseases, notably oral malignant and premalignant lesions, while the unit at Downe in Kent is continuing research on a vaccine against caries. There is collaboration and cooperation with the Medical Research Council.

In 1982 the RCS England established its Hunterian Institute, to coordinate the educational and research activities of the College.

Each Royal College issues its own journal, predominantly devoted to surgical papers, but with others of dental interest from time to time. The most prestigious is the *Annals of the Royal College of Surgeons of England* [488], which is widely read in both the medical and dental professions.

The Colleges' interest in the history of medicine stems from the nineteenth century, when museums began to assume importance. The RCS England maintains the Hunterian Museum, which also incorporates the Odontological Society Collection. The extensive collection of instruments and artefacts of the late J. Menzies Campbell, dental historian at the University of Edinburgh, was presented to the RCS Edin. by Dr. Campbell, and made available for viewing in 1965.

Canada and Australasia each have a Royal College with similar functions to those in Britain.

References

American Association of Dental Schools. *Admission requirements of US and Canadian dental schools*. 1619 Massachusetts Avenue NW, Washington, DC 20036: AADS. Annual.

Also includes general information on dentistry in North America, and sources of finance. Useful for students and administrators.

American Association of Dental Schools. *Advanced dental education: recommendations for the 80s: final report of the task force*. Washington, DC: AADS, 1980. 63pp.

American Dental Association. *Dentistry in the United States: information on education and licensure*. Chicago: ADA, 1981. 29pp.

Details on the training and registration system, for the guidance of foreign dentists.

Barmes, D. E. and Infirri, J. S. 'WHO activities in oral epidemiology'. *Community dentistry and oral epidemiology* **5** (1977): 22–9.

Binder, H. B. 'The State boards for dentistry; now and in the future'. *New York State dental journal* **49** (1983): 92–5.

British Dental Association. *The advance of the dental profession: a centenary history 1880–1980*. London: BDA, 1979. 288pp.

British Dental Journal. *Educational directory*. Every two years. London: BDJ. Published in the September issue and also available as a separate booklet.

Gives information about dental schools, dental organizations, and some useful addresses for further information.

British Dental Students' Association. *Directory of dental house-officer appointments in Great Britain and Northern Ireland*. London: BDSA. Annual. Available from the British Dental Association.

British Postgraduate Medical Federation. *Annual list of courses in the four Thames regions*. London: BPMF. Annual.

Brown, W. E. 'The present status of United States dental education'. *Journal of dental education* **45** (1981): 628–34.

Campbell, J. M. 'An outline of dental history'. *British dental journal* **129** (1970): 523–7, 578–82.

Careers Research and Advisory Centre. *Dentistry degree course guide*. Cambridge: Hobson's Press. Every two years.

A comparative review of courses at British dental schools provided by an independent organization, for prospective students.

'Centenary review'. *British dental journal* **149** (1980): 3–32.

Eight papers which discuss changes in the past hundred years in various fields of dentistry.

Council for Postgraduate Medical Education in England and Wales. *Careers in dentistry*. London: CPME, 1980. 48pp.

Provides guidance on the opportunities and training requirements for each branch of dental practice.

Council for Postgraduate Medical Education. *Guide to postgraduate degrees, diplomas and courses in dentistry*. 2nd ed. London: CPME, 1983. 26pp.

Information on higher education and courses in different subjects in Britain.

Ennis, J. *The story of the FDI, 1900–1962*. London: Fédération Dentaire Internationale, 1967. 238pp.

European Economic Community. 'Dental directives'. *British dental journal* **145** (1978). Supplement to issue dated 17 October. 16pp. Also *see* 'Commentary on the EEC dental directives'. *British dental journal* **145** (1978): 143–6.

Fédération Dentaire Internationale. *Basic fact sheets*. 2nd ed. London: FDI, 1981. Unpaged.

Information on over one hundred countries.

Hindley-Smith, D. 'The General Dental Council: its origins, purposes and functions'. *British dental journal* **128** (1970): 345–9, 411–14.

Journal of dental education. 1936–. Washington, DC: American Association of Dental Schools. Monthly.

Leatherman, G. H. *The FDI 1900–1980*. Chicago: Quintessence, 1981. 51pp.

McCluggage, R. W. *A history of the American Dental Association: a century of health service*. Chicago: American Dental Association, 1959. 520pp.

Nuffield Foundation. *Dental education: the report of a committee of enquiry*. London: Nuffield Foundation, 1980. 115pp.

Orland, F. J. *The first fifty year history of the International Association for Dental Research*. Chicago: University of Chicago, 1973. 417pp.

Santangelo, M. V. 'The history and development of United States dental education'. *Journal of dental education* **45** (1981): 619–27.

Van Reenen, J. F. 'The role of the academic, voluntary and statutory bodies in the profession: a point of view'. *Journal of the Dental Association of South Africa* **36** (1981): 631–2.

World Health Organization. *World directory of dental schools, 1963*. Geneva: WHO, 1967. 282pp.

2 Dental Information: Its Origins and Utilization

The first book devoted entirely to dentistry, the *Artzney Buchlein*, was published in 1530, but the dental journal was not initiated until 1839, when the *American journal of dental science* was founded. Growth was such that in the United States alone, over 550 books were published during the nineteenth century, and there were thirty-one current periodicals in 1900 (Foley, 1950). In 1982 the *Index to dental literature* [17] included papers from over 250 journals devoted to dentistry, of which more than ninety emanated from the United States. Today, textbooks and monographs summarize accepted knowledge and practices, but because of the long delay between completion of a manuscript and eventual publication they are not appropriate vehicles to communicate new developments or research findings. For these the journal is pre-eminent.

It would be hard to estimate the precise number of dental books currently published each year but a comparison of figures may give some indication. The 1982 *Index to dental literature* lists approximately 250 books and reports over fifty pages in length, of which nineteen are not in English. (Foreign-language editions of books already available in English are not normally listed in the *IDL*.) The *Indice de la literatura dental en castellano* [19] for 1980–81 lists about forty books including translations.

The French list of books in print, *Les livres disponibles*, 1982, gives some 240 dental books in French under the headings of 'Dentistry', 'Prosthetic dentistry' and 'Orthodontics'; but as these are titles currently available, and not just new publications, no direct comparisons can be made.

2.1 Journals

The dental journal is an up-to-date, easily accessible means of communication between members of the profession, and is the accepted mode of publication for the widespread dissemination of results of original research.

Journals which are general in scope are today primarily issued by national or local associations, for example *Journal of the American Dental Association* [74] or *Ontario dentist*, although commercial publishers do continue to produce a few titles of broad interest, such as *Dental update* [69]. The days of the important proprietary journals owned by dental manufacturers and epitomized by the excellent *Dental cosmos* (1859–1936) and *Dental items of interest* (1879–1953) are now past, as it was doubted whether this genre of publication was in the interest of the profession; there was the danger of overt or covert advertising and abuse of sponsorship. There has been a trend towards specialization throughout dentistry, and the journal literature has reflected this. Most titles today are, therefore, published directly by or on behalf of specialist societies, as will be seen in the appropriate chapters.

Issues are most commonly monthly, bimonthly or quarterly, the frequency often increasing with a title's success. A few titles appear weekly, for example the *Chirurgien-dentiste de France* [106] and *Information dentaire* [107], while the *British dental journal* [62] is published twice a month.

The author of this *Keyguide* has made an analysis using the online database Medline to identify the number of dental papers published in various countries during the period 1975–79, and the results are as follows:

USA	19,547
Germany (East and West)	7,334
Great Britain	5,394
France	4,337
Switzerland	1,519

Although these figures must be treated with caution since they do not take into account Medline's indexing policy or number of papers per journal, they do give an approximate indication of the size of output from various countries. It must also be borne in mind, however, that journals today often are international in scope; thus, the *Journal of clinical periodontology* [565], the official publication of eleven national periodontology societies throughout Europe, includes papers from these and other countries, and is actually published in Denmark. Its publisher, Munksgaard in Copenhagen, issues some half-dozen highly regarded specialist dental titles with international scope.

The majority of well-known journals are published in English. The key Scandinavian titles, such as the *Scandinavian journal of dental research* [89], switched to English during the 1970s. Riordan and Gjerdet (1981) studied borrowing patterns at the University of Bergen's dental library and concluded that 70 percent of loans were items in the English language. Local material was used to supply news or topical information, and became obsolescent more quickly.

Bilingual countries such as Canada and South Africa publish in both their national languages.

2.2 Books

Whereas the journal is used to communicate new ideas and developments, the textbook provides a convenient exposition of established knowledge. The student is doubtless a major user of the standard textbook and the general practitioner will refer to practical manuals and texts for revision, or to investigate a speciality with which he is not familiar. As with journals, English is the predominant language of publication, but since the international market is of considerable importance, many titles are routinely translated into other languages, notably German, French, Spanish, Italian and Japanese.

With the advances in printing techniques, today's texts are, like the journals, more lavishly illustrated than thirty years ago. In fact, a popular type of text today is the colour atlas, with photographs of anatomical features, and clinical and pathological conditions.

Books are available at all technical levels for the undergraduate, postgraduate and clinician. Cross-disciplinary works are not unusual; for example one may find symposia monographs on *The borderland between caries and periodontal disease*, or treatises on surgical orthodontics.

2.3 Utilization of the Literature

The British Library initiated a survey on the provision and use of medical literature, in which two of the groups of readers studied were hospital dentists and general-practice dentists (GDPs) (Ford, 1979).

The reasons for seeking information varied between these two groups although, as shown in *Figure 2.1*, keeping up to date and researching clinical problems were significant for both. The hospital dentists, however, rated teaching and preparing publications and lectures as more usual reasons than clinical problems. An interesting conclusion from the survey was that hospital dentists had more information needs than the doctors or biochemists working in hospitals, and that they were more likely to be involved in research, teaching, publication and administration than the doctors or biochemists.

Respondents were also asked about their use of different information sources; the dentists' replies are shown in *Table 2.1*. 'Index journals' presumably refers to the *Index to dental literature*. 'Browsing', as far as GDPs were concerned, would also include 'References in journals'; the GDPs were not asked about the latter specifically since they do not have the same ease of access to libraries as their hospital colleagues. Both groups relied heavily on journals for their information,

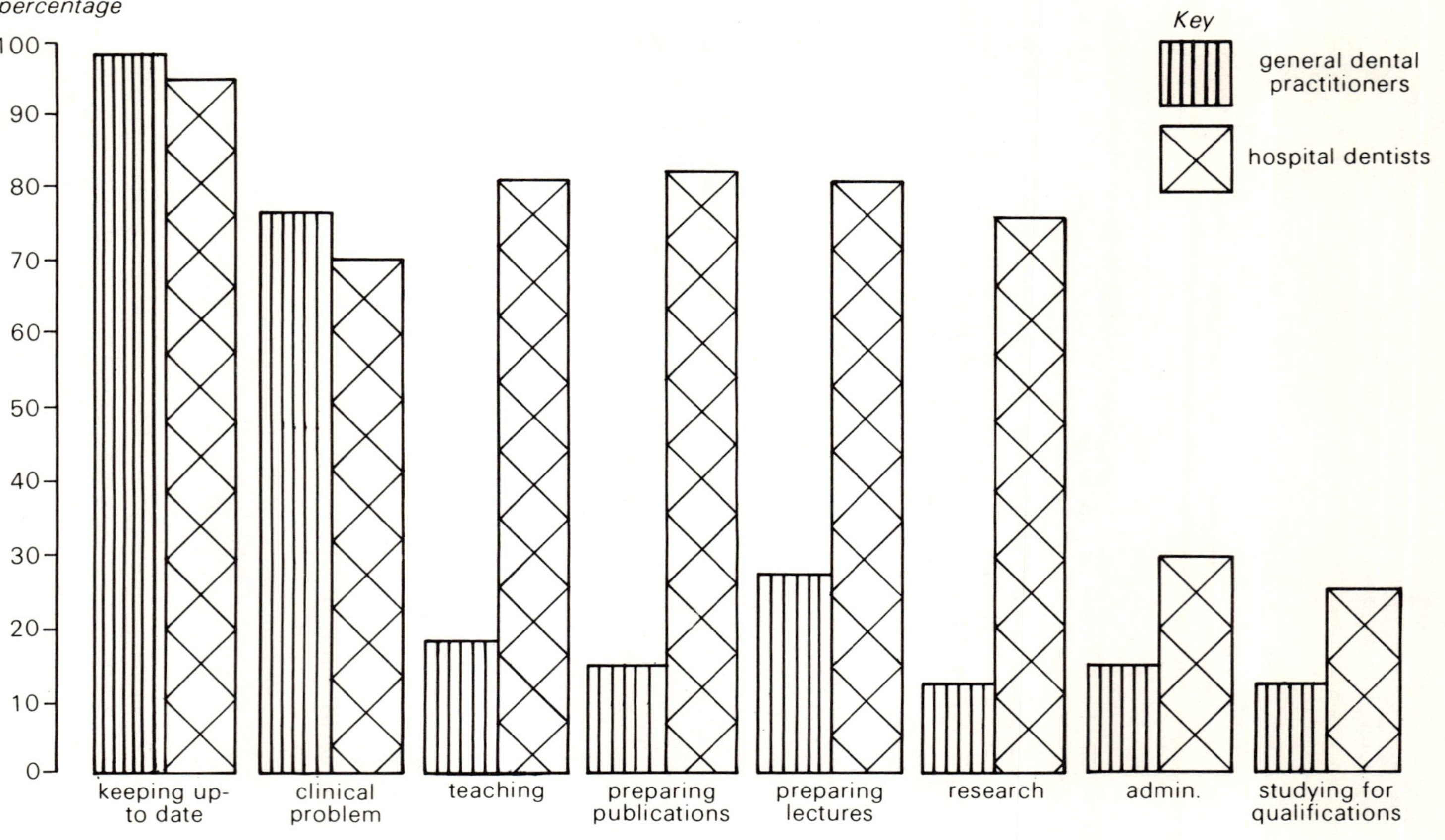

Figure 2.1 Reasons for seeking information.

(Adapted from Ford, G. *Provision and use of medical literature: summary report and conclusions*. Boston Spa, West Yorkshire: British Library, 1979).

Table 2.1 Use of different reference sources

	Hospital dentists		*General dental practitioners*	
	Never (%)	*Frequently*	*Never (%)*	*Within previous month*
Medline	51.6	3.2	84.7	1.2
Abstracts	15.0	21.7	78.5	10.1
Index journals	16.7	36.7	74.7	11.4
Refs. in journals	4.8	46.0	not asked	
Specialist bibliographies	45.5	1.8	73.2	10.1
Review articles	6.2	28.1	59.5	34.2
Colleagues	4.8	19.0	60.7	31.7
Browsing	6.5	12.9	49.0	35.5
Librarian	39.7	7.9	73.4	5.1
Official circulars	32.3	6.5	58.2	7.6

Adapted from Ford, G. *Provision and use of medical literature: summary report and conclusions.* Boston Spa: British Library, 1979.

with colleagues also having an important role. The use of Medline has probably now increased since the survey was undertaken, because a greater number of libraries have access to online terminals, and knowledge of the facility is more widespread.

Journal clubs may be found in dental schools or at postgraduate medical centres. Although detailed arrangements vary from one institution to another, a characteristic of a club is that individuals present to their colleagues papers of interest from recent periodicals, thus making known a range of current literature, often from sources that would not otherwise have been seen by the participants.

2.4 Literary Style

Style and presentation of dental literature follow the same principles as medical writing. There are, however, texts available specifically intended for dental authors. Craddock's small book (1968) is the only British manual, and deserves to be better known; it is an excellent text. There are American works by Easlick *et al.* (1974), whose manual is predominantly devoted to grammar and stylistic matters, and Darby and Bowen (1980), who discuss writing and research methodology. For the publisher, the American Dental Association has produced a practical guide edited by Nolen (1981).

The problems inherent in revising manuscripts to conform with the different house styles of various journals faced by authors submitting papers for publication have attracted the attention of publishers, and led to an important time-saving development. Following a meeting in Vancouver, Canada, in 1978, an international committee of medical editors was formed, and a series of uniform technical requirements for manuscripts was adopted by a number of journals. Slight revisions have since been made, but by mid 1982 150 journals, including some dental titles, had agreed to accept papers prepared in accordance with the requirements. The criteria are officially entitled *Uniform requirements for manuscripts submitted to biomedical journals*, but are commonly known as the 'Vancouver style', and were published by the International Committee (1982) in the *British medical journal*, together with a list of journals that accept papers prepared according to the requirements. Topics covered by the specifications include preparation of the manuscript, abstract, text and references. The numerical system of reference citation is advocated, in which references in the text are numbered consecutively and listed in that order at the end of the paper. Included in the details for each reference are the title of paper and last page number—useful features for readers, and ones that had not previously been given in many reference lists. The Harvard system, whereby references are arranged by author (as in this book), is therefore being superseded in many journals.

For prospective postgraduate students, Kelly (1981) has written a very useful summary of the points to be remembered when preparing and writing a thesis, advice also appropriate for other, similar research reports.

2.5 Dental Libraries

Separate dental library collections are decreasing in number, as larger general medical libraries are today more economical than small, specialized ones. In general, dental libraries or collections are found in dental schools or national associations, and the British situation, described below, is typical of that found in many other countries.

2.5.1 Dental Libraries in Britain

While many medical libraries have dental literature in their stock, only a handful actually specialize in the subject, and the majority are in the dental schools. There are at present sixteen undergraduate schools in the United Kingdom, plus one postgraduate establishment, the Institute of Dental Surgery in London. Smaller dental collections are found in postgraduate medical centres, particularly those connected to hospitals carrying out oral surgery or with large dental departments and in armed forces libraries. The libraries of the Royal College of Surgeons of England and Royal Society of Medicine include dental literature to serve the members of the Faculty of Dental Surgery, and Odontological Section respectively. The British Dental Association has the largest collection.

Undergraduate Schools

Dental school librarians are not usually autonomous, but are assistants under their medical school librarian's jurisdiction. Their degree of independence and their status vary considerably from one school to another. Some schools have separate dental libraries, such as those of Cardiff and Bristol; others, for example Edinburgh and Leeds, have the dental stock included in an integrated medical school library. Where there is no separate dental library, there is less likely to be a member of the library staff specifically responsible for the subject field. Integrated or not, these collections serve undergraduates, postgraduates and teaching staff, plus the staff of the local dental hospital.

Postgraduate Level

There is one establishment in Britain devoted entirely to higher education: the Institute of Dental Surgery, which is a part of the British Postgraduate Medical Federation, a school of London University. It was established in 1950. Students here are mainly on taught MSc or Fellowship in Dental Surgery courses, lasting one or two years, and most come from overseas. Many of the teaching staff have honorary contracts with the associated Eastman Dental Hospital, and clinical, non-teaching, hospital staff use the library as well as the academics. The Institute of Dental Surgery library has two full-time staff, and although its readership may be smaller than in an undergraduate school, it is probably more intensively used.

British Dental Association

The British Dental Association (BDA) has the most comprehensive dental library in Britain, and was founded in 1920, forty years after the establishment of the Association itself. Current holdings include 10,000 monographs, 2,000 pamphlets, 500 subject packages, 200 current journals, and a historical collection of over 500 titles. Since readers are from all spheres of dental practice, coverage is of every aspect of the subject field, and from elementary to research level. As readers are scattered throughout the whole of Britain, and may also be working overseas, there is an extensive postal enquiry and loan service. There are four members of staff. The history and scope of the BDA library are described by Spencer (1981). The BDA is the major British back-up library for older or obscure dental literature and coordinates contacts between other dental libraries.

2.5.2 Libraries in Other Countries

In the United States there are more dental schools than in Britain and therefore more libraries; one of the largest, with an extensive historical collection, is that of the Northwestern University Dental School in Chicago.

The most important library in the USA, however, is the Bureau of Library Services of the American Dental Association (ADA), which serves its own members and acts as a national and international resource centre. Library facilities were first offered to ADA members in 1927, in the form of loans, bibliographies and package libraries (collections of reprints on specific subjects).

These traditional services continue to be provided, but in far greater volume. Now photocopying is a common practice, to some extent replacing loans, and audiovisual material falls within the scope of the Bureau. The stock currently comprises some 37,000 monographs, 900 serial titles and over 2,000 different subject packages. As a department of the world's largest national dental association, it has resources and functions beyond those of the smaller national dental libraries in other countries: for instance, responsibility for the *Index to dental literature*, and the preparation of indexes to various journals such as *Journal of the American Dental Association*. Some leaflets and pamphlets are issued by the Bureau for the benefit of readers and other librarians with less extensive acquisitions programmes; these include *Books and package libraries for dentists* [34], lists of current journals, an *Accessions list* [23] and *Basic dental reference works* [33]. The staff complement is nineteen, of which nine are professional posts. The development of the Bureau has been described by Washburn (1978).

Since the provision of dental literature throughout the world broadly follows the British and American pattern, other collections will not be described. Details of Dutch dental libraries are given by Napjus (1983). A worldwide listing of dental collections is published in the *Index to dental literature* (1980). Although there are some omissions (for instance, the Institute of Dental Surgery in London, and, surprisingly, the ADA itself), this is a useful indicator of the existence of libraries, and their size, in different countries. Arrangement is by country, giving addresses, number of monographs and serial titles held and number of current periodical titles received.

American medical libraries are listed in the *Directory of health science libraries in the United States* (1979), British ones in the *Directory of medical and health care libraries in the United Kingdom* (1982). A more specific guide to British dental collections is *Library resources for dentistry* (1983), which lists twenty-four libraries, most, but not all, serving dental schools.

A selected list of libraries is given in Part III of this book.

The (American) Medical Library Association has a dental section, established in 1933, to link persons interested in the field and to contribute to the management of dental collections. No formal dental group exists in Britain as there are insufficient numbers of people to make one viable. Most dental librarians belong to the Library Association's Medical, Health and Welfare Libraries Group, and there is much informal cooperation.

Journals of particular interest to librarians in the field are the *Bulletin of the Medical Library Association* and *Health Libraries review*, the latter published by Blackwell for the Library Association's Medical, Health and Welfare Libraries Group.

2.6 Classification Schemes and Subject Headings Used in Libraries

The one classification scheme devised specifically for dentistry is that of A. D. Black, originator of the *Index to dental literature* [17], and it is used in the early volumes of the *Index* for the subject arrangement of journal articles. The second edition, published in 1975, is used by the American Dental Association's Bureau of Library Services, and, in a modified format, by the British Dental Association's library. Black's is the one scheme to provide in its schedules sufficient detail for these large, specialized collections; extensive holdings on dentistry classified by other schemes usually necessitate making additions to the schedules and notation. Black's notation is numerical, but all numbers are prefaced by the letter D, as is demonstrated by the extracts in *Tables 2.2b* and *2.3b*. All classification schemes suffer to some extent from the problems of 'distributed relatives', where related topics are classified at distant numbers by the nature of the scheme. In Black's case, this results in the physiological and pathological aspects of the hard and soft tissues being separated. For example, Dental pulp (i.e. its physiology), is classified at D 124, while Endodontics (treatment of the pulp), is at D 24; Gingival histology is at D 125, Periodontal membrane at D 125, Oral mucosa at D127, while Periodontal diseases are at D 64.

There is an increasing trend away from home-made schemes, and those which are lesser-known or not kept up to date, towards others used nationally or internationally, notably the schemes of the National Library of Medicine (NLM) and the Library of Congress (LC), both emanating from the United States. These have significant advantages, such as the regular appearance of new

Table 2.2a Comparison of classification schemes: conservative dentistry

Library of Congress	
RK 500	Operative dentistry
501	General works
510	Anaesthesia
512	Special anaesthetics A–Z, e.g. N55 Nitrous oxide
515	Cavity preparation
517	Fillings, inlays
.519	By material, e.g. A4 Amalgam
Dewey	
617.67	Cavities (caries)
.672	Cavity preparation
.675	Fillings and inlays
National Library of Medicine	
WU 300	Operative dentistry: general works
350	Cavities. Cavity treatment
360	Inlays
CANDO	
WD 32	Operative dentistry
WD 39a	Materials
WD 80	Caries

Table 2.2b Comparison of classification schemes: conservative dentistry

Black		
D 2		Operative dentistry
D 21		Instruments and appliances
	211	Impression materials and technique
	212	Control of saliva, rubber dam
D 22		Filling teeth (includes cavity preparation)
		Filling materials (physical properties at D 151)
	221	Gold and platinum
	222	Amalgam
	223	Cement
	224	Temporary fillings
	225	Metallic fillings, other than gold and amalgam
	226	Acrylic resins and other synthetic resins
D 23		Inlays
	231	Gold inlays. Casting
	232	Other metallic inlays
	236	Acrylic resins
	237	Porcelain
D 24		Endodontics (four subdivisions)
D 25		Bleaching teeth. Discolorations
D 26		Fractures of teeth and correction through operative procedures

N.B. Crowns and bridges are classified under Prosthetic Dentistry

Table 2.3a Comparison of classification schemes: orthodontics

Library of Congress	
RK 521	General works
523	Disorders of occlusion. Malocclusion
525	Disorders of dentition. Impacted teeth. Unerupted teeth. Therapies
527	General
528	Special
Dewey	
617.643	Orthodontics
NLM	
WU 400	General works
440	Occlusion. Malocclusion
CANDO	
WA 37	Orthodontics

editions reflecting medical progress. These schemes are also attractive from the management and administrative viewpoints, since NLM and LC class numbers are usually provided with the cataloguing in publication details reproduced by the publisher on the back of each title page. Shared cataloguing and computerized systems, such as OCLC or Blaise-Locas, to which many large libraries now subscribe, encourage the use of these popular schemes.

The fourth edition of the *NLM classification* was published in 1978. Its dental class WU is certainly adequate for an undergraduate dental school library, and allows room for additional classes to be inserted. An expansion by Strauss (1973) of the WU class from the third edition, 1964, is still appropriate for some classes in the fourth edition, for instance Oral surgery (*Table 2.5*). To provide for very specific classes does, however, require a complex notation. The Northwestern University Dental School library uses NLM, and the long class numbers needed for some of its acquisitions can be seen in its accessions list, *Titles acquired* [29].

The Library of Congress provides a useful degree of detail in its dental class RK, generally more than NLM (*Tables 2.2a* and *2.3a*), and is certainly adequate for a non-specialist collection. This scheme is often favoured by university libraries with wide-ranging stocks covering all subject fields, and where the

Table 2.3b Comparison of classification schemes: orthodontics

Black			
D 4			Orthodontics
	41		Instruments, appliances and materials
	42		Aetiology of malocclusion
		421	Heredity as a cause of malocclusion
		422	Habits as a cause of malocclusion
		423	Nasal and pharyngeal conditions. Mouth breathing
		424	Retention and loss of teeth as a cause of malocclusion
D 43			Methods of diagnosis in orthodontics
		431	Roentgenology
		432	Photography
		433	Cephalometry
D 44			Classification of cases
D 45			Treatment
		451	Retention
		452	Harmful effects in orthodontic treatment
		453	Reaction of pulp, periodontal membrane and alveolar bone to orthodontic treatment
		454	Extraction in treatment
D 46			Preventive orthodontics. Space maintenance
D 47			Growth and development of the face and jaws
		471	Measurement of teeth and jaws
		472	Effect of endocrine disturbances

Table 2.4a Comparison of classification schemes: periodontology

Library of Congress		
	RK 361	General works
	371	Alveolar abscess
	375	Other abscesses
	381	Pyorrhea
	401	Gum diseases
	410	Gingivitis
	440	Diseases of alveolar process
	450	Other diseases
Dewey		
	617.632	Periodontics
National Library of Medicine		
	WU 240	Periodontium. Alveolar process. Gingiva (periodontics)
	WU 242	Periodontics and related diseases
Black		
	D 64	Diseases of investing tissues of the teeth: gingiva, periodontal membrane, alveolar process. Includes treatment (Physiological aspects classified at D 125, D 126)

classification of medical stock has to be compatible with the library holdings *in toto*. LC is usually used to supplement NLM for material beyond the scope of the latter scheme. The notation is similar, with letters and numbers.

The Dewey Decimal classification is traditionally a public library scheme, where there is little need for specificity in medicine. Broad classes are the norm, with no provision for further subdivisions, except at the expense of a long notation. Dentistry is assigned to class 617.6, with a further one or two decimal numbers for different aspects of the subject field (*Tables 2.2a* and *2.3a*).

A unique approach to the classification of medical literature is provided by the French scheme *CANDO Médical et Pharmaceutique: classification alphanumérique de la documentation*, of which the fourth edition was published in 1984. The dental section, class W, has been published and discussed by Chevallier (1973). This is a faceted scheme, with letters to represent organs or features and numbers to depict the particular aspect studied, plus the occasional use of lower-case letters for further detail. Subdivisions relate mainly to anatomical parts, such as WB Teeth, WF Mouth, WG Gums. Emphasis is on disease states rather than treatment, with only single numbers for Orthodontics (WA 3) and Prosthetics (WB 39), but a detailed breakdown for periodontal disease (*Table 2.4b*).

The *International classification of diseases* and its separately published excerpt *Application of the ICD to dentistry and stomatology* [219], described in Chapter 6, could be used for library classification, although their main purpose is for diagnostic

Table 2.4b Comparison of classification schemes: periodontology

CANDO			
WE	Periodontium	WG	Gingiva
01	General works	01	General works
16	Morphology	16	Anatomy
16u	Morphology of cementum	18	Physiology (gingival fluid)
16v	Morphology of periodontal ligament	38	Surgery
16w	Morphology of alveolar bone	38j	Surgical exposure of wisdom teeth
17	Embryology	38n	Electrosurgery
18	Physiology	45	Pathology
19	Histology	46	Pathological symptoms (pigmentation of gums)
19u	Cementum	48	Pathological syndromes
19v	Periodontal ligament	49	Gingivitis
19w	Alveolar bone	51	Toxic gingivitis
32	Surgery (periapical curettage, apical resection)	52	Infectious gingivitis
33j	Iontophoresis	54v	Syphilitic chancre
45	Periodontal pathology	56	Tuberculosis
49	Perodontitis, pericementitis	60	Tumours (epulis) (*see also* WF 60 Mouth: tumours)
52	Infection: pyorrhea alveolaris	61	Benign gingival tumours
52c	Abscesses of dental origin, periapical abscess	62	Malignant tumours
79m	Arthrosis of the periodontium	65t	Gingival haemorrhage (*see also* WA 65t Oral haemorrhage)

and epidemiological records. For a clinician's personal collection of literature or audiovisual material in the field of oral surgery or medicine, this scheme might also be appropriate, although, like the CANDO one, it deals with pathology rather than therapy, and in addition excludes the broader fields of conservation and prosthetics.

Lists of subject headings are not as varied as classification schemes. *Library of congress* (LC) headings are frequently used in subject catalogues, but there is a trend towards the use of *Medical subject headings* (MESH), as used in *Index medicus*. A fuller discussion of MESH is given in Chapter 4; suffice it to say here that there is an obvious advantage in having an in-house catalogue that has headings compatible with printed and on-line bibliographies. Outside North America, modifications to spelling and terminology are commonly made, such as anaesthesia instead of anesthesia, dental surgeries rather than dental offices. In specialized collections, such as that of the BDA, 'dental' as an entry word may be dropped.

LC and MESH headings are frequently given with cataloguing in publication data, allowing a comparison between them, for instance:

LC	MESH
Dental public health	Public health dentistry
Prosthodontics	Dental prosthesis
Mouth—Diseases—Diagnosis	Diagnosis, oral

Table 2.5 NLM classification: oral surgery

NLM			*Strauss expansion*	
WU	600	General works		
			603	Instruments
	605	Tooth extraction		
			607	Atlases
	610	Maxillofacial injuries. Mandibular injuries. Fractures and dislocations of the jaw		
	640	Dental implantation. Tooth reimplantation. Transplantation		
			680	Traumatic, industrial and emergency oral surgery

References

Chevallier, J. 'Classification de la bibliographie stomatologique'. *Revue d'odonto-stomatologie* **20** (1973): 175–83.

Craddock, F. W. *Dental writing*. 2nd ed. Bristol: John Wright, 1968. 95pp.

Darby, M. L. and Bowen, D. M. *Research methods for oral health professionals: an introduction*. St. Louis: C. V. Mosby, 1980. 193pp.

'Dental collections around the world'. *Index to dental literature* (1980): pp. vii–xxvi.

Directory of health science libraries in the United States. Edited by A. M. Rees and S. Crawford. Chicago: Medical Library Association, 1979. 360pp.

Directory of medical and health care libraries in the United Kingdom and Republic of Ireland 1982. 5th ed. Compiled by W. D. Linton. London: Library Association, 1982. 228pp.

Easlick, K. A., Craig, R. G., Russell, A. L. and Seger, S. I. *Communicating in dentistry: sources and evaluation of information and preparation of manuscripts, oral reports and proposals for research*. Springfield, Illinois: Charles C. Thomas, 1974. 228pp.

Ford, G. *Provision and use of medical literature: summary report and conclusions*. Boston Spa: British Library, 1979. 17pp.

Foley, G. P. H. 'Advances in dental literature, 1900–1950'. *Journal of the American Dental Association* **40** (1950): 769–89.

International Committee of Medical Editors. 'Uniform requirements for manuscripts submitted to biomedical journals'. *British medical journal* **284** (1982): 1766–70.

Kelly, M. J. 'Preparation of a mastership thesis'. *Annals of the Royal College of Surgeons of England* **63** (1981): 286–9.

Library resources for dentistry. 2nd ed. Typescript. London: 1982. 23pp. Available from the BDA Library.

Napjus, J. S. L. van Hecht Munting. 'A short history of dental libraries in the Netherlands'. *Index to dental literature* 1983, pp. vii–xiv.

Nolen, C. *Publishing the professional journal or newsletter: an editor's guide.* Chicago: American Dental Association, 1981. 185pp.

Riordan, P. J. and Gjerdet, N. R. 'The use of periodical literature in a Norwegian dental library'. *Bulletin of the Medical Library Association* **69** (1981) 387–91.

Spencer, E. M. 'The Robert and Lilian Lindsay Library of the British Dental Association'. *Index to dental literature* 1979, pp. vii–xii.

Strauss, C. D. 'A suggested expansion of the NLM classification scheme for dentistry'. *Bulletin of the Medical Library Association* **61** (1973): 328–32.

Washburn, D. A. 'A short history of the American Dental Association Bureau of Library Services'. *Index to dental literature* 1978, pp. vii–xiii.

World Health Organization. *Application of the 'International classification of diseases to dentistry and stomatology' (ICD-DA).* 2nd ed. Geneva: WHO, 1978. 150pp.

3 Who, What, Where?

Finding out about individuals and organizations can be straightforward, complicated or almost impossible, depending on the subject field or country of interest. Directories which exist for the specialities are discussed in Part II, and only general sources are discussed here.

3.1 General Directories

Three European countries—France, West Germany and Italy—have general dental directories. These simplify matters considerably, since they contain a diverse range of information, much of which can be understood by an enquirer who does not speak the language concerned.

The French *Annuaire dentaire* [187], published each year by Chabassol, is arranged in three parts. The first contains information on the dental trade; that is, manufacturers and their products, and on dental laboratories. The middle section comprises legislative and organizational information, including addresses of government departments, regional societies and speciality organizations, and dental schools. Finally there is a directory of dentists arranged by name with a geographical index. Each section is printed on different-coloured paper: green, pink and white respectively.

The *Deutsche zahnärztliche Adressbuch* [188] appears at approximately six-year intervals, the twelfth edition being published in 1978, the thirteenth due in 1985. It is therefore less up to date than its French equivalent, but is better than no directory at all. As well as a dentists' list arranged by region with a name index, it gives names and addresses for national and local organizations and German journals. Also included is a list of dental schools throughout the world, and the addresses of national and international dental associations.

The *Annuario dentale italiano* [189] is a newcomer to the field, the first edition having been published in 1983. As well as being a directory of dentists, it lists Italian dental schools, technicians' training schools, addresses of some national and international organizations and a selection of the world's journals.

For other countries data are more diffuse; directories of dentists may exist but, as in the case of Britain, no comprehensive list of societies. General reference books, as opposed to those specifically related to dentistry, may be relevant tools as will be demonstrated in due course. Serendipity, or else systematic scanning of relevant journals, may be the only way to find information. National journals such as the *Journal of the American Dental Association* [74] and the *British dental journal* [62] contain valuable details in their news, information and advertisement sections. Through these features, for example, may be found addresses of societies which are publishing notices of meetings, or of manufacturers who have placed trade advertisements.

When there is no obvious published source of information, a dental school library or the national dental association may be able to provide an answer; or, alternatively, suggest a possible source. As in any subject field, vast arrays of facts, figures and specialized knowledge are in people's heads. The lists of dental schools, national associations and societies in Part III are but one step towards finding an answer.

3.2 Directories of Individuals

Because dentistry is a closed profession, and registration is a prerequisite to being allowed to practise, most countries have available some kind of published list of registered dentists. France, West Germany and Italy have commercially produced general directories, as already mentioned, and a substantial part of all three is taken up with alphabetical and geographical listings of dentists registered in those countries.

For any country, the most comprehensive list of dentists is that held by the national or state registering bodies. In Britain it is mandatory for dentists to register with the General Dental Council (GDC) in order to practise, and a *Dentists register* [193] is published in accordance with the Dentists Act each year by the GDC. The *Register* comprises an alphabetical list of dentists giving full names, qualifications and the dates they were awarded, and addresses. Most are personal, as opposed to practice, addresses; telephone numbers are not given. Up to 1983 there are three alphabetical name sequences; after the main list are shorter ones for the 'Foreign' and 'Commonwealth' dentists; that is, dentists who obtained their basic dental degree outside Britain. Following the 1983 Dentists Act, and a modification to the legislation, these two sequences, often forgotten, have been incorporated into the main list. The local list is divided into broad regions: England, Wales, Scotland, Ireland, overseas, with each group arranged alphabetically by town. The *Register* has been published annually since the first Dentists Act in 1878, and is therefore valuable for retrospective searching.

As its name implies, it is intended as a list of names only, and therefore gives no extraneous information about individuals, and little on other aspects of dentistry in Britain. It does include a table showing the numbers of dentists registered each year from 1921 to date, but since retired dentists, and British dentists practising abroad, can still choose to be registered, it does not purport to indicate the exact number of dentists practising in Britain. Also included in the *Register* is the text of the Dentists Act, and the GDC's own 'Notice of guidance to dentists', which advises on ethical and disciplinary conduct.

By contrast, registrable bodies in Australia are at the level of individual states, and each may maintain records of practitioners within its boundaries. Victoria and Western Australia publish lists of registered dentists in their respective *Government gazettes* [182, 183]; Queensland issues two lists, published by its government printer, one of general practitioners, the other of specialists [180, 179].

The South African Medical and Dental Council issues a combined annual list of doctors and dentists.

National dental associations may publish membership lists, but these will be less comprehensive than those produced by registration bodies, since membership of a professional organization is not mandatory. One of the most substantial sources in this category is the American Dental Association's *American dental directory* [198]. This large tome is issued annually, and its bulk comprises a list arranged by state then town, with names, addresses and telephone numbers. There follows an alphabetical name index. Since some 90 percent of American dentists belong to the ADA its national listing is valuable.

Membership lists produced by other national organizations are inevitably only a fraction of the size from the point of view of simple numbers, but are no less valuable. The Australian dental directory [178] for example, published annually by the Australian Dental Association, may be more widely available than the official state lists, and includes approximately 90 percent of dentists in the continent. The Swedish and Swiss dental associations also publish annual membership lists. Details of individual lists are given in Part II.

Not all national organizations issue lists of members, however, and cost can be a determining factor, influencing the production of a directory, or the frequency with which it is issued. The 1983 updating of the Canadian Dental Association's *Directory*, for example, was not produced, for economic reasons. The British Dental Association made available lists of members for the years 1897–1936 but today does not consider the cost justifiable.

In place of a special list, sometimes the appropriate details are included in the association's journal. This is not feasible when the membership is large, but for a smaller organization can make the publication of a list of members a viable proposition. Many American state or regional associations follow this practice, for instance Michigan. The New York Academy of Dentistry, too, includes a membership roster in the first issue of *Annals of dentistry* each year. The Royal Australasian College of Dental Surgeons publishes a list of fellows in its annual *Annals* [181] and the Fédération Dentaire Internationale gives the names and addresses of members each year in the *International dental journal* [176]. Larger organizations may use the same means of publication, but issue their directories less regularly. For instance, the Alpha Omega Fraternity published a membership directory in a 1983 issue of *Alpha omegan* [175], the first time for seventeen years!

Other sources may play a part in identifying or locating individuals, for example university calendars. The *Medical directory* [194], issued annually, includes British dentists who also have a medical qualification; these will be primarily oral surgeons and anaesthetists. As well as addresses and qualifications, details of present and former professional posts are listed.

General biographical directories, such as *Who's who* or *American men and women of science*, may include eminent dentists, but by and large do not include many members of the profession. For retrospective searching, the *Lives of the Fellows of the Royal College of Surgeons of England* [195] includes entries for dentists who were Fellows of the RCS. Five volumes are currently available, covering the years 1843–1973. *Who's who in dentistry* [200], in two small volumes, gives short biographical sketches of U.S. and Canadian dentists who were prominent in the profession at the time of publication, that is, 1916 and 1925.

Biographical entries may also be found in dictionaries.

3.3 Organizations and Institutions

National dental societies in France, West Germany and Italy are listed in their respective directories, previously described, although the *Annuario dentale Italiano* is not comprehensive in this respect. For the United States, the *American dental directory* [198] publishes a list of national dental organizations in the USA, giving the name and address of the secretary or director of over ninety specialist societies. It also lists officials of the state dental associations, which are important regional organizations.

Contact points for specialist societies in New Zealand are given in each issue of the *New Zealand dental journal* [84], while for Australia, the Australian Dental Association's *Directory* [178] may be consulted.

Unfortunately there is no central listing of dental societies in Britain, although the *Medical directory* [194] includes a handful in its list of British medical organizations, and is worth checking when this source is easily accessible. It is hoped, therefore, that this *Keyguide* will alleviate the problem of identifying British societies, by providing details in the selective guide in Part III. A feature of most specialist organizations, especially in Britain, is that their members are scattered throughout the country, and they have no centralized headquarters. This is in contrast to the position of some of the large American societies, which have administrative premises of their own, a number being based in the ADA building in Chicago. Officials of most societies, especially in Britain, are honorary officers undertaking their duties in their own time, and there may be a regular turnover of contact points and addresses. It must therefore be borne in mind that although correct at compilation, the details of officers given in the list of organizations in Part III are subject to change. Nevertheless, the list will serve as a guide to the existence of particular organizations. The appropriate speciality or a general journal should be scanned for the most up-to-date information.

Names and addresses of international organizations are given in the *American dental directory* [198]; this annually published listing may be consulted to update the information given in Part III.

Dental schools are usually attached to general universities, these being covered by the standard reference guides *World of learning* and *Commonwealth universities yearbook*, the latter including in each entry the names of senior staff in each faculty. For convenience, addresses of dental schools are given in Part III; a list of United States accredited schools is also given in the *American dental directory*. Calendars and prospectuses of individual institutions will provide information on staff, facilities and courses.

Dental hospitals are linked to the schools, but large general hospitals may have dental departments. The British *Medical directory* [194] includes a section on National Health Service hospitals, arranged under regional health authority, and for each hospital indicates the various departments and the senior staff in each. It is therefore possible to check whether a particular hospital has, for example, an orthodontic or oral surgery department and the names of the consultants in them.

3.4 The Dental Trade

The range of items which the dentist needs to carry out his profession includes, at one extreme, the extensive fittings of the surgery itself, such as the patient's chair, lighting and cabinets, to sets of hand instruments and face masks. A variety of materials for different types of fillings and impression procedures are required, plus drugs and anaesthetics. The dental trade is responsible for the manufacture and supply of these goods, which are constantly being redesigned, redeveloped or even superseded by newer products.

Today the manufacture of dental equipment and supplies is predominantly in the hands of large companies whose products are exported throughout the world; Scandinavia and Australia, for example, do not undertake extensive development of new materials, but rely considerably on imports, mainly from the United States. The national or local distributor therefore plays a vital role in the supply of goods to the dentist, and it is common for the practitioner to order his requirements from a dental supply house rather than individual manufacturers.

The trade relies heavily on direct mail and journal advertising to publicize its products; journals may also carry short press notices of new materials or equipment such as the trade news section in the *British dental journal*. National trade associations have been formed in many countries, such as the Verband der

Deutschen Industrie in West Germany and the British Dental Trade Association, to encourage high professional standards; their existence is noted in the FDI's *Basic fact sheets* [217] but addresses are not given. Trade shows, organized by the trade associations themselves, or as adjuncts to dental congresses, are popular.

Directories of traders or manufacturers are available for a number of countries, but not necessarily as separate publications. For France, the first section of the *Annuaire dentaire* [187] has three relevant lists: an alphabetical index of manufacturers and suppliers with their addresses, a list of trade names with the manufacturers' names, and a subject list of products. The German journal *Dental echo* [202] carries a subject directory of equipment and supplies each month giving names and addresses of firms, but has no alphabetical index of companies. For Britain, the most comprehensive source is the *Dental technician yearbook and directory* [204] which has a product directory and list of manufacturers and traders.

The oral hygiene industry has a special position in the trade since it is selling its products, such as toothbrushes and toothpaste, to the public as well as dealing with the dental profession. This sector of the trade may promote dental health education projects, and issues a multiplicity of leaflets and other educational material. British manufacturers in this field may be members of the Cosmetics, Toiletry and Perfumery Alliance.

3.5 Research

In most countries, research is the province of dental schools, although not exclusively so. A limited amount of work is done in industry, in government institutes, independent institutions, the hospital and community dental services and by individual practitioners. In Britain it is the staff and students of the dental schools who are numerically the largest body of research workers, fitting their investigations into the teaching and clinical timetable. Finance is, in the majority of cases, ultimately from government sources, since the universities themselves are funded by the Department of Education and Science, but there is no central directive as to which areas of dentistry or which individual projects should be supported. Comparatively little funding is provided by outside sources, in contrast to some other medical specialities, where a considerable proportion of the necessary costs are met by commercial firms, pharmaceutical companies, private bequests or charitable foundations—cancer research being a case in point. Nevertheless, limited funds are provided by the drug and oral hygiene industries, charities, and health authorities.

Outside the dental schools research activity is limited, but nevertheless is still operational. The Laboratory of the Government Chemist includes in its scope the investigation of dental materials and has a short section on dental research in its annual report. The Medical Research Council, which has a number of specialized units throughout Britain, has dental units based at the London Hospital

Medical College, and at Bristol Dental School, and also issues grants for other projects. Close links are retained between the MRC and the Royal College of Surgeons of England, which, as was stated earlier, supports two research units from its own funds, one in central London, the other in Kent. These are currently investigating periodontal diseases, and the immunological aspects of caries.

The oral hygiene industry conducts its own research, for instance into the formulation of toothpastes, but much of this remains confidential, at least until a product has been launched.

Research in the United States is for the most part undertaken in dental schools. Ayer *et al.* (*c.* 1980) conducted a survey of dental researchers in 1979 and found that some 69 percent of research took place in academic institutions, almost 54 percent specifically in dental schools. Trailing far behind as research locations were government institutions (14 percent), hospitals (6 percent) and industry (5 percent). For most of the respondents to their questionnaire, Ayer *et al.* found that research was a secondary activity, teaching being the principal occupation. The breakdown of major subject areas of interest was as follows: dental materials 17.2 percent, periodontology 11.8 percent, craniofacial biology 9.8 percent, behavioural science 8.4 percent, mineralized tissues 7.8 percent, microbiology 7.2 percent and cariology 7 percent.

It is significant in the context of this chapter to note that no single source listing individual research workers was regarded as sufficient when identifying individuals to whom the questionnaire should be sent. Ayer *et al.* were of the opinion that the American Association for Dental Research roster provided the most complete single listing, but they also used additional sources. A list of trainees and fellows was supplied by the National Institute of Dental Research; names given in *Dental research in the US and other countries* [207] and authors of *IADR abstracts* [77] were included as well. The results of the survey make interesting reading, and provide an insight into various facets of research activity in the United States.

The National Institute of Dental Research (NIDR) is a major research body. Founded in 1948, it is one of the speciality centres of the National Institute of Health, which themselves are part of the United States Government's Department of Health and Human Services. The NIDR is responsible for funding and conducting research in a range of dental subject fields, and providing training for potential research workers. *Figure 3.1* indicates the structure and subject interests of the Institute. At NIDR headquarters in Bethesda, Maryland, there is a staff of some 100 investigators, while extensive research sponsored by the NIDR is carried out at academic institutes and government agencies through its Extramural Program and the National Caries Program.

Projects in these two categories account for the greater part of the NIDR budget, and a range of grant and contract funds are available for research and training. Nevertheless, despite its importance in the dental field, the NIDR has the smallest financial allocation of any of the NIH institutes, and has insufficient

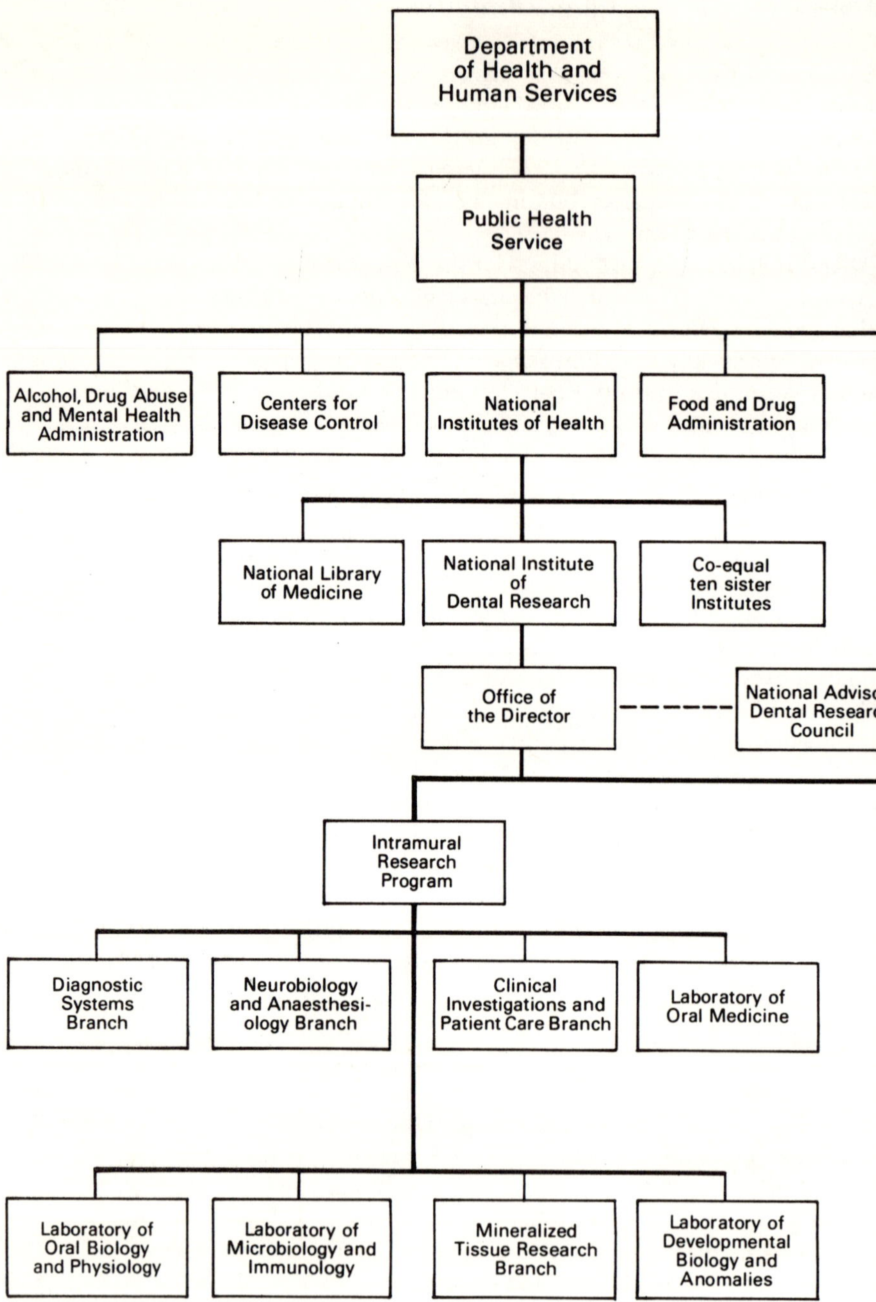

Figure 3.1 Structure of the National Institute of Dental Research.

(Adapted from *Journal of the American Dental Association* **106** [March 1983], pp. 306–7, and reproduced by courtesy of the American Dental Association).

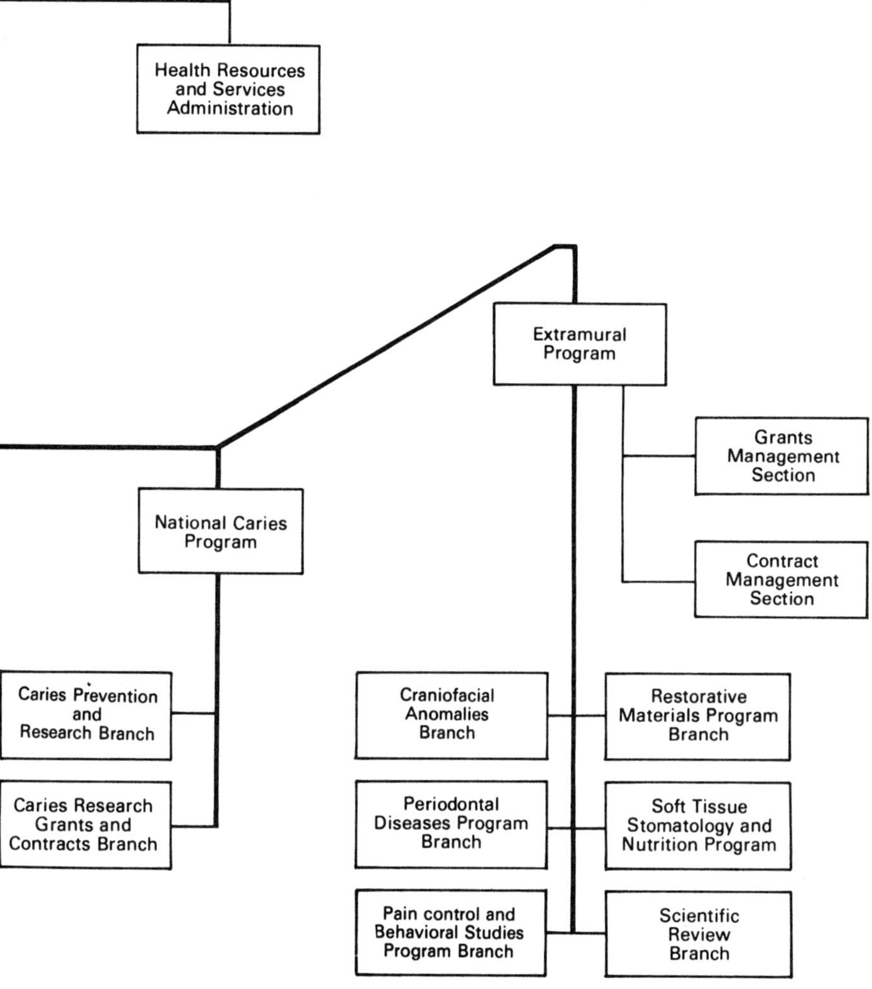
Health Resources and Services Administration
Extramural Program
Grants Management Section
Contract Management Section
National Caries Program
Caries Prevention and Research Branch
Caries Research Grants and Contracts Branch
Craniofacial Anomalies Branch
Restorative Materials Program Branch
Periodontal Diseases Program Branch
Soft Tissue Stomatology and Nutrition Program
Pain control and Behavioral Studies Program Branch
Scientific Review Branch

funds to sponsor all applicants for its grants. Researchers are therefore being encouraged to apply to private foundations for funds, as described by Verrusio and Gibson (1982) in the ADA's *Journal*.

An excellent presentation entitled 'NIDR, 1983' describes the activities of the different departments of the Institute.

Two regular publications emanate from the NIDR. The *Selected list of technical reports in dentistry* [245] is, as its name implies, a bibliography of technical reports prepared by researchers with NIDR funding which have been submitted to the National Technical Information Service for publication. Most of these reports are also published in the journal literature as conventional research papers and are thereby identified in the usual way. *NIDR abstracts* [10] is a monthly production with informative abstracts of research papers in basic and applied sciences rather than dentistry itself.

Research in American government institutions may be only a small proportion of the whole, but it is nevertheless significant. Three bodies involved are the National Bureau of Standards, which operates principally in the area of dental materials, the Naval Dental Research Institute and the Army Institute of Dental Research. The history of the latter is described by Cutright and Daniel (1977). Founded in 1922, research in this institution is primarily, although not exclusively, related to military aspects of dentistry.

The American Association for Dental Research is the North American section of the International Association for Dental Research, which was described in Chapter 1, Section 1.4.2. It is a force for the promotion of research, with an extensive membership.

In Canada, some 60 percent of funds for dental research are provided by the Medical Research Council, yet dentistry accounts for only 2 percent of the total MRC research allocation. Provincial funding accounts for some 16 percent, private industry and charitable foundations 3 percent each, and US agencies 4 percent. The University of Toronto received some 46 percent of the 1978 total funds. Jones (1982), who cites these figures, is critical of the low proportion of MRC funds allocated to dentistry, and wishes to encourage more research by faculty members. He is also dissatisfied with the existing concentration of subjects which receive most funds, these being periodontology, microbiology and neurophysiology, and he argues for a greater expenditure on research into dental materials.

Research in Australia is carried out in the dental schools, the Institute of Dental Research at Sydney and the Australian Dental Standards Laboratory, the latter being recognized internationally as a leading centre in materials research. The Institute of Dental Research, established in 1946, is concerned chiefly with biological aspects of oral disease, for example immunology and pathology. It receives financial support from the World Health Organization and the NIDR, as well as from Australian sources. As in other countries, research is funded mainly from the university budgets, although other sources include the National Health and Medical Council, the Australian Research Grants Commission and the Australian Research and Education Trust. However, inevitably there are many more applications for grants than funds available.

In Norway, a specialized research function is carried out by the Nordiske Institutt for Odontologisk Materialprovning (Scandinavian Institute of Dental Materials), which develops new materials and techniques, and tests materials on the Scandinavian market.

The role of the International Association for Dental Research and its constituent divisions was discussed in Chapter 1, Section 1.4.2. Less well known is the Groupement International pour la Recherche Scientifique en Stomatologie et Odontologie, based in Belgium, and predominantly a European organization. Its quarterly *Bulletin* contains articles published mainly in French, but by authors from a range of countries. Klees (1981) briefly describes the origins of the Groupement.

3.5.1 Research Directories

Britain is fortunate in having a regularly produced source in *Research in British universities, polytechnics and colleges* (*RBUPC*) [211], published annually by the British Library. The second of this three-volume work is devoted to biological sciences, section 9 being dental science. Under each institution is given the name of the investigator, the subject, and the years during which the project is being undertaken. Keyword and name indexes are provided.

The *Medical research directory* [209], published by Wiley in 1983, includes dentistry as section 31 of forty-five subject sections. The details provided for each project are similar to those in *RBUPC*, but since the scope is not restricted to academic institutions, the Laboratory of the Government Chemist, the Medical Research Council and the Royal College of Surgeons of England are included. It is searchable online via Data-Star.

Medical research centres [210], produced by Longmans, has worldwide coverage of research centres in 140 countries, in the fields of dentistry, nursing, pharmacy, psychiatry and surgery. *European research centres* [208] from the same publisher covers science, technology, agriculture and medicine. Under each entry is given the full name, address, list of activities and head of department.

For the United States and Canada, Bowker has published *Research programs in the medical sciences* [212], which lists organizations alphabetically, but the most useful American publication is now unfortunately defunct. The NIDR used to compile *Dental research in the US and other countries: a catalog of dental research projects during the fiscal year* [207]. This was arranged in broad subject groups, with descriptive summaries of some 2,000 projects and details of the names and institutions of the researchers. Owing to the phasing out of the Smithsonian Science Information Exchange, with whose help it was compiled, and publication cutbacks generally, the last issue to be published covers the fiscal year 1980.

The *Grants register* [214] can be useful for identifying potential sources of funding, since it gives details of research and travel grants available in the USA, the UK and the Commonwealth. With each award given are notes on purpose, duration, eligibility and application dates.

For the United States, the *Foundation grants index* [213] lists grants of $5,000 and above, awarded by some 400 organizations.

References

Ayer, W. A., Gift, H., Green, D. B., Howe, A. and Grossman, B. C. *Dental researchers in the United States*. Chicago: American Dental Association, [*c.* 1980]. 95pp.

Cutright, D. E. and Daniel, J. L. 'The US Army Institute of Dental Research: 53 years of dedicated research and education'. *Military medicine* **141** (1977): 45–8.

Jones, D. W. 'A materialistic look at dental research in Canada'. *Journal of the Canadian Dental Association* **48** (1982): 533–8.

Klees, L. 'Quelques souvenirs des débuts de GIRSO'. *Bulletin du Groupement International pour la Recherche Scientifique en Stomatologie et Odontologie* **24** (1981): 75–80.

'NIDR 1983: new directions for improving the nation's health'. *Journal of the American Dental Association* **106** (1983): 304–13.

Verrusio, C. A. and Gibson, W. A. 'Funding for dental research'. *Journal of the American Dental Association* **105** (1982): 680–3.

4 Keeping Up To Date with Current Information

4.1 Introduction

Dentistry, like any other contemporary discipline, is subject to changes. New materials are developed which in turn may necessitate modifications in clinical techniques. Equipment and instruments are continually under assessment. Not only may clinical or technical progress affect the profession, but broader political or social factors. Government legislation—for instance on health and safety at work, or dismissal of staff—will have implications for the business side of dentistry. An individual in any sphere of the profession, whether an academic research worker or general practitioner, needs to have access to up-to-date information, although the means by which it is provided may vary according to the needs or interests of the person concerned. At one extreme is the comprehensive, systematic approach, with monthly bibliographies provided automatically by a computerized database, according to a personally tailored search formulation. At the other is the casual browsing through periodicals practised by an individual when time permits or merely when he feels so inclined.

In Britain there is no legal requirement for dentists to keep up to date in professional matters, although various voluntary means of doing so are popular. Courses on specialist and general topics are numerous. Married women dentists in Britain are encouraged to join the Dentists' Retainer Scheme, a means of keeping in touch with the profession while unable to practise because of family commitments. Sarll and Holloway (1982) investigated factors affecting the adoption of new methods and techniques by general practitioners, and found three significant influences: membership of professional organizations, attendance at scientific meetings and subscription to journals.

Researchers and students are generally more motivated to use systematic methods of remaining in touch with new developments than general practitioners, and are therefore more likely to use abstracts, indexes and other published lists, as shown by Ford (1979) in the British Library survey discussed in Chapter 2, section 2.3.

Abstracting and indexing services are described in Chapter 5, since they are more valuable for systematic searches covering a period of years than for identifying current references. Discussion here is primarily confined to the three major tools which are used for keeping up to date, the *Index to dental literature*, *Index medicus* and *Dental abstracts*.

4.2 Index to Dental Literature

The main bibliographical tool is the *Index to dental literature* (*IDL*) [17] for both current awareness and retrospective searching. Because the *IDL* is central to any discussion related to identifying published papers in dentistry, it will be described at this point with reference to its use for finding both new and historical material. This important index lists periodical articles back to 1839, when the first dental journal was published. Early volumes cover five-year, then three-year periods, until 1950 when annual volumes commenced. The *IDL* is now published quarterly by the American Dental Association (ADA), the issues cumulating and the final quarter for each year being the annual cumulation.

Subject entries for the years 1839–1938 are under broad classified headings, the system being a modification devised by A. D. Black (the originator of the *IDL*) of the Dewey Decimal classification (*see* Chapter 2, section 2.6). Black provided more detail and simplified the notation, so that the Dewey number for dentistry, 617.6, became D. Thus 617.61 Dental anatomy is D1; 617.62 Operative dentistry is D2, etc. Non-dental material included in the *IDL* is classified under conventional Dewey numbers. Within each class, arrangement is alphabetical by journal. A comprehensive subject index is printed on pink pages in the centre of each volume and is an essential feature for today's user, who is unlikely to be familiar with the classified arrangement. An author index completes each volume. The early history and underlying concepts behind the classified arrangement have been described by Black himself (1921).

In 1939 a dictionary arrangement combining author and subject entries was introduced, the choice of subject headings being based in part on those used in *Quarterly cumulative index medicus*. Subheadings were used extensively; by 1964 the heading 'Caries, dental' listed 500 papers and had ten subdivisions, including the cumbersome 'diet in relation to' and 'fluoride for prevention', which today are presented more succinctly, and 'incidence', which was further subdivided by country, a feature regrettably not present in current volumes.

From 1965 the ADA has cooperated with the National Library of Medicine to produce the *IDL*, the latter's production facilities for *Index medicus* being used. The most obvious changes apparent to the user are the split into separate subject and author sequences, and the introduction of MESH headings; that is to say, Medical Subject Headings, the structured, controlled vocabulary used in *Index medicus*. There are, however, disadvantages arising from the adoption of a subject-heading system intended for the whole of medicine, particularly for the new or casual user. Many headings begin with the word 'Dental', e.g. 'Dental amalgam', 'Dental caries', or with 'Tooth', e.g. 'Tooth extraction', 'Tooth, impacted'. Subtle distinctions in the use of some headings may not be apparent to even the more experienced searcher, e.g. between 'Community dentistry' and 'Public health dentistry'. Long-standing anomalies still remain, e.g. 'Tooth root', 'Root canal therapy', and yet for the root canal itself 'Dental pulp cavity'. Some problems related to terminology can, however, be overcome when searching online by use of free-text entry words.

Cross-references in the main body of the index are sparse; there is a 'List of dental descriptors' at the front of each volume, which gives some '*see*' and '*see also*' references, but which could nevertheless benefit from expansion. For example, there is no reference to indicate that papers on fissure sealants, a commonly used term, are indexed under 'Pit and fissure sealants'. As a final source for identifying appropriate search headings there is the annual MESH volume itself, issued with each January *Index medicus*, in which should be scanned free tables A14 (Anatomy—jaws and teeth), C6 (Procedures and technics, dental) and E7 (Mouth and tooth diseases). It should be noted that some headings listed in MESH as 'minor descriptors', that is to say, not used as headings in the printed *Index medicus* (for instance, 'Activator appliances'), *are* used in *IDL* as subject headings. Users from outside North America should take into account variations in spelling and terminology, for example an*e*sthesia; dental offices (British equivalent, dental surgeries). It is ADA policy to index papers under an average of three different headings. A familiarity with MESH headings for the researcher is vital, not only for making optimum use of *IDL* and *Index medicus* but also library catalogues, since many collections now use this scheme for subject indexing. Extracts from MESH are reproduced in *Figures 4.1–4.4*.

Coverage for many years was restricted to English-language journals, but in 1952 papers written in English in foreign-language titles were included, and, from 1962, journals written in European languages. Today coverage is of some 9,000 journals in over forty languages, including Russian and Japanese, and a significant factor regarding inclusion is availability at the ADA or National Library of Medicine libraries. An analysis by country of origin of journals indexed is shown in *Figure 4.5*.

As shown in *Figure 4.6*, approximately two-thirds of papers in the *Index* are in English with the German language in second place. There is inevitably a bias towards American journals as regards coverage of minor titles and speed of

DENTAL CAVITY PREPARATION
E6.323.325

DENTAL CEMENTS
D25.339.291+ D26.16.275
72; was CEMENT, DENTAL see under DENTAL MATERIALS 1963-64; POLYCARBOXYLATE CEMENT was see under ACRYLIC RESINS 1977-81, was see under ACRYLATES 1975-76
XU GLASS IONOMER CEMENTS
XU POLYCARBOXYLATE CEMENT
XR CEMENTATION

DENTAL CEMENTUM
A14.254.646.267 A14.254.860.232
X CEMENTUM

DENTAL CLINICS
N2.278.192.250
65
X CLINICS, DENTAL
XR ORAL HEALTH
XR PREVENTIVE DENTISTRY

DENTAL CROWNS see CROWNS

DENTAL DEPOSITS
A12.300+ C7.793.208+
65

DENTAL DEVICES, HOME CARE
E6.186.250 E6.761.726.292
E7.222.250
72
XR ORAL HYGIENE

DENTAL ENAMEL
A14.254.860.268+

DENTAL HEALTH SURVEYS
E6.208+ G3.890.160+
N1.224.458.251+
72
XU DENTAL PLAQUE INDEX
XU ORAL HYGIENE INDEX
XR ORAL HEALTH

DENTAL HIGH SPEED EQUIPMENT
E6.186.376 E7.222.376
65

DENTAL HIGH SPEED TECHNIC
E6.216
65

DENTAL HYGIENISTS
M1.526.485.67.105.376 N2.350.84.200.110
65

DENTAL IMPLANTATION
E4.833.800.310+ E6.231+
E6.780.314+ E6.892.800.310+
65
X DENTAL PROSTHESIS, SURGICAL

DENTAL IMPLANTATION, ENDOSSEOUS
E4.833.800.310.310+ E6.231.310+
E6.780.314.310+ E6.892.800.310.310+
77
X ENDOSSEOUS IMPLANTATION
XU BLADE IMPLANTATION

DENTAL IMPLANTATION, ENDOSSEOUS, ENDODONTIC
E6.231.310.360 E6.397.345

Figure 4.1 A typical extract from MESH.

(Reproduced by courtesy of the National Library of Medicine.)

C7 - DISEASES-ORAL

MOUTH AND TOOTH DISEASES (NON MESH)

MOUTH AND TOOTH DISEASES (NON MESH)	C7	
MOUTH DISEASES	C7.465	
BEHCET'S SYNDROME	C7.465.75	C11.941.879. C17.66
BURNING MOUTH SYNDROME •	C7.465.114	
CANDIDIASIS, ORAL	C7.465.130	C1.703.160.
DENTAL FISTULA	C7.465.187	
OROANTRAL FISTULA	C7.465.187.577	
DRY SOCKET	C7.465.227	
HEMORRHAGE, ORAL	C7.465.316	C23.542.544
GINGIVAL HEMORRHAGE •	C7.465.316.446	C7.465.714. C23.542.544.
JAW, EDENTULOUS	C7.465.340	
MOUTH, EDENTULOUS	C7.465.340.630	
JAW, EDENTULOUS, PARTIALLY	C7.465.360	
LEUKOEDEMA, ORAL •	C7.465.385	
LIP DISEASES	C7.465.409	
CHEILITIS	C7.465.409.215	
HERPES LABIALIS	C7.465.409.466	C2.256.466. C17.838.424.
LIP NEOPLASMS	C7.465.409.640	C4.588.546.
LUDWIG'S ANGINA	C7.465.433	C1.539.535
MELKERSSON-ROSENTHAL SYNDROME	C7.465.466	C10.772.204.
MICROSTOMIA •	C7.465.497	C16.131.314.
MOUTH NEOPLASMS	C7.465.565	C4.588.546
LEUKOPLAKIA, ORAL	C7.465.565.429	C4.588.546. C4.834.512.
PALATAL NEOPLASMS	C7.465.565.666	C4.588.149. C4.588.546. C5.500.69
NOMA	C7.465.604	

Figure 4.2 MESH tree structures: extract from table C7.

(Reproduced by courtesy of the National Library of Medicine.)

E6 - PROCEDURES AND TECHNICS-DENTAL

DENTISTRY

DENTISTRY	E6	G2.163		
ANESTHESIA, DENTAL	E6.45	E3.155.141		
HYPNOSIS, DENTAL	E6.45.481	E3.155.141.	E3.155.675.	
BONDING, DENTAL	E6.95			
ACID ETCHING, DENTAL •	E6.95.100			
DENTAL CARE	E6.170	N2.421.196		
DENTAL CARE FOR HANDICAPPED	E6.170.310	N2.421.196.		
DENTAL EQUIPMENT	E6.186	E7.222		
DENTAL ARTICULATORS •	E6.186.210	E7.222.210		
DENTAL DEVICES, HOME CARE	E6.186.250	E6.761.726.	E7.222.250	
DENTAL HIGH SPEED EQUIPMENT	E6.186.376	E7.222.376		
DENTAL INSTRUMENTS	E6.186.501	E7.222.501		
MATRIX BANDS •	E6.186.501.630	E7.222.501.		
DENTAL HEALTH SURVEYS	E6.208	G3.890.160	N1.224.458.	
DENTAL PLAQUE INDEX •	E6.208.250	G3.890.160.	N1.224.458.	
DMF INDEX	E6.208.266	G3.890.160.	N1.224.458.	
ORAL HYGIENE INDEX •	E6.208.576	G3.890.160.	N1.224.458.	
PERIODONTAL INDEX	E6.208.720	E6.721.658	G3.890.160.	N1.224.458.
DENTAL HIGH SPEED TECHNIC	E6.216			
DENTAL IMPLANTATION	E6.231	E4.833.800.	E6.780.314	E6.892.800.
DENTAL IMPLANTATION, ENDOSSEOUS	E6.231.310	E4.833.800.	E6.780.314.	E6.892.800.
BLADE IMPLANTATION •	E6.231.310.340	E4.833.800.	E6.780.314.	E6.892.800.
DENTAL IMPLANTATION, ENDOSSEOUS, ENDODONTIC	E6.231.310.360	E6.397.345		

Figure 4.3 MESH tree structures: extract from table E6.

(Reproduced by courtesy of the National Library of Medicine.)

inclusion. Core journals are normally indexed within six months, most others within a year, but some foreign-language items may not be indexed until two years after original publication.

Medical articles relevant to dentistry but from non-dental journals have been included since 1965, when the NLM's resources became available. Coverage of relevant scientific or technical literature, e.g. in the field of materials, is weak, however, since there is no other back-up source. Papers in journals such as *Surface technology* or *Journal of polymer science* will not be included, although coverage of biomedical literature is satisfactory. Approximately 39 percent of the papers indexed each year are from non-dental journals, but with a lower percentage of foreign-language material; 29 percent of the items from non-dental journals are in languages other than English, whereas 48 percent of papers from dental journals are in other languages.

Although the majority of entries are for journal papers, letters and editorials are indexed if considered sufficiently important. Book reviews, abstracts and obituaries are excluded, although they were indexed in the early years. Useful preliminary sections are found in each volume. The 'List of dental books' comprises English-language works, arranged by author or title, with a trend towards the latter for multi-author works. Dissertations are listed by country, subject and author, and there is also a 'Bibliography of dental reviews', with MESH and author sequences.

Although ostensibly the *Index* appears quarterly, the annual cumulation may

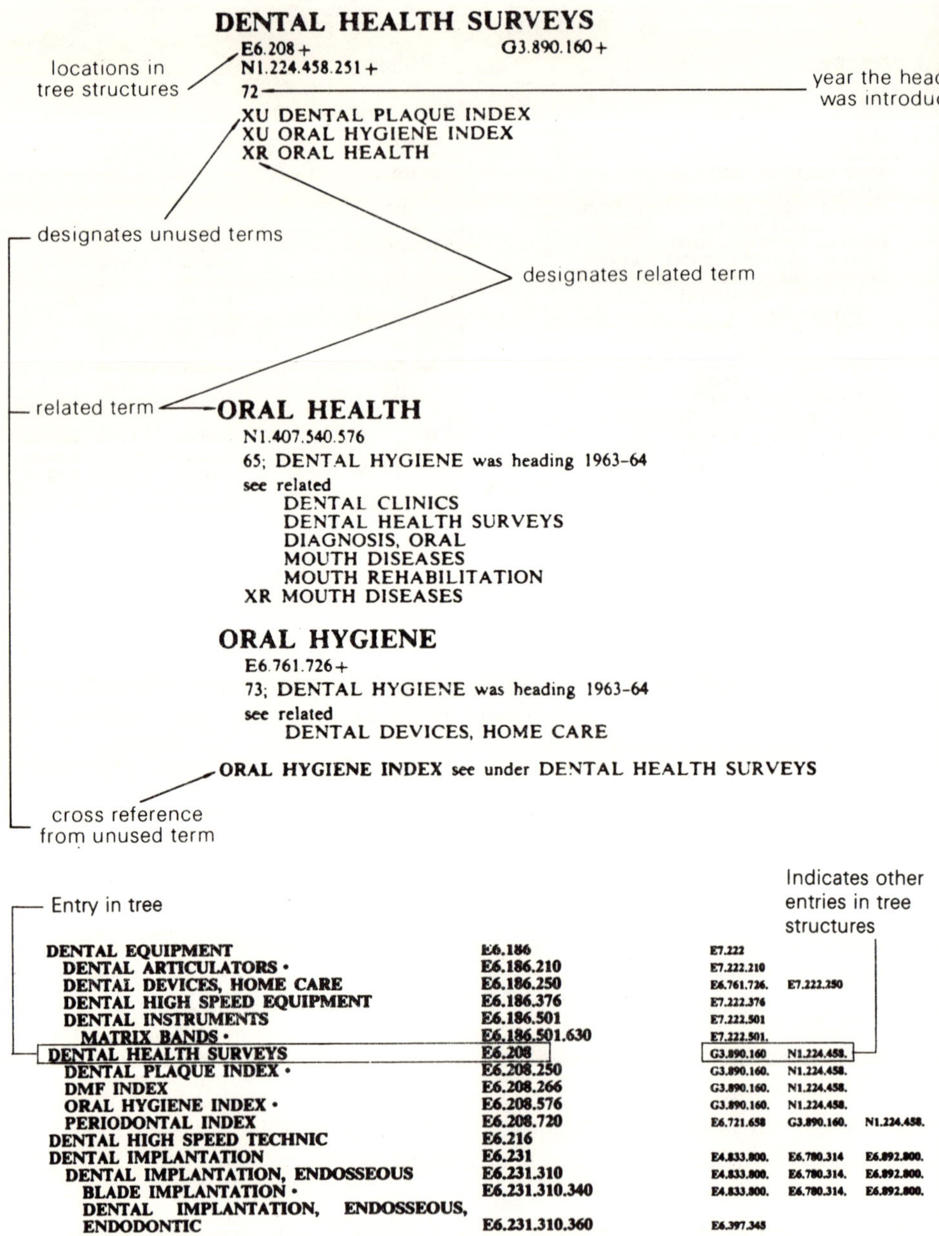

DENTAL EQUIPMENT	E6.186	E7.222		
DENTAL ARTICULATORS •	E6.186.210	E7.222.210		
DENTAL DEVICES, HOME CARE	E6.186.250	E6.761.726.	E7.222.250	
DENTAL HIGH SPEED EQUIPMENT	E6.186.376	E7.222.376		
DENTAL INSTRUMENTS	E6.186.501	E7.222.501		
MATRIX BANDS •	E6.186.501.630	E7.222.501.		
DENTAL HEALTH SURVEYS	E6.208	G3.890.160	N1.224.458.	
DENTAL PLAQUE INDEX •	E6.208.250	G3.890.160.	N1.224.458.	
DMF INDEX	E6.208.266	G3.890.160.	N1.224.458.	
ORAL HYGIENE INDEX •	E6.208.576	G3.890.160.	N1.224.458.	
PERIODONTAL INDEX	E6.208.720	E6.721.658	G3.890.160.	N1.224.458.
DENTAL HIGH SPEED TECHNIC	E6.216			
DENTAL IMPLANTATION	E6.231	E4.833.800.	E6.780.314	E6.892.800.
DENTAL IMPLANTATION, ENDOSSEOUS	E6.231.310	E4.833.800.	E6.780.314.	E6.892.800.
BLADE IMPLANTATION •	E6.231.310.340	E4.833.800.	E6.780.314.	E6.892.800.
DENTAL IMPLANTATION, ENDOSSEOUS, ENDODONTIC	E6.231.310.360	E6.397.345		

* Asterisks indicate minor descriptors given as cross-references in printed indexes, but searchable on-line.

Figure 4.4 MESH entries: content and relationships.

(Reproduced by courtesy of the National Library of Medicine.)

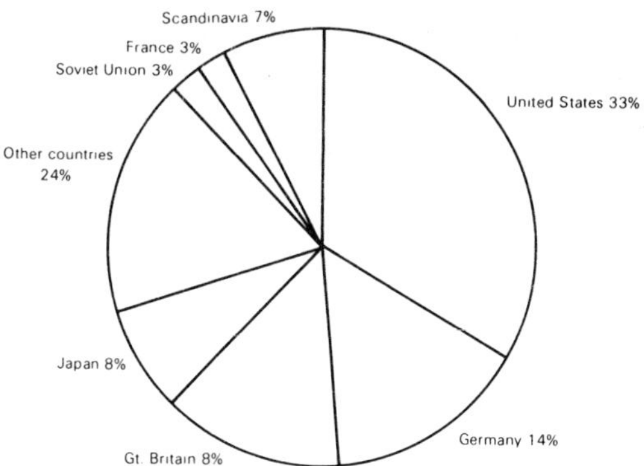

Figure 4.5 *Index to dental literature*: country coverage 1980–83.

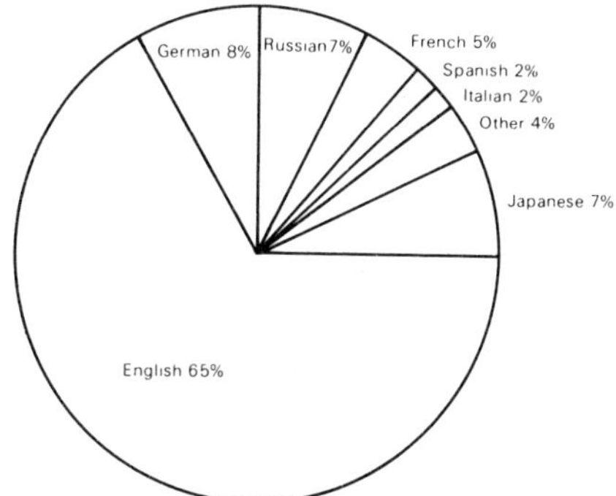

Figure 4.6 *Index to dental literature*: language coverage.

Table 4.1 Time lag before inclusion in Medline

British medical journal (weekly)	3 months
British dental journal (twice a month)	5 months
Journal of the American Medical Association (weekly)	2 months
Journal of the American Dental Association (monthly)	4 months
Presse médicale (twice a month)	3 months
Information dentaire (weekly)	6 months
American journal of surgery (monthly)	2 months
Oral surgery, oral medicine, oral pathology (monthly)	3 months
American journal of diseases of children (monthly)	2 months
Journal of dentistry for children (bimonthly)	3 months
Pediatric dentistry (quarterly)	6 months
American journal of orthodontics (monthly)	2 months
Journal of clinical orthodontics (monthly)	4 months

not arrive in Britain before June of the following year, followed a few weeks later by the January–March issue for the current year.

Since *IDL* is a specialized bibliography produced under the *Index medicus* umbrella, it is included in the NLM's Medline database, and is therefore available online back to 1966. Medline is therefore extremely useful for retrieving up-to-date references, for current-awareness purposes. However, inclusion of papers from dental journals is not as fast as from medical ones, as shown in *Table 4.1*. Nevertheless, it is an important means of identifying references not yet listed in the printed *IDL*.

When searching Medline it is possible to use *IDL* as a search parameter; that is, to specify that references from the *IDL* only, as opposed to the whole database, be listed. However, using this facility will exclude journals also covered by *Index medicus* as well as *IDL*, such as *Journal of the American Dental Association*, the *British dental journal* and the *Journal of prosthetic dentistry*. Although that may be the intention of searchers who have already scanned *Index medicus* but not *IDL*, the strategy should obviously not be used when it is necessary to identify all the significant papers on a topic, since references in many core journals will be missed.

One way to overcome this problem of specifying the concept of dentistry as a whole is to enter the number for the tree tables E6 (Mouth and tooth diseases) and C7 (Procedures and technics, dental), parts of which are reproduced in *Figures 4.2* and *4.3*. This procedure is, however, best used for a limited time span, or when the other search parameters have been sharply defined, and is not always practical for a large file, owing to the high recall.

Further information on Medline and the host systems from which it is available is provided by Norris (1984). Papers describing the use of Medline to search the dental literature have been written by McKee and McKee (1979) and Sinclair (1982), while Glaser (1984) discusses terminological problems encountered by the librarian and means of overcoming them when searching online. An uncritical historical review of the *Index* is given by Howard (1972), but Ring (1971) supplies a more realistic account.

Despite its shortcomings, the *IDL* is the most comprehensive bibliographical tool in the field, and indispensable for any library using dental literature. A sample page is reproduced as *Figure 4.7*.

4.3 Index Medicus

Index medicus, the most important bibliographical tool in medicine, and to which the *Index to dental literature* is so closely linked, has been issued in its present format since 1960. Each monthly issue has subject and author sections, like its dental cousin; there is an annual cumulation. Part 2 of the January issue comprises the important MESH (Medical Subject Headings) volume, which includes an alphabetical list of headings with cross-references, categorized lists of headings, and information on new or altered headings. *Index medicus* [18] covers about sixty

INDEX MEDICUS 63

Puberty gingivitis in insulin-dependent diabetic children. I. Cross-sectional observations. Gusberti FA, et al. **J Periodontol** 1983 Dec;54(12):714–20

PUBERTY, PRECOCIOUS

PATHOLOGY

Peutz-Jeghers syndrome associated with precocious puberty. Solh HM, et al. **J Pediatr** 1983 Oct;103(4):593–5

PUBLIC HEALTH

EDUCATION

Guide to materials for use in teaching clinical nutrition in schools of medicine, dentistry, and public health. Read MS. **Am J Clin Nutr** 1983 Nov;38(5):775–94

PUBLIC HEALTH ADMINISTRATION

The Michigan Department of Health: an acorn sprouts. Jones DA. **J Mich Dent Assoc** 1983 Oct;65(10):463–4

PUBLIC HEALTH DENTISTRY

Proceedings of a forum on the use of fissure sealants in public health programs. Sponsored by the Dental Health Section, American Public Health Association. **J Public Health Dent** 1983 Summer;43(3):198–247
The cost of sealant application in a state dental disease prevention program. Calderone JJ, et al. **J Public Health Dent** 1983 Summer;43(3):249–54
The use of pit-and-fissure sealants in community public health programs in Tennessee. Hardison JR. **J Public Health Dent** 1983 Summer;43(3):233–9
The use of fissure sealants in public health programs: a reactor's comments. Stamm JW. **J Public Health Dent** 1983 Summer;43(3):243–6
Dental therapists in Botswana. Eriksen HM, et al. **Odontostomatol Trop** 1983 Jun;6(2):69–74
[Aspects of social dentistry and the role of behavioral sciences in dentistry] Roefs AJ. **Ned Tijdschr Tandheelkd** 1983 Jul–Aug;90(7–8):364–7 (Eng. Abstr.) **(Dut)**

EDUCATION

Effect of extramural experiences on dental students' attitudes. Grantham EV, et al. **J Dent Educ** 1983 Oct; 47(10):681–4

TRENDS

The microscope and the telescope [editorial] Dunning JM. **J Public Health Dent** 1983 Summer;43(3):196–7

PUBLIC RELATIONS

Does your office portray a positive image? Boyer GL. **Dent Econ** 1983 Sep;73(9):81–4

PULPITIS

COMPLICATIONS

An evaluation of dental pain using visual analogue scales and the Mcgill Pain Questionnaire. Seymour RA, et al. **J Oral Maxillofac Surg** 1983 Oct;41(10):643–8

DIAGNOSIS

A new technique of selective anesthesia for diagnosing acute pulpitis in the mandible [letter] Farber JP. **J Endod** 1983 Oct;9(10):454

DRUG THERAPY

Histological investigation of the effect of a controlled-released anti-inflammatory drug on exposed inflamed dog pulps. Wijnbergen-Buijen van Weelderen M, et al. **Biomaterials** 1983 Jul;4(3):165–9

ETIOLOGY

[Effect of advancing periodontitis on the dental pulp] Yanagimura N, et al. **Nippon Shishubyo Gakkai Kaishi** 1983 Jun;25(2):324–39 (Eng. Abstr.) **(Jpn)**
[Treatment of complicated caries in sailors in the pre-voyage period] Blagochinnyĭ VE, et al. **Voen Med Zh** 1983 Aug; (8):54–5 **(Rus)**

MICROBIOLOGY

Death of an African elephant from probable toxemia attributed to chronic pulpitis. McGavin MD, et al. **J Am Vet Med Assoc** 1983 Dec 1;183(11):1269–73

PATHOLOGY

Vascular reactions in the dental pulp during inflammation. Tønder KJ. **Acta Odontol Scand** 1983 Aug;41(4):247–56
Histological investigation of the effect of a controlled-released anti-inflammatory drug on exposed inflamed dog pulps. Wijnbergen-Buijen van Weelderen M, et al. **Biomaterials** 1983 Jul;4(3):165–9
Reduction in pulpal inflammation beneath surface-sealed silicates. Tobias RS, et al. **Int Endod J** 1982 Oct; 15(4):173–80
Death of an African elephant from probable toxemia attributed to chronic pulpitis. McGavin MD, et al. **J Am Vet Med Assoc** 1983 Dec 1;183(11):1269–73

PHYSIOPATHOLOGY

Vascular reactions in the dental pulp during inflammation. Tønder KJ. **Acta Odontol Scand** 1983 Aug;41(4):247–56

PREVENTION & CONTROL

Reduction in pulpal inflammation beneath surface-sealed

Figure 4.7 Part of a typical page from *Index to dental literature*.
(Reproduced by courtesy of the American Dental Association.)

dental journals, and is useful to update the *Index to dental literature*. The 'List of journals indexed' in the latter marks with an asterisk titles also included in *Index medicus*.

This indexing service has a history, albeit not continuous, that dates back to 1879, the year it started publication. A concise review of its development is given by Sutherland (1984) but a brief résumé is in order here, in view of its importance for retrospective searching.

Series 1, 1879–99, and series 2, 1903–20, were published monthly, with subject entries in a classified order and annual author and subject indexes. Series 3,

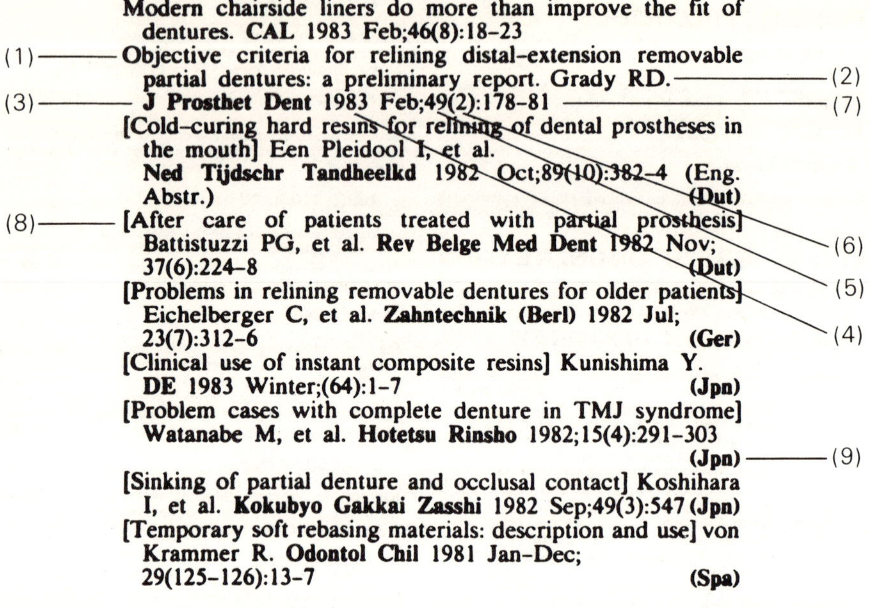
DENTURE REBASING

Modern chairside liners do more than improve the fit of dentures. CAL 1983 Feb;46(8):18-23
(1) Objective criteria for relining distal-extension removable partial dentures: a preliminary report. Grady RD. (2)
(3) J Prosthet Dent 1983 Feb;49(2):178-81 (7)
[Cold-curing hard resins for relining of dental prostheses in the mouth] Een Pleidool I, et al. Ned Tijdschr Tandheelkd 1982 Oct;89(10):382-4 (Eng. Abstr.) (Dut)
(8) [After care of patients treated with partial prosthesis] Battistuzzi PG, et al. Rev Belge Med Dent 1982 Nov; 37(6):224-8 (Dut) (6) (5) (4)
[Problems in relining removable dentures for older patients] Eichelberger C, et al. Zahntechnik (Berl) 1982 Jul; 23(7):312-6 (Ger)
[Clinical use of instant composite resins] Kunishima Y. DE 1983 Winter;(64):1-7 (Jpn)
[Problem cases with complete denture in TMJ syndrome] Watanabe M, et al. Hotetsu Rinsho 1982;15(4):291-303 (Jpn) (9)
[Sinking of partial denture and occlusal contact] Koshihara I, et al. Kokubyo Gakkai Zasshi 1982 Sep;49(3):547 (Jpn)
[Temporary soft rebasing materials: description and use] von Krammer R. Odontol Chil 1981 Jan-Dec; 29(125-126):13-7 (Spa)

(1) title of paper
(2) author
(3) abbreviation of journal title
(4) year
(5) volume
(6) part number
(7) pages
(8) square brackets indicate paper is not in English
(9) language of the paper

Figure 4.8 Elements of entries in *Index to dental literature*.

1921–27, changed to quarterly issues, and an alphabetical subject-heading sequence. There were annual author, but no subject, indexes. For the period 1879–1927 it supplements the *Index catalogue of the library of the Surgeon General's office* [40], described in the next chapter, by providing an author guide to the periodical literature.

Quarterly cumulative index medicus (*QCIM*), published from 1927 to 1956, was the result of a merger between *Index medicus* and the *Quarterly cumulative index to medical literature*, the latter having been initiated by the American Medical Association in 1916. Delays in publication were primarily responsible for its demise, since it was not fulfilling the need for up-to-date indexing of newly published material.

The *Current list of medical literature*, 1941–59 was intended to meet the demand for a rapid indexing service, which the *QCIM* was failing to do, and which was considered a priority for assisting medical officers during the war years. Publication was weekly, then, from 1950, monthly, and was the forerunner of today's

Current contents publications since it arranged journal titles alphabetically, and then listed the details of the paper in each issue. Author and subject indexes were issued twice a year. For the years 1957–59 it is the only medical indexing tool, its companion having ceased publication in 1956. The *Current list* itself finished in 1959, when new indexing arrangements were finalized, and the NLM started to publish *Index medicus* in its present format.

4.4 Dental Abstracts

A monthly publication produced by the American Dental Association since 1956, *Dental abstracts* is intended for the practising dentist. Some 200 journals are scanned and 100 unsigned but informative abstracts published each month, arranged in broad subject groups. Seventy percent of material is from the United States; foreign-language material is rarely included. Photographs and diagrams from the original papers are sometimes included, and an author's address is given for every paper. Each issue and volume has an author index. Unlike many abstracting services, *Dental abstracts* [5] is up to date, with delays of only three to nine months between publication of the original and the abstract. It is therefore a useful current-awareness tool.

Like *Dental abstracts, The dentaletter* [27] aims to provide an updating service for general practitioners. As its name suggests, it has a newsletter format, each issue containing signed, informative abstracts of between fifteen and twenty articles from English-language journals, some six months after the publication of the original.

4.5 Contents Lists

There are two 'current contents'-type publications whose specific function is current awareness in dentistry. The library of the Royal Dental College at Arhus in Denmark produces a monthly *Accessions* list [31]. Despite its name, it does not necessarily relate to books, but is a typed list of contents of journals received by the library, written in English, French, German or a Scandinavian language. Also listed are dental papers in non-dental journals, such as *Acta anatomica.*

The other title solely in the dental field is *Periodicals digest in dentistry* [30], which appears monthly, reproducing the actual contents pages of some forty titles per month, predominantly from the United States. A useful feature is its reprints service, whereby copies of papers listed in the *Digest* may be ordered by readers.

Current contents [25] itself includes dental titles in the *Clinical practice* and *Life sciences* editions, both weekly. Each issue of *Current contents* includes a list of the journals included that week, a keyword index, and address list for first authors. Published in the United States by the Institute for Scientific Information, *Current contents* may reach British libraries before the journals included in it, since, unlike most printed material, it is shipped airmail. Coverage of dental journals is greater in the *Clinical practice* edition, which includes some thirty titles, as opposed to about a dozen in *Life sciences.*

4.6 Information on Newly Published Books

New books are listed most comprehensively in American sources. The *Index to dental literature* has an author/title sequence in each issue cumulating throughout the volume. Titles are predominantly English-language. The American Dental Association Bureau of Library Services issues a monthly *Accessions list* [23], also arranged by author, which includes dissertations and some American publications not easily available elsewhere. The library of the Northwestern University Dental School publishes a classified list called *Titles acquired* [29] approximately every two months, with NLM class numbers given for each item. There are separate sections for books, pamphlets, bibliographies, theses and periodicals.

British medicine [24], published monthly since 1972, lists new books, pamphlets and audiovisual presentations emanating from Great Britain, and gives contents of journals from Britain and elsewhere.

Most journals review new books, but inevitably are selective in coverage and their reviews may not appear until long after the books have been published. Two of the most useful journals carrying reviews are the *British dental journal* and the *Journal of the American Dental Association*, since their coverage is wide, and the reviews are the most timely to appear, often within a month or two after publication of the books themselves.

Publishers and bookshops can be useful sources of information on new and forthcoming books. Most publishers issue annual catalogues of titles in print; many also distribute regular newssheets or booklets describing new books. Blackwell, for instance, issues a bimonthly list. Mailing shots may also be distributed in journals or sent direct to prospective purchasers.

There is a contrast in practice between British and North American publishers, in that the former do not regularly take extensive advertising space in journals, although a publishing house may advertise its books in one of its own journals. In America, however, it is usual practice for publishers to have full-page advertisements to promote a selection of their titles.

Booksellers may offer alerting services to potential purchasers. The well-established London firm H. K. Lewis issues an annual *Medical booklist* [41], arranged by subject, which is supplemented by *Lewis's quarterly list* [28], giving details of new titles and editions. Neither publication identifies publishers but bibliographical details are to an excellent standard of accuracy. Lewis's do not routinely list books published by Quintessence, a limitation to be noted by prospective users from the dental profession.

4.7 Trade Literature

Mailing shots of trade literature are normally sent by manufacturers of equipment or drugs direct to practitioners. Libraries see comparatively little of this kind of material, although it is common to find loose advertising material in some journals. Obviously trade literature will keep a reader informed of new products, but the manufacturer's vested interest in promoting his wares must be taken into account when evaluating the usefulness of this type of literature. Too often trade leaflets concentrate on glossy pictures rather than facts and figures.

4.8 Conferences

Conferences and courses in dentistry are advertised in the press. The most comprehensive source for North America and events of international interest is the *Journal of the American Dental Association.* Each issue includes three listings: ADA constituent societies; meetings inside the continental USA; and meetings outside the continental USA, itemizing events for the next three months. The April and October issues, however, list future events for the forthcoming year and beyond, arranged chronologically within the three sections [220].

The *Zahnmed Kongress Kalender* [221] issued annually by Demeter Verlag includes details of some 700 conferences held in Germany and elsewhere.

Events of general interest in a particular country are advertised in the appropriate national journals. In Britain, those with the highest readerships are the *British dental journal* and the newspaper-format *Dental practice.* Specialist events attracting participants from a large number of countries are publicized in the appropriate speciality journals.

References

Black, A. D. 'The development of the *Index* and its use'. *Index to dental literature* 1916–20: ix–xiii.

Glaser, J. '*Index to dental literature* and Medline: a guide to searching the dental literature'. *Medical reference services quarterly* **3** (1984): 1–16.

Howard, J. W. 'A half century of dental indexing'. *Journal of the American Dental Association* **84** (1972): 1315–29.

McKee, A. M. and McKee, J. D. 'Using computers to search dental literature'. *Journal of the Maryland State Dental Association* **22** [2]: (1979): 91–8.

Norris, C. 'Mechanised sources of information retrieval'. In Morton, L. T. and Godbolt, S. (eds.), *Information sources in the medical sciences.* 3rd ed. London: Butterworth, 1984, pp. 90–119.

On-line Information Centre. *Medical databases.* London: On-line Information Centre, 1983. 53pp.

Ring, M. E. 'Fifty years of the *Index to dental literature*: a critical appraisal'. *Bulletin of the Medical Library Association* **59** (1971): 463–78.

Sarll, D. W. and Holloway, P. J. 'Factors influencing innovation in general dental practice'. *British dental journal* **153** (1982): 264–6.

Sinclair, S. A. 'Searching the dental literature by computer'. *Oral health* **72** [9]: (1982): 70–1.

Sutherland, F. M. 'Indexes, abstracts, bibliographies and reviews'. In Morton, L. T. and Godbolt, S. (eds.), *Information sources in the medical sciences.* 3rd ed. London: Butterworth, 1984, pp. 44–69.

5 Finding Out About the Literature of Dentistry

5.1 Guides to the Literature

Whereas some fields, such as biology, have published guides to relevant literature there is no comparable publication for dentistry, and it is this gap which the present book is attempting to fill. Dentistry is a profession allied to medicine, and is treated as a medical speciality in secondary sources such as general medical bibliographies and indexing services. However, it is not a straightforward speciality comparable, say, to orthopaedics, gynaecology or paediatrics, either in terms of organization or range of work. Although there are hospital and academic dentists, as explained in Chapter 1, the majority work in general practice, and a significant proportion in the community dental service. The profession is, therefore, more strictly comparable with the medical profession as a whole, with different sections having a variety of information needs; but as far as information sources are concerned, it is a poor relation.

For the librarian unfamiliar with the literature of dentistry, there are brief guides as to what books and journals are currently available. Raskin and Hathorn [45] have published a 'Selected list of books and journals for a small dental library', listing 116 books and twenty journals which are appropriate for an American collection. This list is published in the *Bulletin of the Medical Library Association* and is updated at approximately five-year intervals, the most recent being in 1980. Although librarians from other countries would not disagree over the core journals identified by Raskin and Hathorn, their choice of textbooks would be different.

Providing a British view is the chapter on dentistry by E. M. Spencer, revised by M. A. Clennett, in *Information sources in the medical sciences* by L. T. Morton and S. Godbolt [1], the third edition of which was published by Butterworth in 1984. This is a narrative description, occupying some twenty pages, of books and journals with both general and speciality coverage of particular value to the British reader who is not familiar with the field. The American Dental Association's *Basic dental reference works* [33] is an invaluable bibliography of some 130 reference sources, most of which are relevant to countries outside North America. Journals are not included.

M. L. Darby and D. M. Bowen, in *Research methods for oral health professionals*, 1980 [225], include a chapter on using libraries, and list abstracts and indexes which the dental researcher might need to use, but do not discuss specific books or journals.

The problem of identifying useful sources is exacerbated by two factors: the inadequacy of guidance given to undergraduates at dental schools on the scope and use of dental literature, and the decreasing number of dental, and also medical specialists in libraries. To enlarge on the first point, dental students have comparatively little project or essay work, and their reading is predominantly confined to recommended texts or reading lists. There is therefore little scope or necessity for them to read around or beyond the set references. If a project is undertaken, it is not, in Britain certainly, normally preceded by appropriate guidance from teaching or library staff to the published material available or indexes in the field. Most postgraduate students who studied at the Institute of Dental Surgery in London during the 1970s and early 1980s had never used the *Index to dental literature* before, nor were they aware that such a wide range of journals was published. It is not until he undertakes advanced study, therefore, that the dentist begins to appreciate the variety and level of published sources.

The general practitioner in Britain tends to rely for information mainly on the *British dental journal* and the controlled-circulation periodicals that arrive on his doorstep, although this situation is changing with the advent of vocational training courses for newly qualified dentists, courses which are likely to include a research project. As described in Chapter 3, the general dentist normally does not feel the need for regular perusal of a wide range of literature.

The second factor militating against the optimum use of the literature is the library staffing situation. The librarian to whom the dentist will go for assistance has a responsibility to point the way to pertinent material, and will know that, as in other fields, there is a common pattern of primary and secondary literature, core journals, abstracts and indexes. What he or she may not know are many of the details, and the idiosyncrasies of particular titles, which are only learnt from experience or gleaned from a guide to literature. With the demise of autonomous dental libraries, and the trend towards integrated medical collections, much expertise is being lost. It is to be hoped, therefore, that this *Keyguide* will formalize for the information worker much of the knowledge normally acquired through experience or by serendipity. However, terminology will inevitably remain a problem for the non-dentist.

5.2 Bibliographies

Having noted that few sources outline the important material in the field, we shall now discuss bibliographical sources in more detail. Abstracts and indexes that list mainly material of current interest have been discussed in the previous chapter, although it must be remembered that some, notably the *Index to dental literature*, are equally important for retrospective use. This section concentrates on listings of books.

A bibliography may be defined as a list of references that are in some way related; for instance, they may be on a common subject, or by the same author. So when may a bibliography be justifiably classified as an index? There is no hard and fast answer; generally speaking, however, an index appears at regular intervals and is a guide to material published during a specified period, whereas a bibliography has broader scope. For the purpose of this book, therefore, 'indexes' are defined as recurring bibliographies that deal predominantly with journal papers, whereas lists called 'bibliographies' may cover books, periodical articles, reports, and may be issued at intervals or once only.

To be discussed in this chapter are bibliographies that cover dentistry as a whole, rather than specific aspects or specialities, which are dealt with in Part II, and coverage is mostly of books. As will be seen, some sources emanate from dental institutions and are confined to dental topics while others are more general in coverage, but include a significant dental section. They will be described in two groups, those devoted primarily to dentistry and those with a wider scope.

5.2.1 Dental Bibliographies

The *Index to dental literature* has a 'List of books published' [17] in each issue and volume, based on acquisitions to the ADA Bureau of Library Services. It includes books, reports and pamphlets, and is predominantly of titles in English, being particularly comprehensive for North American material. Indeed, some publications are difficult to acquire outside that continent, while others would not be relevant or of interest in other countries. Arrangement is under author, or the title if the work is a multi-author book, and details given include publisher, edition, number of pages and price. There is no subject index, and no cross-referencing from unused headings to preferred entry terms. Like the main body of the *IDL*, the 'List' cumulates; most items included have been published within the previous eighteen months. Its main uses, therefore, are to identify recent books, and verify details when an approximate year of publication is known.

Also from the ADA Bureau of Library Services comes *Books and package libraries for dentists* [34], a pamphlet listing English-language books published during the previous two years, and arranged in author order. This booklet is intended as a guide to items that are available for loan. Details listed for each book are author, title, edition, publisher, date, number of pages and price. The package libraries, also available for loan, are collections of reprints on specified subjects and cover over 2,000 topics.

Georgetown University's Dahlgren Memorial Library has published *A dental bibliography of selected books, journals and audiovisuals, 1976–1982* [38], which is based on its own holdings but is supplemented by other material included on National Library of Medicine (NLM) databases. Excluded are non-English material, theses and defunct journals. Arrangement is by broad subject. Library class numbers are given for each item.

Many libraries publish lists of new additions, and these are generally regarded as current-awareness listings, since they appear frequently and do not cumulate. The British Dental Association's library issues irregular *Supplements* to its original *Catalogue of dental and allied works published since 1950*, which was issued in 1967. The third supplement, *Books added December 1979–January 1983*, lists some 600 titles in broad subject groups, and is therefore of more value as a subject guide for the past few years than as a current-awareness list.

On the theme of bibliographies produced by dental libraries, mention must now be made of Northwestern University's Dental School Library *Catalog* [44]. A photographic reproduction of the actual card catalogue published in 1978, it comprises eight volumes, with the entries arranged in dictionary form. The Northwestern University Dental School Library, founded in 1896, has one of the largest dental collections in the world; the *Catalog* is therefore an important research tool. Because of its high price, it was not widely purchased in Britain but is held in the Leeds University medical and dental library.

Turning now to other retrospective bibliographies, there are four important listings to be noted. Although they will be discussed in the History of dentistry section in Part II, it is also appropriate to include them here, as they are wide-ranging listings and authoritative works of reference. Taking them chronologically, the first is C. G. Crowley's *Dental bibliography* [352], issued in 1885 by S. S. White of Philadelphia, which lists books by date of publication. T. David's *Bibliographie française de l'art dentaire* [353], published in Paris in 1889 and reprinted in 1970, is a list of books, pamphlets and theses arranged by author. B. W. Weinberger's *Dental bibliography* [357], produced in two small volumes in 1929 and 1932, includes books in that author's own collection and the New York Academy of Medicine's library. J. M. Campbell's *Dental bibliography: British and American, 1682–1880* [351] gives brief details of 723 items, arranged chronologically.

Finally in this section are listings more specialized in nature, albeit still broad enough to fall into the category of general, as opposed to subject, bibliographies.

Dental prostheses 1964–February 1983 [47] is a misleading title for a somewhat costly bibliography of 192 citations from the US National Technical Information Service (NTIS) database. Many items are journal papers which can be retrieved from NLM indexes, but a feature of the list is that it does include NTIS reports not listed in easily accessible sources. Subject coverage includes materials, oral surgery and restorative dentistry.

It is usual for libraries to maintain records of publications emanating from staff employed in their parent institutions. These may be unpublished, listed for internal or restricted circulation, or published in a house journal.

The Institute of Dental Surgery in London produces a typescript list of staff publications for each academic year, arranged by department; whereas each issue of *Guy's Hospital gazette* has a listing of 'Papers by Guy's men', although this covers medicine as a whole, not just dentistry. The Royal Dental College at Arhus in Denmark has published 'Arhus Tandlaegehojkoles videnskabelige produktion 1958–1983' [35], in a 1983 issue of the journal *Tandlaegebladet*. This is a bibliography of theses, books and papers emanating from the College during a twenty-five-year period; most items are published in English.

An interesting review of the non-clinical aspects of dentistry has been undertaken by N. D. Richards and L. K. Cohen [46] in *Social sciences and dentistry: a critical bibliography*, which was published by the FDI in 1971. Narrative reviews are followed by extensive bibliographies on such topics as dental education, utilization of dental services, dentist–patient relations and fluoridation. Volume 2, by L. K. Cohen and P. S. Bryant, is a companion as well as an update. It covers literature published from 1972 to 1982 on some of the topics discussed in volume 1 and, in addition, has chapters on other subjects, such as preventive dentistry, institutional and community aspects, and behavioural factors affecting treatment.

5.2.2 General Bibliographies

The National Library of Medicine's *Current catalog* [43], published since 1966, gives both author and subject approaches, the latter via MESH headings. Current listings are invariably slow but the *Catalog* is valuable for retrospective searching. Published quarterly, it has annual and five-year cumulations. The most recent of these, 1976–80, is available only on microfiche. Predecessors of the *Current catalog* are the *Armed Forces' Medical Library catalog 1950–1954* (six volumes) and the *National Library of Medicine catalog 1955–1959*, and *1960–1965*, which also have six volumes each.

The most important forerunner of the NLM *Current catalog* is the *Index catalog of the library of the Surgeon General's office* , [40] known commonly as the *Index catalog* or the *Surgeon General's catalog*, which covers the years 1880–1950 in five series, the degree of comprehensiveness and scope varying from one series to another. Books, pamphlets and selected journal articles are included, although the fifth series is limited to selected monographs. The *Index catalog* is particularly useful for pre-1930 material in all forms, and for books up to 1950. Arrangement is in dictionary form, with author and subject entries in a single sequence. Foreign-language material is included, but not exhaustively. The history of the *Index catalog* is described briefly by Sutherland (1984) and in detail by Rogers and Adams (1950).

Covering the time span of both the *Index catalog* and *Current catalog* is *Health science books in print 1876–1982* [39], issued by Bowker in four volumes. Inevitably it is a less comprehensive work, and inclusion of dental titles is selective. It can be useful when the other sources are not available, or for quick reference, for instance when the year of publication is not known. Coverage of 1982 material is scanty, presumably owing to an early cut-off date. There is a bias towards American material. Arrangement is by Library of Congress headings, with cross-references from MESH terms wherever these differ. Volume 4 comprises author and title indexes, referring the user to page numbers in the main sequence.

Medical books and serials in print [42], issued annually, has extensive coverage of dentistry, although it must be remembered that the title refers to items in print in the United States. The international nature of publishing does, however, ensure that many titles from other countries are included. There are sequences for author, title and subject, the latter having a number of specific dental headings, such as orthodontics or periodontics, which assist the searcher in identifying titles in a particular field.

General bibliographies, widely available in large libraries, include some dental material. The *British national bibliography* [36], first published in 1950, appears weekly, with four-monthly and annual cumulations, and is useful for current and retrospective searching for British material that may not reach the American listings, since it includes all publications received by the Copyright Receipt Office. Also included are forthcoming books, as notified by publishers. Arrangement is by the Dewey classification, dentistry being found at class number 617.6 and its subdivisions.

The *Cumulative book index* is an American publication that aims to list all books published in English. A dictionary format is used, interfiling author, subject and title entries. Publication is monthly, with annual cumulations.

National bibliographies can be useful for identifying vernacular material, as also can the 'books in print' type of publication, although the ease of subject approach varies in the latter. For example, *Les livres disponibles* lists French titles in print, with the subject section arranged by the Universal Decimal classification (UDC), 616.31 being the number for dentistry. The Italian *Catalogo dei libri in commercio* scatters dental material under various subject headings, such as Bocca (mouth), Denti (teeth), Stomatologia (stomatology) or Odontoiatria (dentistry). By contrast, *Libros españoles* has no separate section for dentistry; the titles are scattered throughout the medical sections such as pathology, clinical medicine and anatomy, while in the German *Verzeichnis lieferbarer Bücher* there is a single author/title sequence, allowing no subject approach.

Booksellers have been mentioned as sources of current information, notably H. K. Lewis in London. This company's annual *Medical booklist* [41] has a section on dentistry in which currently available and forthcoming editions are listed. Lewis's also operate a subscription library and have published a catalogue giving brief details of books included in their stock, which is limited to hardback, English-language titles. The *Catalogue of Lewis's medical, scientific and technical lending library* [37] is not as comprehensive as, for instance, the NLM *Current catalog*, but is useful for quick reference, and as an overview of titles in the field. The original catalogue covers books held in the lending library up to 1972, with three supplements updating it to 1981.

5.2.3 Subject Bibliographies

Because of their specialized nature, subject bibliographies tend to cover periodical articles. The publication of 'one-off' subject bibliographies in book form, such as the extensive works on caries ([309]–[311]), has all but ceased. These were invaluable in their day, before the era of online searching, and when printed abstracting or indexing services were less comprehensive. Now recurring bibliographies have international coverage, and most are available online, so that specialist bibliographies can be easily and speedily produced to meet the demands of a large user group or of an individual. Historical aspects are obviously an exception, but for topics of current interest, retrieval of journal papers from printed or online indexing services is the norm. The NLM Literature Search Service produces printed bibliographies on topics of current interest from its databases, and lists recent searches in *Index medicus*. Copies of these bibliographies are supplied free of charge on application to the Literature Search Service. Most relate to medicine, but it is worth scanning the list from time to time, since dental subjects are occasionally included. An example was 'Dental sealants' in 1983.

5.3 Review Articles

Although online searching has its advantages, notably speed of retrieval and a high recall rate, one disadvantage is the lack of qualitative evaluation. References are retrieved which are, to judge by the titles of the papers concerned, highly relevant, but these articles may be written at the wrong level, for instance for a dental nurse when advanced research material is required, or be in journals which are of dubious quality or difficult to obtain. The searcher scanning printed indexes will, with experience, learn which references he can safely ignore, but may be frustrated by papers with misleading titles which do not discuss what they purport to do.

The review paper overcomes these problems, and for the researcher lucky enough to find a review on the subject in which he is interested, provides a useful short cut in the process of finding relevant publications. It is the author of the review article who has identified, sifted and evaluated the multiplicity of papers, so that subsequent researchers will benefit, knowing that references mentioned in the review are pertinent and of high standard, and that all the appropriate major reports on the subject have been listed. The review article therefore provides a description of the history and development of a subject, and gives an extensive bibliography of significant papers.

Review articles are listed in a preliminary section of *Index medicus* and *Index to dental literature*, entitled *Bibliography of medical* (or *dental*) *reviews*, with author and subject sections. As well as the standard bibliographical data, the number of references cited is given in brackets. Review papers are also included in the main part of *Index medicus* and *IDL*, and can be identified because the number of references cited is indicated.

Oral sciences reviews, published in ten volumes from 1972 to 1977 by Munksgaard, gave authoritative overviews on a range of subjects. Although now some years old, they still provide valuable background material, and extensive lists of classic and significant papers which appeared up to the 1970s. The review articles themselves have been prepared by eminent workers in the field.

The *Journal of the Western Society of Periodontology* [552] carries in each of its quarterly issues a review paper on some aspect of periodontology. Munksgaard journals, in particular the *Journal of oral pathology* [463] and the *Journal of clinical periodontology* [565], quite often carry review papers. Of the general journals, *Journal of the American Dental Association* [74] has a series entitled 'Perspectives', which reviews topics of current interest and also publishes status reports—on techniques, instruments or materials—prepared by the appropriate ADA council. The *SSO Schweizerische Monatsschrift für Zahnmedizin* [132]carries review papers regularly, normally in French or German, and on a wide range of subjects. The literature cited is from English, French- and German-language journals, and the review paper itself has an English abstract.

5.4 Abstracting and Indexing Services in Dentistry

The *Index to dental literature*, the major tool for current and retrospective searching, and *Dental abstracts*, primarily a current-awareness service, have been discussed in the previous chapter. Since *IDL* was, until 1962, limited to papers published in English, other sources to identify material in different languages are valuable.

The most wide-ranging of these supplementary tools are German, the earliest coverage being provided by the *Index der deutschen und ausländischen Literatur und zahnärztliche Bibliographie* [20]. Published between 1902 and 1934, it gives brief details of papers in German and other languages, the first volume having retrospective coverage back to 1847. Papers are grouped by subject, but today the author index is the most usual approach.

For the period 1925–33, *Fortschritte der Zahnheilkunde* [7] provides abstracts of papers published in various languages, these summaries appearing about a year after the original.

From 1934 onwards *Deutsche Zahn- Mund- und Kieferheilkunde* [15] has included a bibliographical section in each monthly issue, many entries being accompanied by short abstracts. The delay in publication of references in this journal, which is still extant today, but minus the '*Deutsche*', must be borne in mind when checking for particular papers; it is three years behind in some cases. Like its predecessors published in the German language, it covers literature from all over the world.

Other sources which can be used to provide a back-up to the *IDL* for vernacular material are confined to particular languages, but are worth checking especially for pre-1961 material. The *Indice de la literatura en castellano* [19] lists books and journal papers in Spanish from 1952 to date. Despite the present coverage of this language by *IDL*, the *Indice* is nevertheless valid as a complementary source today.

From 1950 to 1973 *Odontologisk revy* (now succeeded by the *Swedish dental journal*) published an annual 'Index to the Scandinavian dental literature' [21], grouping papers by subject. The need for this publication diminished as fewer authors continued to publish in their native languages, and as the research-orientated Scandinavian journals themselves switched to English as their principal language of publication during the 1970s.

Still with sources now deceased, *Oral research abstracts* [11] was in its time an excellent tool for the research worker. It was published by the American Dental Association from 1965 to 1978, but regrettably was discontinued for economic reasons. It was far more comprehensive than *Dental abstracts*, which is intended for the practitioner; its scope was international, and it gave high-quality abstracts of the world's journal literature and American patents some one to two years after the originals had appeared. It is primarily of use today for its well-written, informative summaries of papers in journals not readily at hand, and of foreign-language papers.

Sections of *Oral research abstracts* were for some years published in separate annual volumes, entitled *Advances in* . . . ; these were appropriate abstracts from the previous year's monthly issues, and hence were not of value for up-to-date references. Thus *Advances in caries research 1974* would include entries from the 1973 *Oral research abstracts*, that is, of papers published in 1970–72. Other subject fields covered included periodontology, oral surgery, orthodontics, paedodontics and prosthetics.

A current abstracting service and a relative newcomer to the dental field is in the Pascal series, formerly *Bulletin signalétique*, which has been published by the Centre National de Recherche Scientifique in Paris since 1940, covering a wide range of subjects in separately published sections. *Pascal Explore E72 Otorhinolaryngologie, stomatologie, pathologie cervicofaciale* [12] was first issued in 1972 as *Bulletin signalétique* Part 347 covering journals, reports and French theses. Its emphasis is on oral surgery, medicine and pathology, rather than the teeth themselves, but it is up to date, being six to twelve months behind the original. Some 300 indicative abstracts are provided in each monthly issue, those of interest to the dental user being in the subject sections 'Mouth, oropharynx, salivary glands' and 'Face'. For each entry, the title is given in its original language and in French, the address of the first author is provided, and bibliographical details include the ISSN of the journal and the number of references. Brief abstracts are supplied. There is therefore more detail per entry than in the *IDL*, although the scope of the subject field is not comparable.

Finally in this section must be mentioned the *Yearbook of dentistry*. It is not an abstracting service in the accepted sense, but each annual volume provides long abstracts of some 200 papers which the editors have considered to be significant contributions to the past year's literature.

5.5 Abstracting and Indexing Services in Related Fields

Although the *IDL* is the principal tool for current and retrospective searching, it may at times be more convenient or appropriate for the researcher to use other secondary sources, especially when the kind of material sought concerns basic science, rather than clinical dentistry. For this outlook on oral research, *Biological abstracts* may be the tool to choose.

Biological abstracts [2] is an important source for researchers in many fields. It carries over 150,000 abstracts per year, of which over 12,000 relate to the oral cavity. This sizeable recall, however, is of limited use to the searcher interested in the clinical aspects of dentistry, since the abstracts refer principally to anatomical or physiological studies, and on animals rather than humans. *Biological abstracts* is available online as BIOSIS back to 1969.

Excerpta medica [6] is, for many medical specialities, as important as *Index medicus*, since both services carry a significant number of unique entries. There are over forty separately published sections, on such topics as biochemistry, cancer, genetics, pathology and public health, but there is no separate section on the mouth. Clinical dentistry is presently excluded from the scope of this abstracting service, although oral biology and pathology are covered by the appropriate sections, and some 2,000 entries relating in some way to the mouth or teeth are included each year. *Excerpta medica* is available online back to 1974.

To identify the kinds of paper indexed by these two databases a crude interrogation online was made. Each was input with the search strategy 'Tooth or teeth or dental', and a selection of five of the first twenty papers was printed to avoid the possibility of listing consecutive papers in only one or two journals. The results are shown in *Figures 5.1* and *5.2*. A comparison with *Figure 4.7*, a page reproduced from *IDL*, shows the contrast in the type of material included by these databases.

Chemical abstracts [4] may be a relevant tool for a search on materials science, but would not normally be used on a regular basis. The hard-copy versions of *Calcified tissue abstracts* [3] and *Microbiology abstracts* [9] provide useful summaries of papers which, although indexed by *IDL* and by *Index medicus*, would need to be called up on Medline in order to obtain abstracts. A search on psychological aspects of dentistry, which might include dental health education, using *Psychological abstracts* [13] and Medline will reveal a significant number of unique entries, but those identified by the former source are likely to be American dissertations, not necessarily easily available outside North America.

Science citation index [22] is a controversial bibliographical tool, whereby papers are retrieved which cite an article that is known to be relevant. The supposition is that authors are listing references that are closely related to their own work, and also that important papers have not been omitted from reference lists. *SCI* cannot provide the depth of coverage of conventional indexes, but is a useful supplementary tool, especially for cross-disciplinary research. In the case of dentistry, an

Search strategy: Dental or tooth or teeth

Items retrieved:

1 Comparison of electrical thresholds on intradental nerves and jaw opening reflex in the cat. *Acta physiol. scand.* **119** (1983): 399–403

5 Corrosion of the eta' (Cu–Sn) phase in dental amalgam. *J. biomed. mater. res.* **17** (1983): 921–9

10 An unusual case of distal type of lipoatrophy with cavities, stunted somatic growth, painful muscle cramps and hypoplastic uterus. *Clin. neurol.* **23** (1983): 867–73

15 Gap junctions in the epidermis of fetal rats studied by transmission electron microscopy. *J. ultrastruct. res.* **84** (1983): 182–93

20 Intravenous lignocaine in dental anaesthesia. The effect of pretreatment on the incidence of dysrhythmias. *Anaesthesia* **38** (1983): 1066–70

Figure 5.1 Sample search of Excerpta medica.

Search strategy: Dental or tooth or teeth

Items retrieved:

1 Epidermal callosis and silica deposits relations to cuticular transpiration. *Cellule* 1981–1982 (Recd 1983) 267–88

5 Oculo-naso maxillary and neutral anomalies in racoons. *Procyon-lotor. J. wildlife dis.* **19** (1983): 234–43

9 A comparative study on the mouth parts of medically and veterinarily important flies with special reference to the development and origin of the prestomal teeth in *Eyclorrhaphous diptera. Jpn. j. sanit. zool.* **34** (1983): 177–206

14 Validation of age estimation in the harp seal *Phoca groenlandica* using dentinal annuli. *Can. j. fish. aquat. sci.* **40** (1983): 1430–41

20 The first finding of a representative of the family Cetominidae gyrinomimus-notius new species *Osteichthyes cetonimiformes* in the Antarctic waters. *Zool-zh.* **62** (1983): 737–47

Figure 5.2 Sample search of BIOSIS.

example might be the citation of social science literature by authors writing on dental health education; such journals may be beyond the scope of *IDL*.

SCI has been used to conduct analyses of citations in different subject fields. An interesting example is the periodontal study by Brunette, Simon and Reimers (1978), in which analyses were made of citations to the *Journal of periodontology* and *Journal of periodontal research* over a fifteen-year period. These authors found that maximum frequency of citation in both journals occurred two to three years after publication, but that 18 percent of papers from the first journal and 9.5 percent from the latter were not cited at all. Case reports in both journals had a very low citation frequency. The *Journal of periodontal research* was cited more frequently than the *Journal of periodontology*.

More recently Beertsen and Ten Cate (1983) used *SCI* to determine the citation scores of senior staff at the five Dutch dental schools. It was discovered that there was little difference in the results for each school, but that the papers most frequently cited related to basic, non-clinical research.

References

Beertsen, W. and Ten Cate, J. M. 'Analyse van citatiegegevens over onderzoekers werkzam binnen de subfaculteiten tandheelkunde in Nederland'. *Nederlands tijdschrift voor tandheelkunde* **90** (1983): 402–9 (English abstract).

Brunette, D. M., Simon, M. J. and Reimers, M. A. 'Citation records of papers published in the *Journal of periodontology* and the *Journal of periodontal research*'. *Journal of periodontal research*, **13** (1978): 487–97.

Rogers, F. B. and Adams, S. 'The Army Medical Library's publication program'. *Texas reports in biology and medicine*, **8** (1950): 271–300.

Sutherland, F. M. 'Indexes, abstracts, bibliographies and reviews'. In Morton, L. T. and Godbolt, S. (eds.), *Information sources in the medical sciences*, 3rd ed. London: Butterworth, 1984, pp. 44–69.

6 The Literature of Dentistry

6.1 Original Contributions

6.1.1 Serials

The publication of original research is for the most part in journal literature, thereby ensuring that findings can be communicated to a wide audience without undue delay. Speciality journals are highly regarded in this respect, for example *Archives of oral biology* [306], *Caries research* [321] or *Journal of periodontal research* [566], but certain periodicals with a wider scope are equally favoured, notably *Journal of dental research* [77] and, for Scandinavian literature, the *Scandinavian journal of dental research* [89] or *Acta odontologica scandinavica* [60]. Items published in these advanced-level journals have been subject to rigorous scrutiny and criticism before being accepted for publication, and are of high academic standard, such that papers which are published are recognized as significant contributions to dental literature. Needless to say, authors and readers are spread worldwide.

National associations' journals publish research reports, but lay greater emphasis on material of interest to the practising dentist, since the majority of the readership are general practitioners. Therefore the scope of this kind of publication is wide: clinical trials, national or local surveys, case reports, practical hints and reviews, as well as scientific or technical papers. Emphasis is definitely on the clinical, rather than the scientific or theoretical aspects of dentistry, since the general dentist is particularly interested in aspects of research or development that may affect the materials or techniques he uses. This is not to say that specialized research papers are excluded, however.

Journals produced by national organizations offer an appropriate medium for publication of research undertaken in those countries, and papers by foreign authors are rarely included. These national journals reflect current research interests and developments or attitudes in the various countries, and indeed are the first choice of many potential authors submitting manuscripts. It should be noted that most national associations publish a journal, but the international importance is greater for some than others. The *Journal of the American Dental Association* [74], *British dental journal* [62] and *Australian dental journal* [61] are held in especially high regard.

Locally produced journals, for instance those of American state societies or the French regions, publish original research but concentrate on clinical updates or reviews. Obviously there are exceptions that prove the rule, one example being a paper by McInnes on a method of tooth bleaching published in the *Arizona dental journal* in 1966. The technique became a standard procedure, but outside the United States the original reference is virtually unobtainable!

National and local journals carry not only original papers, but also news, information, correspondence and reviews of recent literature. They therefore combine the role of newspaper and recorder. Some countries, such as Sweden and the Netherlands, overcome this by issuing two publications, one for topical information, the other for original papers. The Sveriges Tandläkarförbund issues *Tandläkartidningen* [131] in Swedish twice a month, mainly comprising topical information; its companion the *Swedish dental journal* [91] publishes scientific papers in English.

Important journals which have general coverage, rather than being devoted to a particular speciality, are listed in Part II in two groups: those in English, regardless of country of origin, and those in other languages arranged by country. Since it is not always apparent from some titles whether the journal is a commercial or a society publication, the official organs of national dental associations from selected European countries are identified in the following list.

Austria
Österreichische Zahnärzte-Zeitung [97] (Bundesfachgruppe für Zahn-, Mund- und Kieferheilkunde des Österreichischen Ärztekammer). News.
Zeitschrift für Stomatalogie [98] (Österreichische Gesellschaft für Zahn- , Mund- und Kieferheilkunde). Scientific and clinical material

Belgium
Revue belge de médecine dentaire [100] (Société Royale Belge de Médecine Dentaire)

Denmark
Tandlaegebladet [103] (Dansk Tandlaegeforening)

Finland
Proceedings of the Finnish Dental Society [86]

France
Chirurgien-dentiste de France [106] (Confédération nationale des syndicats dentaires)

German Democratic Republic
Stomatologie der DDR [109] (Gesellschaft für Stomatologie der DDR)

German Federal Republic
Deutsche zahnärztliche Zeitschrift [111] (Deutsche Gesellschaft für Zahn-, Mund- und Kieferheilkunde). Scientific and clinical papers
Zahnärztliche Mitteilungen [112] (Bundesverband der Deutschen Zahnärzte). Clinical and news

Greece
Hellenic stomatological annals [114] (Hellenic Dental Association)

Italy
Rivista italiana di stomatologia [121] (Associazione Medici Dentisti Italiani)

Netherlands
Nederlands tandartsenblad [123] (Nederlandse Maatschappij tot Bevordering der Tandheelkunde)

Norway
Norske tannlaegeforenings tidende [125] (Norske Tannlaegeforening)

Poland
Czasopismo stomatologiczne [126] (Polish Dental Association)

Spain
Revista de actualidad estomatológica española [129] (Consejo General de Colegios de Odontólogos y Estomatólogos de España)

Sweden
Swedish Dental Journal [91] (Swedish Dental Association). Scientific and clinical
Tandläkartidningen [131] (Swedish Dental Association). News

Switzerland
SSO Schweizerische Monatsschrift für Zahnmedizin [132] (Schweizerische Zahnärzte Gesellschaft)

Commercially published journals have an equally important role. Some titles, such as the *International endodontic journal* [341], are produced by a specialist society but published and distributed by a commercial publisher, while others are entirely funded by the publishing company itself, for instance the *Journal of dentistry* [78]. In the American field, the *Journal of prosthetic dentistry* [81] and *Oral surgery, oral medicine, oral pathology* [486] are official organs of various specialist societies, but are published by the C. V. Mosby Company and carry extensive advertising to offset their costs. Most contributors to these two journals are American, but the titles are widely read on an international scale, and are core journals in any dental library. On the British side, the *Journal of dentistry* [78], published by John Wright, and the *Journal of oral rehabilitation* [80], by Blackwell, are highly regarded and also have worldwide readerships; in both of these journals advertising matter is minimal.

6.1.2 Guides to Serials

Selected lists of English-language and foreign-language periodicals with general coverage are given in Part II. Most published guides to dental journals identify current and/or defunct titles, but do not indicate their academic level, which has to be inferred from the actual title; annotations regarding scope and level are therefore included in the Part II listings as appropriate.

To identify current titles a variety of sources are available. Each volume of the *Index to dental literature* includes an alphabetical list of titles indexed [58], but since this includes non-dental journals from which only a few papers may have been included, it is not always the most convenient listing to use. *Medical books and serials in print* [56], annually produced by Bowker, has a substantial section for serials currently published, and includes a 'dentistry' subheading. This is a reasonably comprehensive alphabetical list, with more information per entry than in the *IDL*, including publishers' addresses. Comparable with the Bowker list is the well-known *Ulrich's international periodicals directory* [59], which lists dentistry as a subheading under medicine, and provides details of current journals. *Ulrich* can be searched online using Dialog.

For retrospective coverage, or for listing by country, there is *Index der zahnärztlichen Zeitschriften der Welt* [57] by Schmidt and Schmidt. Since this reference book was published, in 1970, there have been numerous alterations and additions to the periodicals listed, but it remains a valuable source for information on dead titles and name changes, and where geographical listings are required.

Other tools for retrospective use are the *World list of scientific periodicals*, valuable for identifying changes of name and obscure titles, and *World medical periodicals*, which provides subject and geographical approaches. Both these tools are now too out of date to be useful for identifying current material.

Kowitz [55] is preparing an annotated guide to English-language journals, which will be a valuable addition to the reference literature.

6.1.3 Theses

Theses are substantial documents, sometimes comprising two thick volumes, detailing original work undertaken for research-based degrees, such as the PhD or MPhil. Dissertations or reports are also submitted by candidates for MSc degrees, but in this instance the written report forms only a part, rather than the whole, of the candidate's submission. These reports are therefore much shorter, and are variable in quality and academic standard. MSc reports are nowadays a fast-growing form of literature, numerically speaking, but are less frequently cited or exploited for reasons which will become apparent.

Access to theses can be problematical. Although they are available for reference in the library of the author's university, they may not be available for home reading. Inter-library loans of theses in Britain from the awarding institution are made on the strict understanding that the report does not leave the library of the requesting institution, a stipulation that continues to cause dissatisfaction in many a potential borrower. This problem is mitigated to some extent now that most British universities make their doctoral theses available to the British Library for microfilming so that copies are more easily accessible, but this facility does not extend to reports submitted for master's degrees, or theses from other countries. UK master's reports may not even reach the library of the awarding university, but are sometimes retained in departments.

The availability of American theses is normally less of a problem, since most can be supplied in hard copy or on microfilm from the publishers of *Dissertations abstracts*, University Microfilms.

Because of these problems in identifying and obtaining theses, it is common practice for authors to rewrite their material for submission as conventional journal articles, usually with a note appended to the effect that the paper is based on a thesis. Although an amount of detail may be lost, a series of research papers based on a PhD thesis will make available to a wide readership a major proportion of the investigation. MSc reports too may be published as journal articles, often as a joint paper by student and supervisor. Scandinavian theses are frequently published as journal supplements, for example to the *Proceedings of the Finnish Dental Society* [86] or the *Swedish dental journal* [91] and, unlike their European or American equivalents, the submitted theses in these cases are based on research results that have already been published.

Theses may be summarized in journals, as for example in the *Journal of the Nihon University School of Dentistry* [79]. This journal publishes in each issue, in English, single-page abstracts of dissertations accepted at the school. Similarly, the annual English supplement of *Nederlands tijdschrift voor tandheelkunde* [124] includes Dutch theses. *Information dentaire* [107] has abstracts of one or two French theses in most issues, while the *American journal of orthodontics* [517] includes occasional doctoral or MSc dissertations.

6.1.4 Finding Out About Theses

The most comprehensive listing, with international coverage, is in the *Index to dental literature* (*IDL*) [135], which includes some 900 titles per year. Details of the title, year, degree and awarding institution are given in the author sequence; two other approaches are by subject, under MESH headings, and by country. The list is compiled on the basis of information submitted voluntarily to the American Dental Association, and does not claim to be complete; French theses, for instance, are not regularly listed. For most other countries, however, the listing is a reliable source.

Dissertation abstracts: Section C, *European abstracts* [136] has a disappointing level of coverage for dental theses, but does have the merit of supplying abstracts for the ones that are included. Other listings are on a national or regional basis, such as Aslib's *Index to theses* [142], a well-known reference source issued twice a year, which lists theses accepted by institutions in Great Britain and Ireland, arranged in subject groups. Theses prepared in dental faculties are listed under the heading *Pathology and clinical medicine: dentistry, odontology*, but the subject index may reveal other relevant works prepared under the aegis of a different faculty or department, such as psychology, anaesthesia, or materials science. A comparison with *IDL* for 1982 shows that in that year the former included twenty-nine British theses and the latter twenty-three; similar coverage considering the delay in inclusion in both publications, which may be up to two years. Since 1977 Aslib have also prepared *Abstracts of theses*, a microfiche production containing abstracts of selected theses. The inclusion of a thesis in the *Abstracts* is noted in an appropriate entry in the *Index to theses*.

American dissertations are covered by publications from University Microfilms. *Dissertations abstracts* [145] itself is the best-known, but others are *American doctoral dissertations* [143] and *Masters abstracts* [146]. Listings as far as dentistry is concerned, however, are far from comprehensive, but theses that are included will be found under the heading 'Health sciences: dentistry', with subject index entries as appropriate.

French theses may be identified through the subject approach in the *Thésindex dentaire* [139], issued by the library of the University of Clermont-Ferrand, which prepares similar publications for medicine and pharmacy. Precise titles of theses are not given, but subheadings under each entry word indicate the general scope of each item. The 1982–83 volume, the ninth in the present series, includes entries for 1,720 theses. Each is entered under several subject headings, with the basic information of author, year, university and university thesis number being indicated in each entry. Cross-references to preferred and related headings are given. The publication has no author index.

Regular listings of Scandinavian theses can be found annually in *Acta odontologica scandinavica* [140], arranged by country, from 1977 onwards. Supplement 73 of the journal is a cumulative listing, from 1907 to 1975.

6.1.5 Reports

Report literature plays a minor role in clinical dentistry, being a less significant form of publication than in some other fields. Scientific research is communicated in the conventional journal literature where it is more easily accessible, and is routinely recorded for subsequent, and hopefully easy, retrieval by abstracting and indexing services. Reports, so-called 'grey literature', are notoriously difficult to identify and acquire. This said, the field does have a body of report literature that should not be ignored, notably on organizational aspects of the profession.

Although normally rewritten as journal papers, reports of a clinical or research nature are submitted to the National Institute of Dental Research by grant and contract holders and these are listed in the annual *Selected list of technical reports* [245]. The US Naval Dental Research Institute also produces reports on clinical topics. Other bodies produce report literature of either ephemeral or longer-lasting value, usually related to policy, administration and the provision of dental care rather than the clinical aspects of the field. Documents issued by national dental associations are normally publicized, if not actually published, in their own journals; for instance, the British Dental Association (BDA) notes its reports in the *British dental journal* [62]. The variety of publications which can be regarded as reports can be demonstrated by recent BDA publications. In 1983 a glossy briefing paper was prepared entitled *NHS dental treatment: what it costs and how the cost has risen*, a document issued free of charge to individuals and organizations concerning the rise in National Health Service charges to patients. The typescript *Dental manpower requirements to 2020* was noted in the *British dental journal* as being available on application to BDA headquarters, but this document was reprinted some months later in a Department of Health and Social Security report on manpower [584]. In 1982 the BDA published *Computers in general dental practice*, in conjunction with a computer firm; this was a priced publication.

A greater number of reports are issued by the American Dental Association (ADA), mostly on administration, policy and planning, but also with some topics of more direct interest to the general practitioner. Recent ADA titles include *The role of the health professional in the delivery of caries prevention*, in 1983; *Status report on the delivery of prosthodontic care by non-dentists in the USA and Canada*, in 1984, and *Dental marketing planner*, 1983.

Investigations by government bodies or independent foundations are noted in the dental press. Examples of publications in this category are the *Enquiry into dental education*, prepared and published by the Nuffield Foundation (1980) and *Towards better dental health*, the report of the Dental Strategy Review Group, issued by the Department of Health and Social Security in 1981. Government reports with a more general remit may also be of interest, for instance the *Report* of the Royal Commission on the National Health Service (1979) published by HMSO and more recently the *NHS management enquiry* (1983) by R. Griffiths, available only in typescript, but summarized in the *British medical journal*. The now famous *Inequalities in health* by Sir Douglas Black (1980) was virtually unobtainable from government sources, but has subsequently been republished in book form by Penguin.

International organizations issuing report literature in the dental field are the Fédération Dentaire Internationale and the World Health Organization. The former issues technical reports on materials and techniques, short documents which appeared originally in the *International dental journal* [72], while WHO includes dental subjects from time to time in its Technical Report series. Other WHO publications, frequently in typescript, may be issued from regional offices, such as the regional office for Europe in Copenhagen, which has a EURO series.

Local or regional health authorities may also publish report material, such as prevalence studies on oral disease, or studies on the provision of primary care in their area. Wessex Regional Health Authority, for instance, has issued *Filling gaps: dental health in Wessex* (1982).

Annual reports of appropriate bodies can contain worthwhile information, and their appearance is at least predictable. Examples are the *Gibbs report*, produced by Elida Gibbs whose 1982 and 1983 annual reports give facts and figures relating to oral health in an easy-to-assimilate format, and the Laboratory of the Government Chemist, which includes a dental section.

Reports and conference proceedings suffer from nomenclature problems. Some are known by the name of the issuing body, such as the Council of Europe's *Role and training of auxiliary dental staff in the member states*, others by author or editor. Government reports, especially those issued by committees with long names, or on behalf of several departments, tend to fall into this category. Two British examples are the Körner reports, issued in the 1980s from the Department of Health and Social Security's Steering Group on Health Services Information, and the *Final report* of the Interdepartmental Committee on Dentistry, known as the Teviot report, issued in 1946. In some cases a report is identified by its title or subject, like *Computers in general dental practice: report of the tripartite working party*, issued by the DHSS but prepared by the BDA, DHSS and Dental Estimates Board. Acronyms too cause problems: the 'NACNE report' is in fact a *Discussion paper on propsals for nutritional guidelines for health education in Britain*, prepared by the National Advisory Committee on Nutrition Education and published by the Health Education Council in 1983, and of interest to dentists concerned with prevention.

As previously mentioned, this type of material can be hard to identify, since much of it, notably unpriced publications or typescript material, never reaches the conventional bibliographies, such as *BNB* [36] or the NLM *Current catalog* [43]. The book section in *IDL* [17] is worth searching, as it includes a good deal of literature that is not strictly 'books', mainly North American pamphlets and reports, but also some items from other countries. The listing is by author.

Dental literature may occasionally be found in *British reports, translations and theses* [141], which covers acquisitions at the British Library Lending Division, but better sources are *British medicine* [24], described in Chapter 4, section 4.6, and *Health service abstracts* [26], a monthly production from the library of the Department of Health and Social Security. This covers mostly journal papers, but governmental and other documents are also included. Arrangement is by subject.

6.2 Reference Books

Dentistry has not in past years been the subject of an encyclopaedia, although Harris's dictionary [152], to be discussed in section 6.2.1, might almost be regarded in this category. Jablonski (1982) considers that encyclopaedias are a dying breed, as knowledge in all areas is increasing, and cannot feasibly be contained in one publication and yet remain up to date and valid. Only the general encyclopaedias have a future; in scientific fields they are being superseded by dictionaries. The German publishing firm Hüthig apparently does not agree, since it is producing a four-volume work that it is advertising as an encyclopaedia, entitled *Die zahnärztliche Versorgung* by R. Hilger, T. Jung and H. Spranger [52]. These authors discuss the foundations of dentistry, conservative dentistry, periodontology, oral surgery, prosthetics and orthodontics, and the final volume is a dictionary.

A number of directories, which may also be considered appropriate for this chapter, are discussed in Chapter 3.

6.2.1 Dictionaries

English-language dental dictionaries have a lengthy history, the first dating back to 1849, ten years after the first dental journal was founded. In that year Chapin A. Harris published his *Dictionary of dental science, biography, bibliography and medical terminology* [152]. This and the following three editions were more akin to an encyclopaedia, in that lengthy expositions appeared under a number of entries. F. J. S. Gorgas edited the fifth and sixth editions, this last appearing in 1898, trimming the content so that the long entries became more succinct.

Three dictionaries, all American, were published during the first half of the twentieth century. L. P. Anthony's *Dictionary of dental science* [147] and L. Ottofy's *Standard dental dictionary* [156] appeared within a year of each other, in 1922 and 1923 respectively. W. B. Dunning and S. E. Davenport's *A dictionary of dental science and art* [150] followed in 1936. None of these achieved a second edition, despite the fact that they were productions of a high standard. They are still useful today for historical words and phrases, biographical information and illustrations. Occasionally too, general practitioners may use terminology which is now obsolete, but is identifiable in the older dictionaries.

Turning now to modern dictionaries in everyday use, Boucher's *Current clinical dental terminology* [148] was first published in 1963, a cumulation of specialized glossaries produced for specific subject fields. The third edition, entitled *Clinical dental terminology*, by T. J. Zwemer, was published in 1982. As a quick reference tool, it is easy to use, and has a thorough cross-referencing system. The entries themselves are concise and informative.

A newcomer to the field is S. Jablonski's *Illustrated dictionary of dentistry* (1982) [155], an exhaustive listing whose title belies its scope, which far exceeds dentistry. Many terms from medicine, science and technology are included, as well as

American trade names, notably of drugs, and the dictionary is therefore a sizeable tome. It has been criticized on account of this so-called extraneous material, but should be regarded as a medical dictionary compiled for the dental profession, and used as such. Presumably because of the large number of entries, and the economics of publication, a small typeface was chosen. Extensive use is made of subheadings; this feature combined with the small print means that careful scanning may be required to find the appropriate part of a long entry. These, however, are minor criticisms of an excellent work, and the dictionary is most certainly to be recommended as a standard reference tool for any dental collection or serious researcher's personal library.

It must be pointed out that like all North American works, 'Boucher' and 'Jablonski' have drawbacks for the user from other countries. Spelling, for instance, is a critical feature in a dictionary, and there are variations, for example an*ae*sthesia or an*e*sthesia; there are differences in terminology, for example 'bridgework' and 'fixed prosthodontics', and also in the scope of particular terms or phrases (compare the definitions of the British Standards Institution and Jablonski for 'occlusion'). Nevertheless, these two are the most comprehensive listings in English currently available.

Dictionaries produced in Britain are intentionally restricted in scope and coverage. An invaluable source for all people concerned with dentistry is J. E. H. and C. G. Fairpo's *Heinemann modern dictionary for dental students* (1973) [151]. This pocket-sized production has brief entries of one or two sentences, and is especially useful for newcomers to the field, dental assistants and non-dentists, but the research worker may find it less helpful. A new British production aimed at the same level of user is being prepared by Harty and Ogston.

The International Organization for Standardization and the British Standards Institution include terminology in their remit, and the BSI has issued a second edition of its BS 4492 *Glossary of dental terms* (1983) [149]. The aim of this publication is to promote the acceptance and use of words and phrases that have been approved as being accurate and precise, and to discourage the usage of others which are nonspecific, imprecise or out of date. The *Glossary* is arranged by subject field—prosthodontics, orthodontics, conservative dentistry, periodontology, dental materials, basic dental sciences, paedodontics and dental radiology—listing words or phrases in each speciality with a short definition. Where two terms have the same meaning, a preferred term may be indicated. Obsolete or ambiguous words are identified, and may be indicated as 'deprecated'. This publication is particularly helpful for the British user who is unfamiliar with the terminology of dentistry, and for the author who needs a precise, correct phrase.

The International Organization for Standardization has published a *Dental vocabulary* (1983) [154], but this is restricted in scope to materials, instruments and equipment. Brief definitions are supplied in English and French sequences.

Subject glossaries will be described in the various sections of Part II, but it is appropriate to mention here the 'Glossary of prosthodontic terms' [630], produced by the Academy of Denture Prosthetics and published in the *Journal of prosthetic dentistry* in 1977. This valuable listing is of interest to all workers in the field of restorative dentistry generally, and provides short definitions of words used in a range of subject fields.

General medical dictionaries should not be forgotten, the most comprehensive British title being *Butterworth's medical dictionary* (second edition 1978). *Dorland's illustrated medical dictionary* (twenty-sixth edition 1981) is a popular American text.

The French language has two small dental dictionaries, but nothing specifically on dentistry to match Jablonski in scope and comprehensiveness. L. Verchère and P. Budin's *Dictionnaire des termes odontostomatologiques* [161] (second edition 1981) has more entries and more detail per entry than L. Roucoules's *Terminologie fondamentale en odontostomatologie* [159], issued in 1977, although the latter includes numerous line drawings (of which the former has none) and more biographical entries. M. Goudaert and P. Danhiez's *Dictionnaire pratique d'odontologie et de stomatologie* (1983) [158], despite its name, is not a dictionary in the accepted sense. Entries are made under broad terms, and comprise lengthy essays on the topic and its ramifications. Emphasis is on the pathological and clinical aspects of dental disease.

W. Hoffmann-Axthelm has produced a detailed German-language dictionary, now in its third edition, the *Lexikon der Zahnmedizin* [162]. As well as standard dental terminology, abbreviations, proprietary and proper names are included. German definitions are also provided for certain English words and phrases.

Dictionaries are available for the Spanish and Italian languages, which is to be expected; less predictable, perhaps, given the small population to use them are dental dictionaries in Dutch and in the Scandinavian languages. Lofroth (1984) points out that Swedish inaugural dissertations were published in either Swedish or German during the 1920s and 1930s, but English has replaced both as the language of choice. She found, on investigating Swedish-language journals from 1976, 1956, and earlier years, that English words were being used per se or modified and then incorporated into the Swedish vocabulary even before the First World War. Equivalent Swedish translations were not used, because the translation would be cumbersome, involving more words, or because the English term was convenient to use.

6.2.2 Miscellaneous Reference Books

A unique handbook, intended for the American dentist but with a wealth of information for practitioners in other countries too, is the *Dentists' desk reference* [215], prepared at two-yearly intervals by the ADA Council on Dental Materials, Instruments and Equipment. There is particularly extensive coverage of the various materials used in the mouth and extra-orally, with information on uses, properties and characteristics; also discussed are instruments, dental equipment, hygiene aids, and safety in the surgery. Each section has a list of 'Dos and don'ts', and a note of available products. There is an index to manufacturers, and a general index which includes trade names. The book is a useful quick reference source for facts and figures, although its American origin should be taken into account when noting trade names and manufacturers' addresses. A companion volume on drugs in dentistry is *Accepted dental therapeutics* [575], described in the pharmacology section of Part II.

Of particular value to those who need to record data on oral disease is the World Health Organization's *Application of the 'International classification of diseases' to dentistry and stomatology* [219], commonly known as *ICD/DA*. The second edition was issued in 1978, following the publication of the ninth edition of the *International classification of diseases* in 1975. *ICD/DA* is based on the ninth edition of *ICD*, but certain sections have been expanded to provide more detail. It includes diseases and conditions that occur in, have manifestations in, or are associated in some way with the mouth, but excludes treatment. Diseases of the oral structures are classified under section IX, diseases of the digestive system, class numbers 520–29, in this section covering the oral cavity, salivary glands and jaws. The extent to which the mouth is affected by, or implicated in, systemic disease is indicated by the fact that this section comprises only twelve pages from the total of eighty in the classified sequence. There is a detailed subject index, and two annexes which comprise the International Histological Classification of Oral and Odontogenic Tumours and Allied Lesions, also compiled by WHO.

The *ICD/DA* thus provides a basis for coding data according to a standardized system, allowing the recording of detailed diagnostic information. It makes possible the collection of epidemiological data, and subsequent comparison on an international level. Statistics on oral disease can be compiled locally and nationally, by and for the pathologist, physician and surgeon, and the public health dentist.

The Fédération Dentaire Internationale publication *Basic fact sheets* [217] offers facts and figures on dentistry in 114 countries, based on information received from national dental associations, or ministries of health. The year in which the information was supplied is noted at the top of each country's entry. The following details are supplied for most countries: manpower (dentists, technicians, dental ancillaries); membership of national associations; official journals; membership of organizations of traders and manufacturers; education (number of schools, length of curriculum, annual number of graduates); specialization; licensure; epidemiological surveys; dental practice; fluoridation. Addresses of national organizations are not given. Appendices tabulate the world dental manpower situation, the world fluoridation status and survey auxiliary personnel.

For information on aspects of Britain's National Health Service (NHS), the standard reference book *Hospitals and health services yearbook* [218] includes a range of facts and figures, names and addresses. Hospitals are listed according to regional health authority; other sections cover government departments, suppliers and manufacturers and circulars from the Department of Health and Social Security. From the same organization, the Institute of Health Service

Administrators, is a new production edited by N. W. Chaplin: *Health care in the UK: its organization and management* [216], which provides a degree of detail not found in most other books about the running of the NHS.

6.3 Textbooks and Monographs

When dentistry was a less complex field of knowledge, to encompass the different aspects of the subject in a single text was a more feasible proposition than it is today. Even so, Litch's *American system of dentistry* ran to three volumes in 1886–87, and the second edition of Sir Norman Bennett's *Science and practice of dental surgery* was composed of two volumes in 1931. Nowadays, books which attempt to cover the entire range of dental practice within the confines of a single textbook are the exception, apart from those with their subject content pitched at a superficial level, for instance to meet the needs of dental ancillary staff. Books for dental surgery assistants, for instance, touch on a range of topics, but only in sufficient detail as is necessary for background knowledge or as is relevant to their own duties.

A general work for dentists who wish to expand their knowledge and clinical expertise is Morris, Bohannan and Casullo's *The dental specialties in general practice* (1983) [53]. This has chapters on the various special fields, with the emphasis on procedures and techniques the nonspecialist may wish to add to his own repertoire. It is also useful for specialists in one field who wish to update their knowledge in others.

For the general dentist who requires practical information, an interesting type of literature is the loose-leaf production, housed in ring binders, which can be updated by the addition of new or revised sheets. This type of publication is intended as a reference manual, combining the benefits of a journal's currency and timeliness with a book's convenience and ease of location of relevant material. The American *Clinical dentistry*, edited by J. W. Clark [48] and published by Harper & Row in 1976, set the precedent which has been followed by Kluwer in Britain with *General dental practice* (1978–) [50] and *General dental treatment* (1983–) [51]. These are aimed at the general practitioner, not the academic, and deal with specific problems encountered clinically and administratively. New sections, revisions and updates are sent to subscribers automatically.

At a more academic level Rowe and Johns are editing a multi-volume work entitled *Companion to dental studies* [301], a sister to the successful *Companion to medical studies*, published by Blackwell, with the intention of integrating the clinical and basic sciences for undergraduate and postgraduate students. Three of the four books in the set expound the principles of biological sciences as they apply to dentistry. In volume 1, book 1 covers anatomy, biochemistry and physiology, and book 2 dental anatomy and embryology. Volume 2 will cover clinical methods, pathology and pharmacology, while the final volume is devoted to clinical dentistry. Chapters in volume 3 will deal with all the specialities, and describe disorders of the mouth and masticatory apparatus and their management.

Authoritative coverage of biology and pathology is provided by B. Cohen and I. R. H. Kramer, who have edited contributions from a number of eminent authorities with the needs of advanced students in mind. *Scientific foundations of dentistry* [295] is a companion to others in a series published by Heinemann, which includes titles on anaesthesia, oncology, paediatrics and surgery. The Scientific Foundations series is highly regarded, the dental volume being no exception.

The *Deutscher Zahnärztekalender* [49] is a yearbook highly regarded in the German-speaking profession. Each annual issue includes papers on a wide range of topics, prepared by authorities in the field, and reflecting current thought and practice.

A new yearbook is the *Dental annual* [49A], first issued in 1985. This provides reviews on current practice and research for general practitioners, written by respected British authors.

Apart from these titles mentioned, the reader must use specific texts in each field for an overview of dentistry; individual books are discussed in the subject sections of Part II. A range of titles are available in each speciality to meet the needs of students at all levels, and of practitioners.

Although many publishers issue dental works, a few have established special reputations for high-quality productions both in physical format and in content. In Britain, Churchill Livingstone and John Wright are pre-eminent, and the Scandinavian firm of Munksgaard is also well known for its excellent publications. Among the numerous American companies, Mosby and Saunders each produce a consistent number of respected titles each year.

Information Retrieval, with London and Washington offices, does not issue many dental titles, but publishes on behalf of other organizations specialist conference reports of interest to research workers. Important examples are *Mechanisms of localized bone loss* (1978), edited by J. E. Horton and others, published for the National Institute of Dental Research; *Methods of caries prediction* (1978), edited by B. G. Bibby and R. J. Shern, also for the NIDR, and *Bacterial adhesion and preventive dentistry* (1984) by S. A. Leach and others for the International Association for Dental Research's Research Group on Surface and Colloid Phenomena in the Oral Cavity. Information Retrieval's dental publications are paperback, with perfect bindings, and prepared from camera-ready copy, but their contents are at a high academic level, and the contributors well known in their subject fields.

John Wright have an excellent series, well thought of in the profession, entitled Dental Practitioner Handbooks. The first title in the series was published in 1965; by mid 1984 no. 33 had been issued, with new additions, or revisions to existing titles continuing to be made frequently. Books in this series are suitable for undergraduates, clinicians, and students beginning advanced courses, and are all by British authors. The books themselves are paperbacks, and of a uniform size, and until 1983 were easily recognizable by their distinctive green and white covers, but in 1984 a new design of green and blue was introduced.

The Swiss firm Karger publishes two important monograph series for the researcher and advanced student. Frontiers in Oral Physiology has four titles issued between 1974 and 1983, Monographs in Oral Science having twelve for the period 1972–83, but with a wider remit which includes phosphates, fluorosis and the temporomandibular joint. These two series are described in more detail in the 'Biological sciences' section of Part II.

One of the most prolific publishers of general texts and specialist monographs is the international firm Quintessence. A feature of their publications is the high-quality colour photography used to illustrate clinical conditions and techniques in many of their volumes.

Reference

Lofroth, A-L. 'English influence on Swedish odontological vocabulary'. *Tandläkartidningen* **76** (1984); 457–67.

7 Sources of Special Information

There are occasions when the conventional documentary sources—books and serials—are inadequate or insufficient, and it becomes necessary to use a different type of material, such as a British Standard or an Act of Parliament. These sources have their own idiosyncrasies, mainly concerning identification or acquisition of the material itself, but interpretation is sometimes a difficulty too, if for example they contain statistical data or legal jargon. Specific points will be discussed in relation to the various types of material dealt with in this chapter: government publications, standards, patents, trade literature, statistical data and audiovisual material.

7.1 Government Publications

Central government impinges on the practice of dentistry in varying degrees, according to the country concerned, and government publications correspondingly may be few or plentiful, according to the state involvement with the profession. In countries where private practice is the norm, there may be little government activity other than the passing of a Dentists Act, or the formulation of registration requirements. In the United States, for example, there is less governmental published output relating to the practice of dentistry than in Britain, where most dentists work within the framework of the National Health Service (NHS).

British dentists are dependent on political decisions in respect of the organizational structure of the Health Service as a whole, and for conditions of service and payment. There is a multiplicity of documents emanating from the relevant government department, the Department of Health and Social Security

(DHSS), in relation to the NHS; but the dentist himself will need to be aware of few of these, since they relate in the main to the minutiae of planning and administration. The government has been keeping a watchful eye on the profession, however, since before the inception of the NHS, primarily because of a longstanding manpower shortage which has only now been overcome. In 1946, for example, the Interdepartmental Committee on Dentistry (the Teviot report) looked at manpower, legislation and research, before the assimilation of dental care into the NHS in 1948. In 1956 McNair headed the Committee on Recruitment to the Dental Profession.

Developments in the NHS continue to affect dental practice, thus any general reports relating to its organization may be of interest to the profession. The findings of the Royal Commission on the NHS (the Merrison report) were published in 1979; reorganizations of the structure of the NHS itself were implemented in 1974 and 1982, accompanied by a proliferation of documents. Dentists in the Community Dental Service were directly affected by this most recent reorganization, since a complete staffing tier, which included the area dental officers, was removed.

General practitioners are issued with a loose-leaf *Handbook for general dental practitioners* published by the DHSS, which explains their responsibilities under the various Acts and NHS regulations. They are also affected by other government legislation such as the Health and Safety at Work Act, and employment statutes.

A new Dentists Act was passed in 1983, amending the 1957 Act. Debates in the Houses of Commons and Lords, but no summary of the new Act itself, were reproduced in the *British dental journal*. A consolidating Act was passed in 1984.

Remuneration of dentists and patients' charges are subject to government decision, two perennially contentious issues within the profession itself and among the general public. Recommendations on dentists' rates of pay are presented to government each year by the Review Body on Doctors' and Dentists' Remuneration, whose annual report is published as a command paper by HMSO [234]. The Review Body receives oral and written evidence from individuals and organizations, and makes recommendations for the coming year's fees and salaries for doctors and dentists in general practice, and the hospital and community service. Nevertheless, the government has no obligation to accept the Review Body's findings, or award the increases that it proposes. The Review Body has existed in its present form since 1971, and its annual report contains not only remuneration proposals but information on earnings comparisons, movements in earnings, detailed salary scales, fees and allowances, and chapters on hospital, community and general practitioners. It is therefore an important source of facts and figures on the contemporary situation.

Investigations by the DHSS and governmental departments continue to be made which are of interest to the profession. The Dental Strategy Review Group's report *Towards better dental health* appeared in 1981, a policy document that gave recommendations for discussion between the government and its profession. Topics covered included preventive dentistry, the general and community dental services, and manpower. Studies made on wider aspects of health care also have dental implications, such as the report of the Committee on Child Health Services (the Court report) *Fit for the future*, published in 1976, and *Access to primary health care*, a DHSS report.

The Office of Population, Censuses and Surveys is responsible for the *Adult dental health survey* [645] published in two volumes in 1980 and 1982, and the 1983 *Children's dental health survey* [233]. These reports are described in more detail in Part II.

Clinical matters may come to government's attention, but to a lesser extent than policy or planning. Examples of publications in this category are reports on anaesthesia in 1967, and hepatitis in 1979.

Although HMSO, Her Majesty's Stationery Office, is the official government publisher, shorter but no less important documents may be issued by the departments themselves. Into this latter category come, for example, the Dental Strategy Review Group's report *Towards better dental health*, and the DHSS study *Dental manpower* [584]. These are sold by the DHSS Leaflets Department, and are not available from HMSO. Similarly, in the United States, the official publisher is the US Government Printing Office, but some documents are sold or distributed by departments themselves, such as the National Institute for Dental Research.

Priced reports from HMSO reach the standard bibliographical sources, but departmental productions may not. Since 1980 Chadwyck-Healey have produced a *Catalogue of British official publications not published by HMSO* [243] which eases the difficulties of identifying this elusive group of documents. It is issued bimonthly with annual cumulations. A companion is the *Keyword index* [244], also appearing bimonthly, but available only on microfiche. The HMSO *Annual catalogue* covers the conventional government literature, and *Sectional lists* give notes of HMSO publications which emanate from particular departments and which are currently in print. *Health service abstracts* [26], issued monthly by the DHSS Library, is a useful up-to-date source for both HMSO and non-HMSO documents.

7.2 Standards

The existence of national standards bodies, such as the British Standards Institution, the Deutsches Institut für Normung and the American National Standards Institute, is familiar and their publications well known in the countries concerned, but their connection with dentistry may be less widely recognized. However, dentistry is especially reliant on the quality of its materials, more so than other medical specialities, and therefore it is in the area of materials that the standards organizations are chiefly concerned when it comes to dental work. Plastics, metals, or any other substance that is used in the mouth must be free from side-effects, and must have specified physical, chemical and clinical properties. The dentist using any kind of material needs to be confident that the manufacturer, whether from his own country or another, is selling a reliable product.

The first national standard relating to dentistry was issued in the United States in 1925, following a request by the US Army to the National Bureau of Standards that it set up specifications for the selection and grading of amalgam, for use in the federal service. This popular filling material has been used extensively since the nineteenth century in different formulations, but until the early 1900s had been looked on with disfavour, in part because of its then poor quality. Although G. V. Black had re-established its reputation, the US standard was intended to ensure that a product would be manufactured which would be reasonably priced, and meet the clinical performance criteria of the time. By 1979, eight countries had produced standards in the dental fields, those with the largest numbers being Germany (approx. 60), Japan (approx. 63) and Australia (approx. 55), the others being Canada, France, South Africa, Britain and the United States.

In Britain the British Standards Institution prepares and approves standards in cooperation with the British Dental Association and other organizations or individuals; in the United States the American National Standards Institute (ANSI), the American Dental Association (ADA) and the National Bureau of Standards collaborate. The ADA Council on Materials and Equipment is responsible for establishing ADA specifications, and is the administrative sponsor of a standard formulating committee of ANSI. Once an ADA specification has been formulated, manufacturers can apply to have their products tested. Those that comply with the requirements of the specification are permitted to signify on the label that they have been certified by the ADA. It is usual for ADA specifications to be subsequently adopted as ANSI standards. Since some products fall under the jurisdiction of the Food and Drugs Administration, the ADA works closely with that body and the National Bureau of Standards.

In Australia, the antecedents of the Australian Dental Standards Laboratory date back to 1934, when a materials research laboratory was established at the University of Melbourne. This was taken over by the Department of Health in 1947 and called the Commonwealth Bureau of Standards, adopting its present name in 1974. The Laboratory participates in various dental standards committees, has extensive testing facilities and provides technical assistance to the Australian Dental Association in the production of the latter's *List of certified products*, which names products complying with appropriate standards.

Canada has only recently started to formulate its own national standards, the first being issued in 1979 and six being published by 1982. In Oslo, the Nordisk Institutt for Odontologisk Material Prøvning (the Scandinavian Institute for Dental Materials), founded in 1969, tests materials on sale in Scandinavia to ensure their clinical safety and check that they meet technical requirements. The institute operates by agreement among the governments of Sweden, Norway, Denmark and Finland who each contribute a percentage of the annual funds according to their gross national product.

At worldwide level the International Organization for Standardization coordinates and develops internationally acceptable standards through its technical dental committee, TC 106. The ISO is a nongovernmental organization composed of national standards organizations from eighty-four countries; TC 106 has seventeen participating members and twenty-one observer members. The committee has eight groups working on filling materials, prosthetic materials, terminology, instruments, equipment, toothbrushes, dental implants and dental needles. Each of these has a number of task groups, which are formed specifically to develop particular standards, and are likely to be disbanded once the Draft International Standard (DIS) stage is reached.

Some twenty-four ISO standards have been developed since 1963, plus a further nine adopted which were prepared by the Fédération Dentaire Internationale. The FDI was the original instigator of international dental standards and supported a programme that resulted in the formulation of nine specifications. The FDI's Commission on Dental Products continues to make recommendations for clinical and biological testing, and establishes guidelines for certification. It plays an important role consulting and coordinating with national and international bodies.

7.2.1 Finding Out About Standards

The national organizations regularly issue lists of their publications, for instance the annual British Standards Institution *Yearbook* [240], and are recognized as the appropriate local sources to contact for information on publications of standards bodies of other countries.

The United States National Bureau of Standards has published *Organizations engaged in preparing standards for dental materials and therapeutic agents, with a list of standards* (1980) [242], which describes national bodies and gives titles of the actual standards published. From the same source comes a *Bibliography of publications by the dental medical materials section* (1979) [241]; not actually a list of standards, but background scientific papers.

The text of ADA specifications was published in full in the ADA's *Guide to dental materials and devices*, of which the eighth and last edition was published in 1978. When this publication was succeeded in1981 by *Dentists' desk reference* [215], the specifications were, regrettably, no longer included. Notifications of new specifications and relevant ANSI standards are published in the *Journal of the American Dental Association* [74].

7.3 Patents

The clinical dentist is rarely in need of information on patents, but this type of literature is the concern of the manufacturer of instruments, equipment and materials. The dentist is, however, affected by patents, since they protect the interests of the designers and producers of the innovations which he subsequently uses.

Oral research abstracts [11] included patents during its years of publication, 1965–78, but no dental source routinely lists them today. Stecher, however, has provided abstracts of American patents issued since 1970 relating to materials in *New dental materials*, published in 1980 [405]. The Science Reference Library in London has an extensive range of literature relating to patents, as well as a comprehensive collection of British and foreign patents, and access to online indexing services such as *World patent index* and *Impadoc*.

7.4 Trade Literature

Trade literature too is the province of the manufacturer and distributor. Usually in the form of glossy leaflets, it is mailed direct to dentists and intended to promote the manufacturer's products and encourage sales. Such literature may therefore exclude technical data and prices, but may stimulate requests for back-up references, for instance in relation to the properties of materials or impartial evaluations of products. Trade literature is rarely collected systematically, and is subject to no bibliographical control. Leaflets may not even be dated.

An interesting current development is the recognition of the historical value of such literature. Early catalogues from manufacturers such as Claudius Ash are scarce, but are keenly sought-after by dental historians. Advertisements are routinely excluded from bound journals on the library shelves, but these too are useful historical sources.

7.5 Statistical Data

The dentist can no longer ignore the existence or importance of statistics, be it the methodology, or the facts and figures themselves. Methodological aspects are the special concern of the potential author of a thesis or journal paper, since many publications are required to include a suitable statistical analysis of results in order to be approved by a court of examiners or a journal's referees. The epidemiologist in the field of dental public health must have a good understanding of statistical techniques to interpret his masses of data in an accurate way; on a smaller scale, so too must the researcher conducting a clinical trial. It follows that the reader of the papers and theses containing statistical analyses will also benefit from an understanding of the means by which conclusions have been reached.

Nevertheless, dental students, even at postgraduate level, find the subject hard to grasp, and have demonstrated that they need basic information presented in a way that is easy to understand and assimilate. To cater for this need there are several publications, some specifically dental, others not.

Darby and Bowen's *Research methods for oral health professionals* [225] gives a useful introduction to statistics in Chapter 9, 'Analysis and interpretation of oral health research findings', but the whole book is well worth perusing. Weinberg and Cheuk (1980) have issued a useful *Introduction to dental statistics* [228] while Von Fraunhofer and Murray's *Statistics in medical, dental and biological studies* (1976) [227] takes examples predominantly from the dental field, being written by authors with a dental background. *Design and analysis in dental and oral research* by N. W. Chilton (1982) [224] purports to explain fundamental principles, but is a highly detailed presentation and, although excellent for the advanced researcher, is a daunting tome for the novice. A best-seller, however, is the introduction to medical statistical methodology by T. V. D. Swinscow (1983), *Statistics at square one* [226]. This publication is less than 100 pages in length, but offers clear explanations which are ideal for the newcomer.

Statistical data can be grouped into two broad categories: first, management information on the delivery of dental care, which can include manpower figures and financial aspects, and secondly, epidemiological figures on dental diseases. The first type of information is generally collected at national or regional level at the instigation of central or regional government, or a national association. Clinical data may also be collected on behalf of official authorities but are also likely to be amassed by individuals conducting their own research projects.

The Fédération Dentaire Internationale's *Basic fact sheets* [217] provide data supplied mainly by national dental organizations; for each country figures relate to dental manpower and schools, and references are given to any surveys on clinical conditions that have been conducted. Appendices provide comparative data on manpower and fluoridation status in over 100 countries.

Statistical information may also be provided by the WHO Oral Health Unit databank, mentioned in Chapter 1, section 1.4.2.

7.5.1 Management Data

The system of dental care delivery will affect the kind of figures that are collected, and the body that organizes their collection. In Britain, for instance, the majority of dentists are employed in the National Health Service (NHS), and figures on their numbers, the courses of treatment they provide and breakdowns according to general, hospital and community dental services are collected by government sources, notably the Dental Estimates Board and the Department of Health and Social Security. By contrast, in the United States most dentists work in private practice, and it is the American Dental Association (ADA) that collects and publishes data on manpower and aspects of practice. The nature of the collecting body will also influence the type of statistical information collected. For example, most British practitioners do a limited amount of private, as opposed to NHS, work, and some dentists run practices that are entirely private, having no NHS patients at all. Because the DHSS is not, however, concerned with private practice, it collects no data on this aspect of dental treatment. The principal sources of statistical information for Britain are the appendices to the *Annual report* of the Dental Estimates Board [231], which deals with estimates for treatment which have been submitted by general dental practitioners, and *Health and personal social services statistics* [232], which includes figures for general, hospital and community dental services.

The appendices to the Dental Estimates Board's *Annual report* provide the most detailed breakdown available of treatment undertaken in the General Dental Service in England and Wales. Private treatment and work carried out within the Hospital and Community Dental Services are excluded. The complete report is not publicly available, but the statistical appendices are distributed to dental schools and other interested bodies. It should be noted that these publicly available tables are not lettered consecutively, and there is a time lag of approximately nine months before publication; thus the 1982 figures were issued in September/October 1983.

Appendix A, Estimates received by the Board, gives figures for the total number of estimates received and authorized by the Dental Estimates Board and their cost, for a four-year period. Appendix B is another single-page table, on treatment approved of a more expensive kind than was clinically necessary, the patient paying the additional cost. The next appendix, G, comprises five tables relating to the distribution of dentists practising in the General Dental Service. These give analyses of numbers of dentists and dentist–patient population ratios in Family Practitioner Committee and county areas and by region, distribution according to type of practice, age group and sex, and movement to and from the General Dental Service. The main body of the statistical data is encompassed in appendix H, which has fifteen multi-page tables relating to treatment provided, with figures derived from a 5 percent sample. Treatment is categorized into thirty broad groups, with subdivisions allowing a considerable amount of detail to be specified. Thus in table I, 'Incidence and cost of the various items of treatment', category 2 (x-ray, and report), is split into seven subgroups, according to the kind of x-ray. Tables I and II show numbers of treatments, numbers of teeth and cost under these very detailed treatment categories. Further tables relate to types of estimates, analysis by region, patients' contributions, and patients' age groups.

Appendix J relates to orthodontic treatment, figures again derived from a 5 percent sample, and shows treatment provided and age groups. Only completed cases are included in these two tables; cases which have been discontinued or are still unfinished (orthodontic treatment can last several years) are excluded. Finally, appendix K relates to the administrative costs of the Board itself.

In America, many statistical surveys are undertaken by the ADA, for example the *Survey of dental practice* [581], which is carried out every few years. The Australian Dental Association issues a compendium each year entitled *Facts and figures: Australian dentistry* [229], tabulating data on numbers of dentists, fees, ancillary staff and a range of other topics.

From time to time individual reports may be compiled which offer statistical information, such as the Japan Dental Association's *Handbook of statistical data on dental health* [230], published to coincide with the annual meeting of the Fédération Dentaire Internationale in Tokyo in 1983. The DHSS's 1983 report on *Dental manpower* [584] includes projected figures for British dentists by the turn of the century.

7.5.2 Clinical Surveys

Data on the health status of a population, whether it be national or local, are essential to planners, administrators and clinicians to indicate the nature and level of dental disease and point the way to potential manpower requirements or any special provisions which may be necessary.

Clinical surveys on oral conditions may be carried out on behalf of central or local government by bodies such as the World Health Organization or national dental associations. Individual researchers, notably in the public health field, carry out many of the smaller-scale research projects, publishing their results in journals such as *Community dentistry and oral epidemiology* [649].

In Britain the first dental epidemiological survey to be carried out on a national scale was conducted in 1968 and published two years later, as *Adult dental health in England and Wales, 1968.* It was based on interviews and dental examinations of a random sample, and conducted by the Government Social Survey and the London Hospital Medical College Dental School. Studies followed on *Adult dental health in Scotland*, conducted in 1972, and *Child dental health in England and Wales* in 1973. These reports were to be major sources of data until their successors were conducted ten years later. In 1978 a second adult dental health survey was carried out, on this occasion by the Office of Population Censuses and Surveys (OPCS) in collaboration with the University of Birmingham Dental School [645]. Again, a sample population was selected for interview and examination, but this survey also included Scotland. The two-volume report was published in 1980 and 1982, and showed changes in the state of dental health during the ten-year period, as well as providing an overview of the current situation. This is therefore a prime source of statistical data on oral health in Britain. Similarly, a children's dental health survey was conducted in 1983 [233], but instead of there being a two-year delay before the publication of the report, interim results were published in the *OPCS monitor* in the same year.

Like the 1978 adults' survey, it was conducted by the OPCS and covered Scotland as well as England and Wales, which its 1973 predecessor did not. Of particular note in the findings was that the proportion of five-year-olds with some known decay experience decreased from 71 percent in 1973 to 48 percent in 1983.

7.6 Audiovisual Material

Films and slides have been used in undergraduate teaching for many years, with universities producing in-house material for their own students. These traditional formats are now being supplemented by newer ones, primarily the tape slide and videocassette. The former is particularly suited to individual learning or small groups, and comprises a set of slides accompanied by an audio cassette, which may or may not be synchronized. One advantage of the tape slide presentation is that it requires no special equipment; a slide projector, possibly a screen, and a cassette recorder. Videos, on the other hand, do need a compatible machine, although standardization is approaching, as VHS and Betamax formats are the most commonly produced.

Although the target audience for which most audiovisual presentations are intended is still the undergraduate one, programmes that will be of interest to the practitioner and postgraduate are growing in number, possibly as a result of the trend towards continuing education and the greater accessibility of hardware, for example the home video recorder.

Until recently, production and distribution of dental audiovisual material has been uncoordinated. Many institutions did not publicize their productions or make them available to outside enquirers, possibly because of copyright problems, or patients' confidentiality. This situation is changing, as two organizations, the Graves Medical Audiovisual Library [256] and Oxford Educational Resources [258], have been taking active steps to acquire, publicize and make available audiovisual programmes in dentistry.

The Graves Medical Audiovisual Library is a charitable institution, originally established in 1957 to provide an audiovisual updating service for general medical practitioners. Over the years it has expanded in scope, and now has an extensive collection, mainly of tape slide presentations, for doctors, dentists, nurses and first-aiders. Some programmes are especially commissioned, others acquired following negotiations with the institutions which made them; all are available for purchase or hire. A catalogue is available [248] which is arranged by subject, and which is updated by lists of new titles and newsletters. Some sixty dental titles are available, on all aspects of dentistry. As at mid 1985, only one video on dental topics was held by this library.

Videos are the specialism of Oxford Educational Resources, a commercial organization which is the largest British supplier of videocassettes on dentistry, having in 1983 some eighty programmes in the speciality. These are acquired from the universities, and are available for purchase or hire in various formats. Purchase prices are however more expensive than for tape slides, in early 1984 being in the region of £150–£220, depending on the running time. During the same period about two-thirds of their dental videos were in the field of prosthetics, but new additions on all aspects of the subject are being made. Programmes are available for dentists, students and ancillaries. Films are also available, but in smaller numbers. A subject catalogue gives details of available programmes in all formats.

Other British producers are predominantly in the field of dental health education, thereby providing material for the general public, or for use in the surgery by hygienists or dentists. The principal suppliers in this area, who issue slides, films and videos, are the British Dental Health Foundation [251], the Health Education Council [257], the General Dental Council [254] and Gibbs' Oral Hygiene Service [255]. Interestingly, these organizations are funded and backed by different sources. The British Dental Health Foundation has charitable status and relies for support on the profession. The Health Education Council is in receipt of an annual government grant, while the General Dental Council is the statutory registrable body for dentists. Elida Gibbs, which manufactures oral hygiene aids, is the parent company of the Oral Hygiene Service. All have lists of their material.

7.6.1 Finding Out About Audiovisual Material

As mentioned above, the various producers issue their own catalogues. New British programmes are regularly included in the audiovisual section of *British medicine* [24], which is arranged by subject, and for each programme gives standard information such as title, producer, distributor, running time and an annotation indicating the prospective audience or subject coverage.

The British Life Assurance Trust for Health and Medical Education, commonly known as BLAT, is based at the British Medical Association's headquarters and plays an important role in the promotion of audiovisual material in medicine generally, and the encouragement of high standards. The BMA/BLAT film library issues a catalogue entitled *Medical films* [246A] which not only lists films actually in the library itself, but others available from outside distributors which have been awarded a BLAT certificate, a recognition of a high standard of quality, or which have gained an award in the BMA film competition. Six dental films are included. BLAT has also issued a separate list entitled *Audiovisual teaching/learning materials for practising dentists or those studying at postgraduate level* [246] which includes details of tape slides, films and videos.

The British Universities Film and Video Council has amalgamated two publications, *Audiovisual materials for higher education* and *HELPIS*, to form a single *Catalogue* [247] of material suitable for degree-level teaching. The catalogue itself is on microfiche, having a classified main sequence, plus title and subject indexes. Addresses of distributors are printed in an accompanying booklet. The file is also searchable online via Blaise-line. Some thirty dental titles are included.

The standard American source is the National Library of Medicine's *Audiovi-*

suals catalog [249], available online as AVLINE. From 1971 to 1976 audiovisual material was included in the NLM's *Current Catalog*; the present publication is issued quarterly with annual cumulations. Items are listed under MESH headings and in a title sequence. Unlike entries in *Index medicus* or the *Current catalog*, which are listed without any published qualitative evaluation, programmes in the *Audiovisuals catalog* are scrutinized under a peer review process and put into one of five categories: highly recommended, recommended, not recommended, pending review, or no review. Items in the last category are not appropriate for evaluation; an example is news items. Critical abstracts are attached to most entries. Some 11 percent of the total entries relate to dentistry, according to a survey made by Rowberry and others (1979), with 87 percent of these being suitable for lecture support and 13 percent for self-instruction. Rowberry and colleagues described AVLINE with special reference to dentistry, while a general history and review is provided by Suter and Waddell (1982).

New additions to the collection of the American Dental Association's Bureau of Health Education and Audiovisual Services are listed in the review section of *Journal of the American Dental Associations*, with an annotation.

The *Dental bibliography* [38] of Georgetown University's Dahlgren Memorial Library includes audiovisual material added to the library from 1976 to 1982.

Bibliographies of journal papers from *Index medicus* have been prepared by the NLM. Literature search 78–25 includes ninety-eight citations on the subject *Audiovisual aids in dental education*, May 1974 to April 1978; this is updated by LS 81–27, *Audiovisual aids, computer-assisted instruction and programmed instruction in education for the health professions*, which covers January 1978 to October 1981, and includes twenty-five dental audiovisual citations.

References

Beech, D. R. and Tyas, M.J. 'The Australian Dental Standards Laboratory in 1984'. *Australian dental journal* **29** (1984): 283–90.

Jones, D. W. 'Standards for dental materials and devices'. *Journal of the Canadian Dental Association* **48** (1982): 523–8.

Rowberry, S. H., Sparks, S. M. and Kudrick, L. W. 'AVLINE: a search resource for audiovisual instructional materials'. *Journal of dental education* **43** (1979): 323–6.

Suter, E. and Waddell, W. H. 'AVLINE: a data base and critical review system of a.v. materials for the education of health professionals'. *Journal of medical education* **57** (1982): 139–55.

8 Language Problems

We have seen from previous chapters that English is the predominant language of publication, but this is not to say that papers in other languages are not of equal importance. German and French are the most widespread European languages, but increasingly contributions to the Japanese literature are being recognized as of considerable significance. There is little demand for Russian material in Britain.

Abstracts appended to the papers themselves are the first source to be consulted in a foreign-language paper. Many non-English journals have English abstracts appended; for German papers these are generally very helpful, but the quality of so-called 'English abstracts' can vary from an excellent lengthy summary to a single ungrammatical sentence. East European journals tend to offer short, less helpful abstracts. *Oral research abstracts* [11], published from 1965 to 1978, is a good source of English abstracts for foreign papers, but regrettably is has no successor.

Foreign-language journals may provide summaries in their own language of papers in English, but obviously only a selection of papers will be described. The German *Zahn- Mund- und Kieferheilkunde mit Zentralblatt* [15] provides short abstracts for about half of the entries in its *Zentralblatt* section. Occasionally papers are translated into Spanish or Italian, but this is not a regular occurrence. Some English-language journals routinely provide summaries in French, German or Spanish, for example the *International dental journal* [72] and *Journal of clinical periodontology* [565]. In dentistry there are no routine translating services, and no cover-to-cover translation journals such as exist in some technical fields.

Of the European languages, German and French are the most widespread among dental publications, followed by Spanish and Italian. During the early part of the twentieth century German was a more significant language internationally than today, having been overtaken by English. Swedish dissertations, for example, according to the study by Lofroth (1984) cited in Chapter 6, were traditionally published in German, but now are in English.

The most useful translation aid for these four European languages is the Fédération Dentaire Internationale's *A lexicon of English dental terms* [173]. This lists English words, each entry having a unique reference number, and for each word or phrase gives the Italian, German, French and Spanish equivalents respectively. Cross references are made from alphabetical sequences in the four languages concerned. Thus a typical entry would be:

bridgework 1090
puente *m.*
Bruckenarbeit *f.*
bridge *m.*, pont *m.*, prothèse intercalée *f.*
pont *m.*

The corresponding entry in the Italian listing will be puente B1090.

German terminology is treated in more detail in Bucksch's *Dental-Wörterbuch* [169], which also provides direct translations to and from English but no definitions. The International Organization for Standardization lists English, French and German terms for instruments, materials and equipment in ISO 1942: 1983 *Dental vocabulary* [154].

A multilingual approach is provided by Hadziomeragic in his *Lexicon stomatologicum* [174] which, like the FDI's *Dental lexicon*, has its main sequence arranged by English term, but covers German, Latin and Serbo-Croat.

Japanese literature presents its own set of problems for the would-be reader. Important research has been undertaken in the universities and dental schools and subsequently been published in such titles as *Japanese journal of conservative dentistry* or the *Journal of the Japanese Society for Dental Apparatus and Materials*, sometimes with an English abstract, sometimes without. An initial problem is the identification of the journal itself, since citation may be either of the translated title, as given above, which is commonly adopted by journals in their house styles for reference citation, or of the transliterated title, which for the two journals above would be *Nihon Hozon-Shika-Gaku-Zasshi* and *Shika-Riko-Gaku-Zasshi*. Transliterations are used in the *Index to dental literature*. This form of citation is rarely meaningful to a potential non-Japanese reader; the average orthodontist will not know that 'kosei' is the Japanese term for his speciality. Acquisition of the journal or paper may take time, since Japanese dental journals do not have a wide circulation in the West because of their low usage on account of these language difficulties.

The Japanese have attempted to overcome this predicament in two ways, first by publishing in widely available English-language journals, and secondly by issuing English-language journals themselves. The first solution brings its own difficulties however, since papers in established journals such as *Caries research* or *Journal of dental research* will inevitably cite earlier work, published in Japanese journals—the citations of course being all in English, to mislead the reader into thinking that the cited paper is in English too.

English-language journals are published by the universities or schools, and make research reports available to an international readership. Examples are the *Bulletin of the Tokyo Dental College* [63], and the *Journal of the Nihon University School of Dentistry* [79]. *Dentistry in Japan* [70] is issued annually by the Japan Dental Association, and contains reviews, in English, of the literature published in Japanese specialist titles during the previous year.

It remains to be seen whether Japan will follow the Scandinavian precedent and ultimately switch to English for its scientific and clinical dental journals. If not, there is a definite need for a formalized translation system of this under-used body of literature.

There are no special translation services for dentistry in any language, but the dental schools may well have staff or students with foreign-language skills. For the reader in London, the Science Reference Library offers a Linguistic Aid Service. This is not a formal translating service, but the Science Reference Library has staff with reading knowledge in a variety of languages, who can give a verbal interpretation of the subject matter of technical papers. Further information about the Linguistic Aid Service may be obtained from the Science Reference Library at 25 Southampton Buildings, Chancery Lane, London WC2A 1AW, England (Tel. 01–405 8721).

PART II

Bibliography

Bibliography

General Sources

General Bibliographical Guides *(Chapter 5)*

1 **Morton, L. T.** and **Godbolt, S.** *Information sources in the medical sciences*. 3rd ed. London: Butterworth, 1984. 534 pp.

Abstracting Services *(Chapters 4 and 5)*

2 *Biological abstracts*. 1926–. 220 Arch Street, Philadelphia, Pennsylvania 19103–1399: Biosciences Information Service. Twice monthly.
A classified arrangement with informative abstracts for conference proceedings and papers and over 9,000 periodicals. Each issue has indexes as follows: author, biosystematic, generic, concept and subject, which cumulate twice a year. It is available online as BIOSIS.

3 *Calcified tissue abstracts*. 1965–. 5165 River Road, Bethesda, Maryland 26816: Cambridge Scientific Abstracts. Quarterly.
Covers 5,000 periodicals, plus conference proceedings and reports, having 850 abstracts per issue. These are arranged in broad subject groups with subdivisions. Each issue and annual volume has author and subject indexes. Files from 1978 are available online as part of the Life Sciences Collection database, loaded by Dialog.

4 *Chemical abstracts*. 1907–. Easton, Pennsylvania: American Chemical Society. Weekly.
A vast abstracting service, including journal papers, conference proceedings,

reports, theses and patents, arranged in eighty subject groups. Each issue has keyword, author and patent indexes, each volume (two per year) has in addition general subject, chemical substances and formulae indexes. Files from 1967 onwards are available online as CA-search.

5 *Dental abstracts.* 1956–. Chicago: American Dental Association. Monthly.
Includes 100 abstracts per issue from some 200 English-language journals, appearing within twelve months of the original. Author indexes are provided each month and annually.

6 *Excerpta medica.* 1947–. Amsterdam: Excerpta Medica. Monthly.
A very large, important database for medicine as a whole, but of limited value for clinical dentistry, although oral biology is within its scope. There are forty-three subject sections, published separately.

7 *Fortschritte der Zahnheilkunde.* 1925–33. Leipzig: Thieme.
Published 1,600 informative abstracts each year from the world's literature, plus occasional diagrams and illustrations. Arrangement is by subject groups with author and subject indexes.

8 *Meditsinski referativnji zhurnal.* 1957–. Moscow: Vsesoyuznyi Nauchno-issledovatel'skii Institut Meditsinskoi, Medikotekhnicheskoi Informatsii, SSSR. Monthly.
Section 12: Stomatology.

9 *Microbiology abstracts.* 1965–. Bethesda, Maryland: Cambridge Scientific Abstracts. Monthly.
The subject group 'Human bacteriology' has a subdivision 'dental and oral' which includes about thirty informative abstracts per issue. Each issue and volume has author and subject indexes.

10 *NIDR abstracts.* 1965–. Bethesda, Maryland: National Institute of Dental Research. Monthly.
Some sixty long abstracts per issue, of books, journal papers and conference proceedings; relatively few are from dental journals. Arrangement is by first author; there are no indexes.

11 *Oral research abstracts.* 1965–78. Chicago: American Dental Association. Monthly.
Research-orientated, with 8,000 informative or indicative abstracts per year. Some 1,000 journals from throughout the world were covered, also patents. Author and subject annual indexes.

12 *Pascal explore. E72 Otorhinolaryngologie. Stomatologie. Pathologie cervicofaciale.* 1972–. Paris: Centre National de la Recherche Scientifique. Monthly.
Publishes some 300 short abstracts per issue, in seven subject groups, two being 'Mouth' and 'Face'. These cover journal papers and French theses on oral surgery, medicine and pathology. Monthly and annual author and subject

indexes are produced. Current title adopted in 1984; former title was *Bulletin signalétique*, Part 347.

13 *Psychological abstracts*. 1927–. Lancaster, Pennsylvania: American Psychological Association. Twice monthly.
Covers 1,000 journals, conference proceedings, books, theses and reports, with a surprisingly high amount of dental-related material. Available online from 1967 as PSYCINFO.

14 *Yearbook of dentistry*. 1936–. Chicago: Yearbook Medical Publishers. Annual.
A collection of some 200 lengthy, informative abstracts, selected from about forty journals, with diagrams or illustrations from the original if appropriate. Most material is from the year preceding that of the volume date.

15 *Zahn- Mund- und Kieferheilkunde mit Zentralblatt*. 1934–. Leipzig: Barth. Monthly. More then 550 items in each issue, over half accompanied by a short abstract.
Titles of papers are translated into German if necessary. There is a delay of two to three years before listing. This publication is particularly useful for pre-1961 material not covered by the *Index to dental literature*. Present title adopted in 1974; formerly *Deutsche Zahn- Mund- und Kieferheilkunde*.

Indexing Services *(Chapters 4 and 5)*

16 *Bibliography of Finnish dental literature for the period 1976–1981*. Helsinki: Finnish Dental Society, 1983. 210 pp.
Lists about 1,900 periodical papers in a subject arrangement, and also provides a complete record of Finnish dental dissertations for the period 1891–1981.

17 *Index to dental literature*. 1839–. Chicago: American Dental Association. Quarterly.
The most important indexing service in the field. Issues cumulate, the fourth issue for the year being a bound annual volume. Arrangement has varied over the years:

1839–1938: Classified, with author index
1939–64: Dictionary, with authors and subjects interfiled
1965–: Subject section, arranged by MESH headings, and author index.

From 1965 has included foreign-language material. Delay in appearance of index entries varies from six months to two years, depending on the journal indexed. Included in the Medline database, which is available online from 1966. Each issue includes a 'List of books', being mainly recently published titles in English, arranged in an author/title sequence.

18 *Index medicus*. 1879–. National Library of Medicine. Monthly, with annual cumulations.
Series have been published as follows:

series 1 1879–99

series 2 1903–20
series 3 1921–27
1927–56: entitled *Quarterly cumulative index medicus*, following a merger with *Quarterly cumulative index to current medical literature.*
1960–: present format adopted, that is, with subject entries indexed under MESH headings, and a separate author index.

Available online back to 1966 on the Medline database.

19 *Indice de la literatura dental en castellano.* 1952–. Buenos Aires: Asociación Odontológica Argentina. Every two years.
Indexes original articles, translations, editorials and obituaries from over fifty-two journals published in fifteen countries. Also lists books appearing in Spanish during the period covered. Published annually from 1952 to 1969, then biennially. Some 50 percent of the material currently listed is also in the *Index to dental literature*, but is not included there significantly earlier.

20 *Index der deutschen und ausländischen Literatur und zahnärztliche Bibliographie.* Berlin: Meusser, 1902–34.
Volume 1 has retrospective coverage back to 1847. Entries for periodical articles on dentistry in German or other languages are arranged in subject groups, with author and subject indexes. A valuable tool for foreign material not covered by the *Index to dental literature* during this period.

21 *Index to the Scandinavian dental literature 1950–1972.* In: *Odontologisk revy*, 1951–73.
Some 500 periodical papers indexed each year, arranged in subject groups with an author index. Especially useful for the period 1950–61, not covered by the *Index to dental literature.*

22 *Science citation index.* 1964–. Philadelphia: Institute for Scientific Information. Bimonthly, with annual cumulations.
Each issue includes the following sequences: citation index (list of references cited), source index (author index), permuterm index (keyword subject index) and corporate index (arranged by institution). Cumulations are available thus: 1955–64; 1965–69; 1970–74; 1975–79.

Current-awareness Services

23 American Dental Association. Bureau of Library Services. *Accessions list.* Chicago: ADA, Monthly.
A list arranged by author or title, including books, theses and reports.

24 *British medicine: a monthly guide to the literature.* 1972–. Oxford: Pergamon. Monthly.
Includes new books, pamphlets, official publications, reports and audiovisual material, published in Britain. The contents of British and selected foreign medical periodicals are listed. Books are arranged in broad subject groups;

'Dentistry' is a subject heading, and most entries have annotations and/or a list of chapter headings.

British national bibliography. (See [36]).

25 *Current contents*. 1972–. Philadelphia: Institute for Scientific Information. Weekly.

These well-known current-awareness services include about thirty dental titles but do not have the breadth of coverage of the Royal Dental College library list or of *Periodicals digest in dentistry*. They are however extremely up to date, sometimes listing journals in advance of the receipt of the journals themselves. The appropriate *Current contents* series are *Clinical practice* and *Life sciences*.

26 *Current literature on the health services*. Stanmore: DHSS Leaflets. Monthly.

A subject list of journal papers, reports, chapters in books, health circulars, statutory instruments, etc., prepared in the library of the Department of Health and Social Security. From May 1985, entitled *Health service abstracts*.

27 *The dentaletter*. 1983–. 94 Cumberland Street, #513, Toronto, Ontario M5R 1A3: The Dentaletter Inc. 10 issues per year.

An up-to-date, but highly selective service, providing a small number of informative abstracts of journal papers.

28 *Lewis's quarterly list*. London: H. K. Lewis. Quarterly.

A compilation from one of Britain's largest medical bookshops, of new books and editions, arranged under subject headings that include several dental terms. Details for each entry include most usual bibliographical features, plus book size, price and Lewis's postage costs, but regrettably publishers are not given.

29 Northwestern University Dental School Library. *Titles acquired*. Chicago: NUDS. Bimonthly.

Arranges new books by the National Library of Medicine classification, giving the class number, author, title, place, publisher and date for each item. There are separate sections for pamphlets, bibliographies, theses and periodicals.

30 *Periodicals digest in dentistry*. 1981–. 110 Tiburon Boulevard, Suite 5, Mill Valley, California 94941: Periodicals Digest. Bimonthly.

The only commercially produced current-awareness list for dentistry. Some fifty title pages are reproduced in each issue, mostly English-language journals, and a reprint service is available.

31 Royal Dental College Library. *Accessions*. Arhus, Denmark: RDC. Monthly.

Lists the contents of journals in English, French and the Scandinavian languages, and new books acquired by the Library.

32 *Sumarios de odontologia*. 1964–. São Paulo: University. Bimonthly.

A reproduction of the contents pages of over 100 journals, for distribution primarily in South America. There is a delay of about a year before any journal issue is included.

Bibliographies *(Chapter 5)*

33 American Dental Association. Bureau of Library Services. *Basic dental reference works.* 5th ed. Chicago: ADA, 1983. 25 pp.
An annotated bibliography of dictionaries, indexes, directories, bibliographies and other useful reference books, intended for the librarian or information worker.

34 American Dental Association. Bureau of Library Services. *Books and package libraries for dentists.* Chicago: ADA. Annual.
An author sequence of books published in English during the previous two years, and a list of packages (collections of reprints on a wide range of subjects) available for loan from the ADA Library.

35 'Arhus Tandlaegehojkoles videnskabelige produktion 1958–1983'. In: *Tandlaegebladet* **87** (1983): 559–72.
A bibliography of theses, books and journal papers emanating from the Royal Dental College, Arhus, Denmark. Most items are in English.

36 *British national bibliography.* 1950–. London: British Library. Weekly.
A subject listing of new and forthcoming books arranged by the Dewey classification, dentistry being located at 617.6, with author and subject indexes. Cumulations appear four-monthly and annually.

Campbell, J. M. *Dental bibliography.* (See [351]).

37 *Catalogue of Lewis's medical, scientific and technical lending library.* London: H. K. Lewis, 1975. 2 vols.
An extensive guide to hardback books written in English, up to 1972, with author and subject sections. Publishers are not identified. Supplements cover the periods 1973–75; 1976–78; and 1979–81.

Crowley, C. G. *Dental bibliography: a standard reference list of books on dentistry published throughout the world from 1536 to 1885.* (See [352]).

David, T. *Bibliographie française de l'art dentaire.* (See [353]).

38 Georgetown University. Dahlgren Memorial Library. *A dental bibliography of selected books, journals and audiovisuals, 1976–1982.* Washington, DC: The Library, 1982. 56 pp.
Lists items in the library's stock, plus additional material included in NLM databases. Excluded are foreign-language material, theses, popular works, items of local interest other than referring to Georgetown University, and dead journals.

39 *Health science books in print, 1876–1982.* New York: Bowker, 1982. 4 vols.
Main entries are listed under Library of Congress subject headings, cross-references being provided from MESH headings when necessary. There is an author index.

40 *Index catalogue of the library of the Surgeon General's office, US Army.* Washington, DC: US Government Printing Office, 1880–1961. 61 vols.
Five series were published, listing books, pamphlets, and selected periodical articles in various languages, under subjects and author.

41 *Lewis's medical booklist.* London: H. K. Lewis. Annual.
A selective guide to currently available titles, issued by one of Britain's foremost medical bookshops, arranged by subject. Prices, but not publishers, are given. It is supplemented by *Lewis's quarterly list* [28].

'List of books published'. In: *Index to dental literature.* (See [17]).

42 *Medical books and serials in print.* New York: Bowker. Annual.
An extensive listing of books in print in the United States, with author, title and subject sequences.

43 National Library of Medicine. *Current catalog.* 1966–. Bethesda, Maryland: NLM. Quarterly.
A subject listing, using MESH headings, and author index of new books. Cumulations have been issued for the following periods: 1966–70; 1971–75; 1976–80.
Predecessors of the *Current catalog* are:
Armed Forces Medical Library catalog, 1950–54, 6 vols. published 1955.
National Library of Medicine catalog 1955–59, 6 vols. published 1960 and 1960–65, 6 vols. published 1966.

44 Northwestern University Dental School Library. *Catalog.* Chicago: NUDS, 1978. 8 vols.
In dictionary format, and rich in historical and research material.

45 Raskin, R. B. and **Hathorn, I. V.** 'Selected list of books and journals for a small dental library'. *Bulletin of the Medical Library Association* **68** (1980): 263–70.

46 Richards, N. D. and **Cohen, L. K.** *Social sciences and dentistry: a critical bibliography.* London: Fédération Dentaire Internationale, 1971. 381 pp. Volume 2 is by **L. K. Cohen** and **P. S. Bryant**. London: Quintessence, for the Fédération Dentaire Internationale, 1984. 429 pp.
Narrative reviews are followed by extensive bibliographies.

47 United States. National Technical Information Service. *Dental prostheses, 1964–February 1983.* Springfield: NTIS, 1983.
From the NTIS database 192 citations on a range of subjects broader than the title implies.

Weinberger, B. W. *Dental bibliography.* (See [357]).

General Dental Works *(Chapter 6)*

48 Clark, J. W. *Clinical dentistry.* New York: Harper & Row, 1976. 5 vols. Loose-leaf.

Cohen, B. and **Kramer, I. R. H.** *Scientific foundations of dentistry.* (See [295]).

49 *Deutscher Zahnärztekalender.* 1942–. Munich: Hanser. Annual.

49A *Dental annual.* 1985–. Bristol: John Wright. Annual.

50 *General dental practice.* Edited by J. E. Manning. London: Kluwer, 1978–. Loose-leaf.

51 *General dental treatment.* Edited by J. Rayne. London: Kluwer, 1983–. Loose-leaf.

52 Hilger, R., Jung, T. and **Spranger, H.** *Die zahnärztliche Versorgung.* Heidelberg: Huthig, 1984–85. 4 volumes.

53 Morris, A. L., Bohannan, H. M. and **Casullo, D. P.** *The dental specialties in general practice.* Philadelphia: W. B. Saunders, 1983. 711 pp.

Rowe, A. H. and **Johns, R. B.** *Companion to dental studies.* (See [301]).

Lists of Journals *(Chapter 6)*

54 American Dental Association. Bureau of Library Services. *Dental journals published outside the United States and its territories currently received by the Bureau.* Chicago: ADA, approx. 13 pp. Annual.
A list arranged by title of some 260 journals and their addresses. Typescript.

55 Kowitz, A. *Dentistry journals and serials: an analytical guide.* Westport, Connecticut: Greenwood Press. In press.
An annotated guide to English-language journals.

56 'Medicine: dentistry'. In: *Medical books and serials in print.* New York: Bowker. Annual.
An alphabetical list of current journals in the serials subject index which is reasonably comprehensive, although not entirely up to date, and with some inaccuracies. For each entry is given the ISSN, date of commencement, frequency, publisher and address, an indication of the contents, such as book reviews and abstracts, and where it is itself indexed or abstracted. A useful source of addresses.

57 Schmidt, H. J. and **Schmidt, H. J.** *Index der zahnärztlichen Zeitschriften der Welt.* 2nd ed. Munich: Verlag Neuer Merkur, 1970. 249 pp.
Arrangement is by country, and the coverage includes both current and dead journals. Information provided for each journal is publisher and address, frequency, language, date of first issue and, where appropriate, last issue. Although somewhat out of date, it is still a valuable guide especially for non-English titles omitted from other lists.

58 'Serials indexed'. In: *Index to dental literature.* Chicago: American Dental Association. Annual.
An alphabetical list of abbreviated titles, which gives the full title, the town of publication, and the ISSN of journals that have been indexed in that volume of the *Index to dental literature.* Many titles are non-dental.

59 *Ulrich's international periodicals directory.* New York: Bowker. Annual.
Dentistry is included in the subject arrangement as a subheading under 'Medicine', and current titles are listed alphabetically. The price, publisher's address and frequency are given. Like *Medical books and serials in print* this is an easily accessible, extensive list.

Major English-language Journals *(Chapter 6)*

60 *Acta odontologica scandinavica.* 1939–. Box 2959 Toyen, Oslo 6, Norway: Universitetsforlaget. Bimonthly.
Published for the Acta Odontologica Scandinavica Foundation, which comprises sixteen societies and dental schools. The aim of the *Acta* is to make dental research in Scandinavia known to an international readership. Each issue contains eight to ten research-level papers. From 1977 an annual list of Scandinavian dissertations has been included; the list for 1982 is in a 1983 issue. Between 1940 and 1976 seventy-three supplements have been published, many becoming classics in their own right, but none has appeared since 1976. There is an annual contents list but no index.

61 *Australian dental journal.* 1956–. Sydney: Australian Dental Association. Bimonthly.
Each issue contains about ten clinical or scientific papers, plus correspondence, news and topical information from Australia and overseas. A dozen books are reviewed, but the reviews appear twelve to eighteen months after the books themselves. Trade and classified advertisements are carried. The journal supersedes three state journals, the *Australian journal of dentistry*, the *Dental Journal of Australia* and the *Queensland dental journal*, which voluntarily ceased publication in order that a national journal could be established.

62 *British dental journal.* 1880–. BMA House, Tavistock Square, London WC1H 9JR. Twice monthly. Two volumes per year.
The official journal of the British Dental Association, and the country's leading

general dental journal, containing about six papers per issue. There is a substantial correspondence section, together with general, Association, and trade news, and reports of meetings. The book reviews are particularly timely in comparison with those in other journals. Trade and classified advertisements are carried. Series of articles which have been specially commissioned for the journal may be reprinted as separate booklets, recent examples being 'Occlusion and restorative dentistry for the general practitioner', 'The maintenance of dental equipment', and 'Overdentures in general dental practice'. Each volume has a combined subject/author index, but users should note that entries for 1981 (**151**) to 1983 (**155**) do have inconsistencies and omissions, and feature title rather than subject entries.

63 *Bulletin of the Tokyo Dental College*. 1960–. 1–2–2 Masago, Chiba 260, Tokyo. Quarterly.
Each part includes four to six research-level papers from authors connected with the College. There is an annual contents list but no index.

64 *Bulletin of Tokyo Medical and Dental University*. 1954–. Bunko-Ku, Tokyo. Quarterly.
Of similar scope to its companion above, with some twenty papers per year, and an annual contents list.

65 *Cleft palate journal*. 1964–. 331 Salk Hall, University of Pittsburgh, Pennsylvania 15261. Quarterly.
The journal of the American Cleft Palate Association, with six to eight original papers per issue, correspondence, abstracts from other journals and announcements. There are annual author and subject indexes. Although it is not, strictly speaking, a dental journal, its subject matter is of interest to researchers in the fields of oral anatomy and physiology, orthodontics and oral surgery.

66 *Compendium of continuing education in dentistry*. 1980–. 3131 Princeton Pike, Lawrenceville, New Jersey 08648. 10 issues per year.
This title was established following the expansion of continuing education for general practitioners in the United States. Each part has six to eight clinically orientated papers on current techniques and new developments, book reviews, correspondence and advertisements. It is unique in that it can be used as a home study course in the University of Pennsylvania's Continuing Education Program; credits gained by registered participants who complete and return the self-assessment quizzes appended to each paper are recognized by a number of American states for their own continuing education accreditation programmes.

67 *Dental clinics of North America*. 1957–. Philadelphia: W. B. Saunders. Quarterly.
Each issue is devoted to a particular topic, and includes state-of-the-art reports aimed at the clinician. Themes of 1983–84 issues include materials, photography, paedodontics and removable dentures. Each issue is published as a hardback book, and the final one of each year includes a cumulative index for the previous three years. Editions in other languages are available as follows: German—

Medica Verlag; Greek—Anglo Hellenic Agency, 5 Koumpai Street, Athens 138; Italian—Piccin; Spanish—Nueva Editorial Interamericana; Japanese—Shorin.

68 *Dental practice.* 1969–. Epsom: A. E. Morgan. Twice monthly.
In newspaper format, this is a popular, easy to read update for the British general practitioner on clinical techniques and practice management. It includes short papers, reports on meetings, announcements, book reviews and trade and classified advertisements. There is no index.

69 *Dental update.* 1973–. London: Update Publications. 10 issues per year.
Each issue includes about five papers of particular interest to the general dentist. There is extensive trade advertising. Annual author and subject indexes are published.

70 *Dentistry in Japan.* 1967–. 1–20 Kudan Kita 4 Chome, Chiyoda Ku, Tokyo 102: Japanese Association for Dental Science. Annual.
Intended to make available Japanese research to the English-speaking world, this publication reviews papers from the various Japanese speciality journals and appends lengthy reference lists of the original references cited. Sections cover biology, conservative dentistry, prosthetics, oral surgery, orthodontics, dental health, dental materials and devices, dental radiology, paedodontics, periodontology, anaesthesia, history and practice administration. Other useful features are the names and addresses of officials of thirteen specialist societies, and lists of Japanese dental schools and current Japanese dental journals.

71 *General dentistry. c.* 1953–. Chicago: American Academy of General Dentistry. Bimonthly.
The organ of the Academy, providing continuing education for the general practitioner. Each issue has about twelve short clinical papers, together with advertisements, reviews and trade news. There are annual author and subject indexes. Current title adopted in 1976; former title was *Journal of the Academy of General Dentistry.*

IADR abstracts. (See *Journal of dental research* [77])

72 *International dental journal.* 1950–. Bristol: John Wright. Quarterly.
The official journal of the Fédération Dentaire Internationale, publishing eight to ten papers per issue which have been presented at the FDI annual congress. Papers in each issue normally relate to one or two particular topics. Each article has an informative abstract in French, German and Spanish. There is an annual author/subject index. The first issue of the year includes an FDI directory, giving a list of member associations, national treasurers, life members and the composition of committees.

73 *IRCS medical science: dentistry and oral biology.* 1973–. Amsterdam: Elsevier. Quarterly.
Intended to provide a rapid means of publication, this slim production has short, single-page research reports.

74 *Journal of the American Dental Association.* 1859–. Chicago: American Dental Association. Monthly. 2 volumes per year.

One of the foremost journals in the field, *JADA* publishes clinical and scientific papers, news, information and adverts. It has regular sections thus: letters, scientific articles, clinical reports, brief reports, review articles, publications reviews, Association reports, people and meetings, forthcoming meetings, and legislation and litigation. Under the 'publications' heading come book reviews and annotations, as well as additions to the ADA Bureau of Library Services and the audiovisual collection. 'Association reports' comprise status reports on materials and techniques compiled by the various ADA Councils; these are succinct state-of-the-art reports of especial value to the practitioner. There is a considerable amount of advertising material from the dental trade; classified adverts are also included. Each issue has some 150 pages of text, and full-colour illustrations accompany many papers. The overall appearance is therefore of a glossy, substantial publication. From 1914 to 1921 the title was *Journal of the National Dental Association.* There are author and subject indexes for each volume.

75 *Journal of the Canadian Dental Association.* 1935–. Ottawa: Canadian Dental Association. Monthly.

Scientific and clinical papers are published, mostly in English with French abstracts, although some articles are published in French. News items are bilingual; classified and trade advertisements are carried. There is an annual author/subject index.

76 *Journal of the Dental Association of South Africa.* 1946–. PO Box 2059, Pretoria: Mims. Monthly.

Each issue has one or two scientific or clinical papers, and a 'practitioners' corner' feature. News, book reviews and advertisements are included. Much material is published in both English and Afrikaans. There are annual author and contents indexes.

77 *Journal of dental research.* 1919–. Washington, DC: International Association for Dental Research. Monthly.

Each issue has approximately fifteen papers, grouped in sections: basic biological sciences, clinical science and materials science. No letters or trade advertisements are carried. The journal is one of the most prestigious in dentistry, highly regarded in the academic community. Annual author and subject indexes are published.

Abstracts of the IADR annual meeting and of divisional groups have been published in the *Journal* for a number of years, sometimes as supplements, more recently included in the main pagination. The 'IADR abstracts' themselves relate to the annual general session, and are cited in bibliographies from time to time, although not included in the *Index to dental literature*. 'AADR abstracts' refer to the American Association for Dental Research, which is the American equivalent to a division. 'Divisional abstracts' are those presented at the annual regional conferences throughout the world, for instance British, Japanese or Australian.

It is important to note that although each set of abstracts in a volume has its own author index, from 1979 onwards author entries for IADR abstracts are not included in the main index of the journal.

Locations for the different sequences for recent years are to be found in the *Journal of dental research* as follows:

IADR abstracts (i.e. of general sessions)
1977 session, 1977, **56**, special issue A
1978 session, 1978, **57**, special issue A
1979 session, 1979, **58**, special issue A
1980 session, 1980, **59**, special issue B
1981 session, 1981, **60**, special issue A
1982 session, 1982, **61**, 73–376
1983 session, 1983, **62**, 605–700
1984 session, 1984, **63**, 161–360

AADR abstracts
1977 session, 1977, **56**, special issue B
1978 session, 1978, **57**, special issue A
1979 session, 1979, **58**, special issue A combined with IADR abstracts
1980 session, 1980, **59**, special issue A
1981 session, 1981, **60**, special issue A combined with IADR abstracts
1982 session, 1982, **61**, special issue A combined with IADR abstracts
1983 session, 1983, **62**, 161–320
1984 session, 1984, **63**, 161–360 combined with IADR abstracts

IADR divisional abstracts
1977 session, 1977, **56**, special issue D
1979, **58**, special issue C
1978 session, 1979, **58**, special issue Dd
1979 session, 1980, **59**, special issue Di
1980/81 sessions, 1981, **60**, special issue B
1981/82 sessions, 1982, **61**, 521–624
1982/83 sessions, 1983, **62**, 401–524
1983/84 sessions, 1984, **63**, 486–609

78 *Journal of dentistry*. 1972–. Bristol: John Wright. Quarterly.
About ten original contributions, usually from British authors, are published in each issue. Letters and book reviews are included, although the latter are twelve to eighteen months after the book's publication. The journal succeeds *Dental practitioner dental record* which ceased publication in 1972, and is of interest to clinicians and researchers.

The annual index combines authors and subjects; a contents list is also printed.

79 *Journal of the Nihon University School of Dentistry*. 1958–. 1–8–13 Kanda Sugadai, Chiyoda Ku, Tokyo. Quarterly.
Each issue includes about six research papers, and single-page summaries of doctoral dissertations accepted by the University. There are no indexes.

80 *Journal of oral rehabilitation.* 1974–. Oxford: Blackwell. Bimonthly.
An authoritative, scholarly journal, publishing original comments and research. The subjects covered are conservative dentistry, intra-oral and maxillofacial prosthetics, physical and clinical aspects of materials, and oral physiology and dysfunction. Each issue contains about ten papers; there is no advertising material. An annual author index and contents list are given.

81 *Journal of prosthetic dentistry.* 1951–. St. Louis: C. V. Mosby. Monthly. 2 volumes per year.
Some thirty papers are published in each issue, under the following sections: removable prosthodontics, fixed prosthodontics and operative dentistry, maxillofacial prosthetics and dental implants, temporomandibular joint and occlusion, research and education, dental technology. Advertisements, correspondence and news items are included. This is a major journal, popular on both sides of the Atlantic. Each volume has author and subject indexes.

82 *New York journal of dentistry.* 1931–. 295 Madison Avenue, New York, NY 10017: First District Dental Society. 8 issues per year.
Contains six to eight short papers per issue, together with society and general news and advertisements. There are no indexes.

83 *New York State dental journal.* 1933–. 30 East 42nd Street, New York, NY 10017: Dental Society of the State of New York. 10 issues per year.
Six papers are included in each issue, plus advertisements, news and book reviews. An author/subject index is published.

This New York journal is often confused with [82]; not only their names but also their volume numbers are almost alike, and their content is similar. The *New York journal of dentistry* is published by a local society, however, while the *New York State dental journal* is the organ of the state society.

84 *New Zealand dental journal.* 1905–. Auckland: New Zealand Dental Association. Quarterly.
Includes three to four clinical or scientific papers, news, correspondence, book reviews, and research news and advertisements in each issue, as well as a directory of officials of the New Zealand Dental Association and specialist New Zealand societies. There is an annual author/subject index.

85 *Odontostomatologie tropicale/Tropical dental journal.* 1978–. PO Box 2932, Dakar, Senegal: Secretariat of Dental Health in Africa. Quarterly.
Each part has ten papers and advertisements. The journal is of special interest to African countries; most of the authors are from that continent. Papers are in English or French.

86 *Proceedings of the Finnish Dental Society.* 1904–. Akavatalo, Rautatielaisenkatn, SF–00520 Helsinki 52: Finnish Dental Society. Bimonthly.
Comprises half a dozen scientific papers per issue; there is no index. Until 1971 the journal was entitled *Finska Tandlakarsallskapets Forhandlingar*, and early

volumes were in Finnish; now the majority of articles are in English. Doctoral dissertations from Finnish universities are commonly published as supplements.

87 *Quintessence international dental digest.* 1970–. Berlin: Quintessenz. Monthly.
Early volumes contained shortened reports of papers originally published elsewhere, but since 1975 the journal has become a forum for short original reports. Refereeing was introduced in 1984. Until 1985, papers were arranged in the following sections: oral surgery, restorative dentistry and endodontics; prosthodontics, orthodontics, periodontics and oral hygiene; radiography and photography; practice administration; dental science and research; miscellaneous. Annual contents lists are produced, and an author index. Similar journals, albeit not direct translations, are published in German, French, Italian, Japanese, Greek and Spanish editions.

88 *Restorative dentistry.* 1984–. Epsom: A. E. Morgan. Quarterly.
Supported by the British Society for Dental Research, this journal publishes scientific and clinical papers and case reports. The subject scope includes conservative dentistry (crowns, bridgework, operative dentistry and endodontics), prosthetics, periodontology and the related fields of materials science and technology.

89 *Scandinavian journal of dental research.* 1893–. Copenhagen: Munksgaard. Bimonthly.
The official journal of the Nordiska Odontologiska Föreningen, the Scandinavian division of the International Association for Dental Research, which publishes papers by Scandinavian authors or other workers in Scandinavian laboratories. Each part contains about ten scholarly papers; no other material is carried. Until 1969 the journal was entitled *Odontologisk tidskrift* and was published in the vernacular, but since the change in title in 1970 all articles have been in English. There are annual author and subject indexes and a contents list.

90 *Special care in dentistry.* 1981–. Chicago: American Dental Association. Bimonthly.
The organ of the American Society for Hospital Dentists, the American Society for Geriatric Dentistry and the Academy of Dentistry for the Handicapped. Eight to ten papers on appropriate topics are published, plus book reviews and abstracts from other journals. Annual indexes cover authors and subjects.

91 *Swedish dental journal.* 1977–. Box 5843, S–102 48 Stockholm. Bimonthly.
The scientific journal of the Swedish Dental Association, with five to six clinical or scientific articles per part, accompanied by Swedish abstracts. Between 1977 and 1983 nineteen supplements were issued, on a variety of specialized topics. The journal is a fusion of *Svensk tandlakare tidskrift*, 1908–76, and *Odontologisk revy*, 1950–76. An annual contents list is published, but no index.

Medical Journals of Special Interest

The most important English-language journals that cover medicine as a whole all carry items of dental interest from time to time; for example, a new drug treatment for oral herpes simplex infection, an epidemiological survey of fluoridation in relation to cancer mortality, or, more generally, new developments in medicine which are also of interest to dentists, such as the introduction of a hepatitis vaccine, or reorganization of the National Health Service. In all the journals listed here the correspondence section is an important feature, and often contains letters of dental interest.

92 *British medical journal.* 1857–. BMA House, Tavistock Square, London W1: British Medical Association. Weekly.
The official organ of the British Medical Association, orientated more towards the practicalities of medical care than its companion the *Lancet.* Its coverage of medico-political events is especially important.

93 *Journal of the American Medical Association.* 1848–. 535 North Dearborn Street, Chicago, Illinois 60610: American Medical Association. Weekly.

94 *Journal of the Royal Society of Medicine.* 1907–. 1 Wimpole Street, London W1: Royal Society of Medicine. Monthly.
A scholarly publication, which includes papers presented at meetings of its Section of Odontology. The present title was adopted in 1978; previously it was entitled *Proceedings of the Royal Society of Medicine.*

95 *Lancet.* 1823–. 7 Adam Street, London WC2 6AD: Lancet. Weekly.

96 *New England journal of medicine.* 1812–. 10 Shattuck Street, Boston, Massachusetts 02115: Massachusetts Medical Society. Weekly.

Journals in Languages Other than English *(Chapter 6)*

There follows a selected list of important titles of journals in languages other than English which cover all aspects of dentistry. Those journals that are devoted to a particular speciality are listed in the appropriate subject sections.

Austria

97 *Österreichische Zahnärzte-Zeitung.* 1950–. Vienna: Bundesfachgruppe für Zahn-, Mund- und Kieferheilkunde des Österreichischen Ärztekammer. Monthly.
Publishes news and topical information.

98 *Zeitschrift für Stomatologie.* 1903–. Vienna: Österreichische Gesellschaft für Zahn-, Mund- und Kieferheilkunde and the Bundesfachgruppe für Zahntechnik. Monthly.
The official journal of these two bodies, publishing scientific and clinical papers. The current title was adopted in 1984; it was formerly called *Österreichische Zeitschrift für Stomatologie.*

Belgium

99 *Acta stomatologica belgica.* 1903–. rue des Champs-Elysées 43, B–1050 Brussels: Acta Medica Belge. Quarterly.

Organ of the Société Royale Belge de Stomatologie et de Chirurgie Maxillofaciale, publishing original papers in Dutch, French or English, with English and French abstracts. Present title adopted in 1960; formerly called *Revue belge de stomatologie.*

100 *Revue belge de médecine dentaire.* 1946–. 16 Avenue Ptolémée, B–1180 Brussels: Procom SPRL. Quarterly.

Organ of the Société Royale Belge de Médecine Dentaire, with scientific and clinical papers, news, reviews and advertisements.

China

101 *Zhonghua kouqiangke zazhi (Chinese journal of stomatology). c.* 1960–. 42 Dongsi xidajie, Beijing 1007000: Chinese Medical Association. Quarterly.

Czechoslovakia

102 *Czeskoslovenska stomatologie.* 1900–. Zdravofniche nakladatelstvi n.p., Obshodni oddeleni, Malostranské nám 28, 11802 Prague 1: Avicenum. Quarterly.

Contents page in English; most papers have brief abstracts in English and Russian.

Denmark

103 *Tandlaegebladet.* 1897–. Ameliegade 17, Postboks 143, D–1004 Copenhagen K: Danish Dental Association. Twice monthly.

Journal of the Danish Dental Association. One or two scientific papers per issue, otherwise topical information. Each issue includes a list of specialists, arranged by subject.

France

104 *Actualités odontostomatologiques.* 1946–. Paris: Prelat. Quarterly.

Publishes original papers accompanied by abstracts in English, German, Italian, Portuguese, Russian and Spanish.

105 *Bulletin officiel de l'ordre national des chirurgiens-dentistes.* 1945–. 22 rue Emile Menier, F–75116 Paris: Conseil National de l'Ordre National des Chirurgiens-Dentistes.

Contains political and legislative information.

106 *Chirurgien-dentiste de France.* 1940–. 22 avenue de Villiers, F–75017 Paris: Confédération Nationale des Syndicats Dentaires. Weekly.

Includes clinical papers of interest to the general practitioner, but is especially useful for French dento-political news. Also included are non-dental features, notably on the arts, and classified advertising. Current title adopted in 1962; formerly entitled *Le dentiste de France.*

107 *Information dentaire.* 1919–. 42 rue Vignon, F–75009 Paris: Syndicat National de la Presse Médicale. Weekly.
The commercially produced equivalent to *Chirurgien-dentiste de France* [106], with similar content. Title changed in 1938; formerly called *Semaine dentaire.*

108 *Revue d'odontostomatologie.* 1954–. 11 Cité Charles Godon, Paris: Société Odontologique de Paris. Bimonthly.
Clinical and scientific papers are published. Present title adopted in 1972; former title was *Revue française d'odontostomatologie.* 1972 = **19**, but 1974 = **3**, a new volume numbering system having been introduced in that year. The journal is a successor to the important *Odontologie*, 1881–1953.

German Democratic Republic

109 *Stomatologie der DDR.* 1951–. Berlin: Verlag Volk und Gesundheit. Monthly.
Official journal of the Gesellschaft für Stomatologie der DDR, publishing original reports accompanied by summaries in English and Russian.

110 *Zahn- Mund- und Kieferheilkunde.* 1934–. Leipzig: Barth. 8 issues per year.
Original articles have English abstracts. Half of each issue is devoted to abstracts from the world's dental literature; see Chapter 5, section 5.4.

Federal Republic of Germany

111 *Deutsche zahnärztliche Zeitschrift.* 1946–. Munich: Hanser. Monthly.
Official journal of the Deutsche Gesellschaft für Zahn-, Mund- und Kieferheilkunde, the scientific dental society of West Germany. The title page is given in English, and articles have English abstracts.

112 *Zahnärztliche Mitteilungen.* 1910–. Cologne: Deutsche Arzte Verlag. Twice monthly.
The organ of the Bundesverband der Deutschen Zahnärzte and the Kassenzahnärztliche Bundesvereinigung (the German Dental Association and the Panel Dentists' Association). Includes some clinical material, but predominantly information, news and advertisements. It is intended for the general dentist.

113 *ZWR.* 1968–. Heidelberg: Huthig. Monthly.
A commercially produced journal containing topical information and clinical papers for the general practitioner. A fusion of *Zahnärztliche Welt*, *Zahnärztliche Rundschau* and *Zahnärztliche Reform.*

Greece

114 *Hellenic stomatological annals.* 1957–. Athens: Hellenic Dental Association. Bimonthly.

115 *Odontostomatological progress. c.* 1947–. 70 Mikras Asias Street, Athens: Society of Odontostomatological Research. Bimonthly.
Provides a title page and abstracts in English.

116 *Stomatologia.* 1938–. Athens: Stomatological Society of Greece. Bimonthly.
Title page in English; some papers have short English summaries.

Hungary

117 *Fogorvosi szemle.* 1908–. Revai u. 16, 1065 Budapest 6: Ifjusagi Lapkiado Vallalat. Monthly.
Papers have short abstracts in Russian, English and German.

Italy

118 *Dental cadmos.* 1971–. Milan: Gruppo Editoriale Cadmos. Monthly.

119 *Minerva stomatologia.* 1952–. Corso Bramante 83–85, I–10126 Turin: Minerva Medica. Bimonthly.
Official organ of the Società Italiana di Odontostomatologia e Chirurgia Maxillofacciale. Contents page and abstracts of clinical papers in English.

120 *Odontostomatologia e implantoprotesi. c.* 1978–. Via Boccaccio 43, I–20123 Milan: Odontostomatologia. Bimonthly.
A commercially produced title, with original papers, occasional translations of articles from other languages, and numerous advertisements.

121 *Rivista italiana di stomatologia.* 1932–. Milan: Masson Italia Editori. Monthly.
Journal of the Associazione Medici Dentisti Italiani and the Società Italiana di Stomatologia.

Japan

122 *Journal of the Japan Dental Association.* 1948–. Tokyo: JDA. Monthly.
Entirely in Japanese.

Netherlands

123 *Nederlands tandartsenblad.* 1942–. Postbus 13079, NL–3507 LB Utrecht: Bohn Scheltema and Holkema. Monthly.
Official publication of the Nederlandse Maatschappij tot Bevordering der Tandheelkunde, containing topical information but no clinical papers.

124 *Nederlands tijdschrift voor tandheelkunde.* 1894–. Jacques Veltmanstraat 29, NL–1065 EG Amsterdam: Tijl Tijdschriften. Monthly.
A commercial journal, publishing clinical papers accompanied by English abstracts. An annual supplement in English contained a full translation of about three papers, and gave single-page summaries on twenty theses; this ceased in 1983.

Norway

125 *Norske tannlaegeforenings tidende.* 1890–. Oslo: Norske Tannlaegeforening. 16 issues per year.
Predominantly topical information, but includes some clinical papers.

Poland

126 *Czasopismo stomatologiczne*. 1948–. Warsaw: Polskiego Towarzystwa Stomatologicznego (Polish Dental Association). Quarterly.
Gives contents list and abstracts of papers in English and Russian.

127 *Protetyka stomatologiczna*. 1962–. Dluga 38–40, Warsaw: Pánstwowy Zaklad Wydawnictw Lekarskich. Quarterly.
Provides a contents page and abstracts of papers in English and Russian.

Russia

128 *Stomatologiya*. 1922–. Petroverigskii Per. 6–8, Moscow K 142: Izdatel'stvo Meditsina. Bimonthly.

Spain

129 *Revista de actualidad estomatológica española*. 1940–. Madrid: Consejo General de Colegios de Odontólogos y Estomatología de España. Monthly.
Includes news and original articles. Current title adopted in 1984; previously entitled *Boletín de informatión dental*.

130 *Revista española de estomatología*. 1963–. Casanova 57, Barcelona: Graficas Fomento. Bimonthly.
A commercially published journal.

Sweden

131 *Tandläkartidningen*. 1909–. Stockholm: Sveriges Tandläkarforbund. Twice monthly.
Publishes news, information and some scientific papers.

Switzerland

132 *SSO Schweizerische Monatsschrift für Zahnmedizin*. 1891–. Staffelstrasse 12, CH–8021 Zurich: Berichthaus AG. Monthly.
Official organ of the Schweizerische Zahnärzte Gesellschaft, publishing clinical papers and important review articles in French or German. Abstracts are given in English, and French or German, depending on the language of the original. Also includes *Acta parodontologica* (see the Periodontology section) and *Helvetica odontologica acta*. This journal was published twice a year from 1957 to 1975, and reported research results in English from projects undertaken in Switzerland, and it is continued in *SSO* in the same format. Current title adopted in 1984; previously entitled *SSO Schweizerische Monatsschrift für Zahnheilkunde*.

133 *Swiss dent*. 1980–. Freiestrasse 204, Postfach 239, CH–8032 Zurich: Verlag Felix Wust. Monthly.
Includes original articles, topical information and product news, and is published in German.

Yugoslavia

134 *Acta stomatologica croatica*. 1966–. Subiceva 9–1, 41000 Zagreb: Faculty of

Dentistry of the University of Zagreb and the Stomatological Section of the Medical Association of Croatia. Quarterly.
Gives a contents page and abstracts in English.

Information on Theses *(Chapter 6)*

135 'Dissertations'. In: *Index to dental literature.* Chicago: American Dental Association. Quarterly.
International coverage. Main entry is under author, giving details of title, degree, institution date and number of pages; secondary sequences permit country and subject approaches. Some 900 theses are listed each year, the listing in each quarterly issue of *Index to dental literature* cumulating as in the main sequences of the *Index.*

136 *Dissertations abstracts*; Section C, *European abstracts.* 1976–. Ann Arbor, Michigan: University Microfilms International. Quarterly.

Australia

137 Levine, S. *Subject index of the higher degree and diploma theses of the Faculty of Dentistry, 1928–1979.* Sydney: University of Sydney, 1980. 70 pp.

Finland

138 'Complete list of Finnish dental academic dissertations, 1891–1981'. In: *Bibliography of Finnish dental literature for the period 1976–1981* [16]. Helsinki: Finnish Dental Society, 1983.

France

139 *Thésindex dentaire: index alphabétique des sujets traités dans les thèses de science odontologiques et de chirurgie dentaire, soutenues en France et dans certains pays de langue française.* 1968–. Clermont Ferrand University. Annual.
Each volume includes about 1,500 theses. Entries give an indication of the subject, but not the exact title. There is no author index. From 1968–74 entitled *Catalogue des thèses françaises de sciences odontologiques et de chirurgie dentaire.*

Scandinavia

140 Lofgren, A. B. 'Academic dissertations at the dental colleges and odontological faculties in Sweden, Norway, Denmark and Finland, 1907–1975'. In: *Acta odontologica scandinavica* **34** (1976): supplement 73. 104 pp.
Over 300 dissertations are listed, with country and author arrangements. Published annually in the same journal from 1977.

United Kingdom

141 *British reports, translations and theses.* 1970–. Boston Spa: British Library Lending Division. Monthly.
A subject listing of publications from industry, universities and learned societies, and government publications not published by HMSO, which have been acquired by the BLLD. Until 1981 called *BLL Announcement Bulletin.*

142 *Index to theses accepted for higher degrees by the universities of Great Britain and Ireland.* 1950–. London: Aslib. Twice yearly.

Includes a subject section on dentistry, under the heading 'Pathology and clinical medicine: Dentistry. Odontology'. For each entry are given the author, title, degree and date. MSc reports are not normally included. *Abstracts of theses* is a companion on microfiche only; the presence of an abstract in this format is indicated in the hard-copy entry.

United States

143 *American doctoral dissertations.* 1934–. Ann Arbor: University Microfilms International. Annual.

144 *Comprehensive dissertations index.* 1973–. Ann Arbor: University Microfilms International. Annual. 10 year cumulation 1973–82 available as hard copy or on microfiche.

145 *Dissertations abstracts international.* 1938–. Ann Arbor: University Microfilms International. Monthly.

Covers North American theses from 1861.

146 *Masters abstracts.* 1962–. Ann Arbor: University Microfilms International. Quarterly.

Dental theses in these publications are listed under the heading 'Health sciences: dentistry'.

Dictionaries *(Chapters 6 and 8)*

English

147 Anthony, L. P. *Dictionary of dental science.* Philadelphia: Lea & Febiger, 1922. 324 pp.

Still useful for older terms and biographical details.

148 Boucher, C. O. *Clinical dental terminology: a glossary of accepted terms in all disciplines of dentistry.* 3rd ed. by T. J. Zwemer. St. Louis: C. V. Mosby, 1982. 378 pp.

A standard American dictionary today, but the contents are generally less helpful than in Jablonski [155] for users outside the United States. It is, however, easier to use for quick reference.

149 British Standards Institution. *Glossary of dental terms.* (BS 4492: 1983). London: BSI, 1983. 114 pp.

Not a conventional dictionary, in that words are grouped according to subject field, and not as comprehensive as a general dictionary. A most useful tool however, since it includes terms in common spoken usage, but not found as frequently in the literature. Where two terms have the same meaning, one is indicated as the preferred term. Some entries are indicated as 'deprecated' or 'obsolete'. There is an alphabetical index.

150 Dunning, W. B. and **Davenport, S. E.** *A dictionary of dental science and art.* Philadelphia: Blakiston, 1936. 635 pp.
Helpful for older terms, line drawings, portraits and biographical information.

151 Fairpo, J. E. H. and **Fairpo, C. G.** *Heinemann modern dictionary for dental students.* London: Heinemann, 1973. 422 pp.
A pocket-sized book, with brief definitions and diagrams, useful for the entire dental team. Appendices include tables of arteries, muscles, nerves and veins, and a list of dental periodicals.

152 Harris, C. A. *A dictionary of dental science.* 6th ed. by F. J. S. Gorgas. Philadelphia: Lindsay & Blakiston, 1898. 662 pp.
Title varies from one edition to another. An important early dictionary.

153 Harty, F. J. and **Ogston, R.** *Illustrated concise dental dictionary.* Bristol: John Wright. In press.

154 International Organization for Standardization. *Dental vocabulary.* (ISO 1942: 1983). Geneva: ISO, 1983. 41 pp.
Defines terms used in relation to materials, instruments and equipment, and the testing of these products. The terms and their definitions are given in English and French. The grouping is thus: basic terms (45 entries), materials (75 entries), instruments (230 entries, but those which are self-explanatory are not defined), testing (33 entries). English and French alphabetical indexes are provided.

155 Jablonski, S. *Illustrated dictionary of dentistry.* Philadelphia: W. B. Saunders, 1982. 919 pp.
Much broader in scope than dentistry alone, including many medical, scientific and technical terms, plus American trade names. More comprehensive and usually more informative than Boucher, but the small type and extensive use of subheadings makes it harder to use. Nevertheless, the most exhaustive dictionary currently available.

156 Ottofy, L. *Standard dental dictionary.* Chicago: Laird & Lee, 1923. 480 pp.
Useful for orthodontic nomenclature, and illustration of instruments and orthodontic appliances.

Dutch

157 Tempel, F. J. *Tandheelkundig woordenboek.* Utrecht: Bohn Scheltema and Hokema, 1983. 413 pp.

French

158 Goudaert, M. and **Danhiez, P.** *Dictionnaire pratique d'odontologie et de stomatologie.* Paris: Masson, 1983. 334 pp.
More of a concise encyclopedia, in that entries are for general terms, e.g. cancer de la bouche (oral cancer) with cross-references from more specific terms, e.g., leukoplakie (leukoplakia). Gives more information than other French dictionaries.

159 Roucoules, L. *Terminologie fondamentale en odontostomatologie et lexique français–anglais, anglais–français.* Paris: Maloine, 1977. 257 pp.
Brief definitions in French, with one-word English equivalents. Includes proper names. The English–French lexicons at the end of the dictionary should be used only if no other translating source is available.

160 Sinsoilliez, R. *Lexique des termes de parodontologie, de microbiologie periodontale et buccale et de sciences fondamentales.* Paris: Prelat, 1973. 112 pp.

161 Verchère, L. and **Budin, P.** *Dictionnaire des termes odontostomatologiques.* 2nd ed. Paris: Masson, 1981. 244 pp.

German

162 Hoffmann-Axthelm, W. *Lexikon der Zahnmedizin.* 3rd ed. Berlin: Quintessenz, 1983. 691 pp.
Includes illustrations and photographs.

163 Rehberg, H. *Taschenwörterbuch der Zahntechnik.* Munich: Hanser, 1980. 190 pp.

Italian

164 Hoffer, O. *Glossario della terminologia odontostomatologica.* 2nd ed. Milan: Odontostomatologia, 1983.

165 Verchère, L. and **Budin, P.** *Dizionario di terminologia odontoiatria.* Italian ed. by L. Fonzi. Milan: Masson, 1984. 260 pp.

Scandinavian (see also [168])

166 Bjorn, H. *Nordisk odontologisk ordbog.* Copenhagen: Munksgaard, 1970. 322 pp.
Includes Danish, Finnish, Norwegian and Swedish words.

Spanish

167 Friedenthal, M. *Diccionario odontologico.* Buenos Aires: Editorial Medica, Panamericana, 1981. 537 pp.

Swedish (see also [166])

168 Edward, S. *Odontologisk ordbok.* Box 99, S–267 00 Bjuv, Sweden: Invest-Odont, 1981. 55 pp.

Translating Dictionaries

German

169 Bucksch, H. *Dental-Wörterbuch; dictionary of dental practice.* Munich: Neuer Merkur, 1970. 407 pp.
English–German and German–English.

Japanese

170 Yamauchi, R. *A clinical dental dictionary on English–Japanese bilingual principles with German terminology added.* Tokyo: Shigaku Kyrkai, 1970. 484 pp.
English terms are defined; Japanese translations of definitions and pronunciation are given, plus one-word German equivalents. There is no Japanese–English section.

Spanish

171 Mairie, J. S. F. *English–Spanish, Spanish–English dental vocabulary.* Lancaster, Pennsylvania: Jaques Cattell Press, 1943. 159 pp.

Swedish

172 Petterson, E., Loader, D. and **Nystrom, G. P.** 'Glossary of Swedish dental terms: translation of Swedish expressions to British and American equivalents'. In: *Tandläkartidningen* **71** (1978): 23–29.

Multilingual Dictionaries

173 Fédération Dentaire Internationale. *A lexicon of English dental terms, with their equivalents in Español, Deutsch, Français, Italiano.* The Hague: Sijthoff, 1966. 424 pp.
An indispensable aid for anyone using foreign dental material. The main sequence is in English, with Spanish, German, French and Italian equivalents given for each term. Alphabetical listings in each language refer to the main entry. No definitions are given. A new edition is in preparation.

174 Hadziomeragic, M. *Lexicon stomatologicum: Anglais, Germanicus, Croatico-serbicus–Serbocroaticus; Latinus.* Zagreb: the author, 1978. 527 pp.
Like the FDI *Lexicon*, arranged by English terms, with indexes to the other languages.

Directories: General and Biographical *(Chapter 6)*

International

175 Alpha Omega International Dental Fraternity. 'Directory'. In: *Alpha omegan* **76** [3]: (1983).
The first directory of the Fraternity to be published for seventeen years.

176 Fédération Dentaire International. [Directory]. In: *International dental journal.* Annual.
The first issue of each volume includes a list of names and addresses of member organizations, life members, and members of FDI commissions. The 1984 directory occupies thirteen pages.

177 Groupement International pour la Recherche Scientifique en Stomatologie et Odontologie. 'Liste des membres de GIRSO'. In: *Bulletin*

du Groupement International pour la Recherche Scientifique en Stomatologie et Odontologie **22** (1979): 103–10.
An alphabetical list of members and their addresses.

Australia

178 Australian Dental Association. *Directory.* Sydney: the Association. Every two years. Approx. 150 pp.
As well as giving details of the officials and members of the Association it provides the following information: addresses of dental schools, and names of heads of departments, notes of legislative arrangements in the various states; officials of affiliated specialist societies.

179 Dental Board of Queensland. *Register of dental specialists, Queensland.* Brisbane: the Board. Annual.

180 Dental Board of Queensland. *Register of dentists, Queensland.* Brisbane: the Board. Annual.

181 Royal Australasian College of Dental Surgeons. 'List of fellows'. In: *Annual report and membership list.* Sydney: RACDS. Annual.
Includes some 780 members, arranged by state or country of residence.

182 State of Victoria. 'Dentists' register'. Published as an issue of the *Victoria Government gazette.* Annual.

183 State of Western Australia. 'List of registered dentists'. Published as an issue of the *Government gazette.* Annual.

Canada

184 Canadian Dental Association. *Directory.* Toronto: CDA, 1982. 292 pp.

185 Ordre des Dentistes de Québec. *Annuaire dentaire: dental directory.* Montreal: Ordre des Dentistes de Québec. Annual.

Denmark

Danish Dental Association. Dental specialists are listed in each issue of *Tandlaegebladet.* (See [103]).

Finland

186 *Hammaslaakarit-tandlakare.* Helsinki: Laakinohallitus. Annual. Available from Government Printing Centre, PO Box 516, SF–00101 Helsinki 10.
The official list of registered dentists. Lists of specialists are also given.

France

187 *Annuaire dentaire.* Paris: Chabassol. Annual.
A general directory with various sections: manufacturers, products and laboratories; organizations, including government bodies, national and local societies and dental schools; name and geographic lists of dentists.

German Federal Republic

Deutsche Zahnärztekalender. (See [49])
Gives addresses of dental clinics in German-speaking countries, and details of dental organizations in the Federal Republic.

188 *Deutsches zahnärztliches Adressbuch.* 12th ed. Postfach 15 01 20, D–4600 Dortmund 15: Fachverlag Helmut Arnold, 1978. 1,154 pp.
A commercially produced general directory to the profession in West Germany. It includes names and addresses of national and local organizations, German periodicals, national and international dental associations, and dental schools throughout the world. The bulk of the book comprises a geographic list and name index of dentists in the country.
A new edition is due in 1985.

Italy

189 *Annuario dental italiano.* ptta Guastall 3, I–20122 Milan: Civa. Annual. (1st ed. published 1983).
Provides information on schools, national and international organizations, Italian journals, plus a selection of foreign ones, and trademarks, as well as lists of dentists.

Netherlands

190 *Tandartsengids.* Utrecht: Nederlands Maatschappij tot Bevordering der Tandheelkunde, 1975. 447 pp.
Membership list of the Society.

Sweden

191 *Tandlakare medlemmer i Sveriges Tandlakarforbung.* PO Box 5843, S–102 48 Stockholm: STF. Annual.
Membership list of the Association.

Switzerland

192 **Schweizerische Zahnärzte Gesellschaft.** *Mitgliederverzeichnis.* Geneva: SZG, Annual.
Membership list of the Association.

United Kingdom

193 *Dentists register.* 1878–. London: General Dental Council. Annual.
Gives an alphabetical list of dentists registered with the GDC and therefore entitled to practise in Britain, their addresses, qualifications, dates acquired and awarding university. It includes some dentists who have retired and others who may be overseas. A local list is arranged by town. Until 1983 dentists whose basic qualification was attained outside the United Kingdom were listed in separate 'Foreign' and 'Commonwealth' lists; from 1984 these were combined with the main sequence.

194 *Medical directory.* 1845–. Edinburgh: Churchill Livingstone. Annual.
An alphabetical list of registered medical practitioners, with details of private

and/or professional address, telephone number, present and previous posts. Information is given on hospitals, government departments, medical schools, societies and research institutions. Dentists who also have a medical qualification will therefore be listed with greater detail in this directory than in the *Dentists register*.

195 *Lives of the Fellows of the Royal College of Surgeons of England.* 1843–.
1843–1930 by V. G. Plarr. Bristol: John Wright, 1930. 2 vols.
1931–51 by D. A. Power and W. R. LeFanu. London: Royal College of Surgeons, 1953.
1952–64 by R.H.O.B. Robinson and W. R. LeFanu. Edinburgh: Livingstone, 1970.
1965–73 by J. P. Ross and W. R. LeFanu. London: Pitman, 1981.
Short entries provide biographical information and references to obituaries on important personalities who died during the period covered.

United States

196 American Association of Dental Schools. *Directory of dental and allied educators.* American Association of Dental Schools. Every three years.
Teachers in United States and Canadian schools are listed under school.

197 American College of Dentists. *Fellowship handbook and roster.* Bethesda, Maryland: ACD. Annual.
A list arranged by state, with a name index.

198 American Dental Association. *American dental directory.* Chicago: ADA. Annual.
Gives details of dental schools and their deans in the USA and Canada, state dental associations, US national dental organizations, national and international dental organizations of the world, specialist practitioners, and lists ADA members by state and name.

199 New York Academy of Dentistry. 'Fellowship list'. In: *Annals of dentistry.* Annual.
Appears in first issue of each year.

200 *Who's who in dentistry.* New York: Who's Who Dental Publishing, 1916; 1925.
Two small volumes containing brief biographical sketches of United States and Canadian dentists who were prominent in the profession during the period of compilation.

Trade Directories *(Chapter 3)*

The dental trade supplies clinical and laboratory materials, equipment and instruments for dentists and technicians. Literature relating to the trade mainly comprises advertising documentation produced by the firms themselves and directories of manufacturers and suppliers.

Canada

201 *Dental Guide.* 1450 Don Mills Road, Don Mills, Ontario M3B 2Y7: Southam Publications. Annual.

Issued as a supplement to the journal *Oral health* and intended for a national readership. Addresses are therefore of North American suppliers. The following lists are provided: products (equipment, drugs and suppliers) with names of manufacturers; manufacturers' names and addresses; trade names; business service organizations; Canadian dental associations.

France

Annuaire dentaire. (See [187])
The first section in the directory is devoted to the trade.

Germany

202 'Bezugsquellen-Verzeichnis'. In: *Dental echo.* Turnerstrasse 20, D-6900 Heidelberg: Helmut Haase Verlag. Monthly.

Sources of supply in Germany. A subject index of types of equipment giving the names and addresses of manufacturers or suppliers. A detailed list, occupying some thirty pages.

Italy

Annuario dental italiano. (See [189])
Includes a section on manufacturers.

203 'Aziende odontiatriche italiane'. In: *Odontostomatologia e implantoprotesi* (1983) [7]: 123–224. Milan: Odontostomatologia.

An alphabetical list of Italian manufacturers. For each company is given the address, date of establishment and details of products.

United Kingdom

204 *Dental technician yearbook and directory.* Epsom: A. E. Morgan. Annual.
The only British listing, having a product directory and an index of manufacturers and suppliers.

United States

205 **American Dental Trade Association.** *Directory.* Alexandria: ADTA. Annual.

206 *Dental dealers' directory.* PO Box 3408, Tulsa, Oklahoma 74101: Proofs Magazine. Annual.

Dentists' desk reference. (See [215])
Includes a list of manufacturers.

Research Directories *(Chapter 3)*

207 *Dental research in the United States and other countries: a catalog of dental research*

projects during fiscal year 1980 by federal and nonfederal organizations. Bethesda, Maryland: National Institutes of Health, 1982. Various paging.
Descriptive summaries of over 2,000 projects, mostly undertaken in the United States, are arranged in broad subject groups. In each entry is given the project title, investigator, institution, project number and sponsor. Three indexes list investigators, institutions and supporting agencies.

208 *European research centres: a directory of organizations in science, technology, agriculture and medicine.* 5th ed. London: Longman, 1982. 2 vols.
General arrangement is by country; there are indexes to establishments and subjects. For each organization is provided its full name and address, research activities and names of heads of appropriate departments. In the subject index dentistry is subdivided under 'clinical', 'conservative', 'endodontic', 'paediatric', 'periodontic', and 'preventive'. There is a separate entry for orthodontics.

209 *Medical research directory.* Chichester: John Wiley, 1983. 730 pp.
Titles are provided of current research projects in the United Kingdom, arranged under institution. Dentistry is section 31 of the forty-five subject sections. Details for each entry include the name of the investigator, topic, and department. Indexes cover personal names, subjects and institutions. This publication is very similar to *Research in British universities, polytechnics and colleges* [211], but has a wider institutional scope. It therefore includes the Laboratory of the Government Chemist, the Medical Research Council and the Royal College of Surgeons, which the latter does not.

210 *Medical research centres.* 6th ed. London: Longman, 1984. 2 vols.
A worldwide listing of research centres in 140 countries. Available online via Data-Star.

211 *Research in British universities, polytechnics and colleges.* Boston Spa: British Library Lending Division. Annual. 3 vols.
Volume 2 covers the biological sciences, and section G, dental sciences. Arrangement is by institution then department, and for each project includes the investigator, subject, years of operation and sponsors, if any. There are keyword and name indexes.

212 *Research programs in the medical sciences.* New York: Bowker, 1981. 578 pp.
A directory for the United States and Canada, arranged by organization.

213 *Foundation grants index.* 888 Seventh Avenue, New York, NY 10106: Foundation Center. Annual.
Lists grants of $5,000 awarded by over 450 organizations in the United States. Arrangement is by awarding institution, with subject and recipient indexes.

214 *Grants register.* London: Macmillan. Every two years.
Covers research grants, vacation awards and travel grants available mainly in the United Kingdom and Commonwealth.

General Reference Books *(Chapter 6)*

215 American Dental Association. *Dentists' desk reference.* 2nd ed. Chicago: ADA, 1983. 501 pp.

Facts, figures and practical information on materials, instruments and equipment are presented for the practising dentist.

216 Chaplin, N. W. *Health care in the UK: its organization and management.* London: Kluwer, for the Institute of Health Service Administrators, 1982. 511 pp.

217 Fédération Dentaire Internationale. *Basic fact sheets.* London: FDI, 1981. Loose-leaf, unpaged.

Contains information on dentistry in 114 countries, with particular reference to manpower, education, and surveys of oral conditions.

218 *Hospitals and health services yearbook.* 75 Portland Place, London W1N 4AN: Institute of Health Service Administrators. Annual.

219 World Health Organization. *Application of the 'International classification of diseases' to dentistry and stomatology, ICD/ DA.* 2nd ed. Geneva: WHO, 1978. 150 pp.

Brings together material scattered throughout the 9th edition of the *International classification of diseases* that is related to dentistry, and expands sections where appropriate. French and Spanish versions also available.

Conferences *(Chapter 4)*

Announcements of forthcoming events

220 'Meetings'. In: *Journal of the American Dental Association.* Chicago: American Dental Association. Twice yearly.

In issues for April and October each year. Sections cover (a) ADA constituent societies, (b) meetings inside the USA, (c) meetings outside the USA. Lists are arranged in chronological order.

221 *Zahnmed Kongress Kalender.* Gräfeling: Demeter Verlag. Annual.

The 1984 edition includes some 700 conferences, held worldwide.

Guide to published proceedings

222 *Index of conference proceedings received.* 1964–. Boston Spa: British Library Lending Division. Monthly.

Annual cumulations from 1974.

5-year cumulation 1974–78

10-year cumulation 1964–73

A cumulative *Index* 1964–81 is available on microfiche only.

Statistics *(Chapter 7)*

Bibliography

223 **Central Statistical Office.** *Guide to official statistics.* London: HMSO, 1980. 493 pp.

An invaluable guide to British official and non-official sources of statistical information published during the years 1970–80. Arrangement is in broad subject groups, but the searcher may find that a convenient approach is to check 'dental' or 'dentists' in the subject index. Most dental information is in the chapter on social statistics, but the appendices to the Dental Estimates Board report are not included. Regular and occasional published sources are described with an indication of their scope and frequency.

Books on statistical methods

224 **Chilton, N. W.** *Design and analysis in dental and oral research.* 2nd ed. New York: Praeger, 1982. 443 pp.

This comprehensive text for researchers and serious students applies basic statistics and statistical methods to dental data.

225 **Darby, M. L.** and **Bowen, D. M.** *Research methods for oral health professionals.* St. Louis: C. V. Mosby, 1980. 193 pp.

An introduction for the new postgraduate on research methods in general, but with significant coverage on statistical matters.

226 **Swinscow, T. V. D.** *Statistics at square one.* 8th ed. London: British Medical Association, 1983. 86 pp.

A very popular introduction to medical statistics, originally published as a series of papers in the *British medical journal.*

227 **Von Fraunhofer, J. A.** and **Murray, J. J.** *Statistics in medical, dental and biological studies.* 5 Tudor Cottage, Lovers Walk, London N3 1JH: Tri-med books, 1976. 120 pp.

An introduction to the subject by authors practising in the field of dentistry.

228 **Weinberg, R.** and **Cheuk, S. L.** *Introduction to dental statistics.* Park Ridge: Noyes Medical Corporation, 1980. 184 pp.

Statistical Reports and Surveys

International

Fédération Dentaire Internationale. *Basic fact sheets.* (See [217])

Figures on manpower, dental education, specialists, and public and private practice are given for 114 countries in a standard format. Appendices tabulate manpower statistics and the world fluoridation status.

Australia

229 **Australian Dental Association.** *Facts and figures: Australian dentistry.* Sydney: the Association. Annual.
A report comprising tables on the following subjects: total population, indices of economy, registered dentists, Dental Board registrations, dental schools, auxiliary personnel, private dental practice, fees, government dental services, dental benefit organizations.

Japan

230 **Japan Dental Association.** *Handbook of statistical data on dental health, 1983.* Tokyo: JDA, 1983. 61 pp.
Statistical tables, with information from mostly government sources, are provided thus: oral health conditions, dental clinics, dentists, insurance, salaries.

United Kingdom

231 **Dental Estimates Board.** *Annual report. Appendices.* Eastbourne: the Board. Annual. Typescript.
The report itself is confidential and therefore not available to the reader, but certain appendices are distributed for general use. These give figures relating to the number of patients treated under the National Health Service in England and Wales, and the type and cost of that treatment. Figures for private treatment are not available. This document is the most detailed source for statistics on British dental treatment. Five tables cover the distribution of dentists in the General Dental Service, and fifteen cover dental treatment in the GDS, derived from a 5 percent sample. Figures cover the incidence and cost of various items, such as amalgam restorations, orthodontic treatment, partial dentures, etc., with breakdowns by age group, type of estimate, region. Other tables indicate the number of estimates according to cost and patients' contributions, and according to type of estimate. Figures for any one year are published approximately twelve months later.

Department of Health and Social Security. *Dental manpower: report of the Departmental Study Group.* (See [584])
Includes figures for supply and demand projections for the next twenty years. A substantial part of the document comprises the British Dental Association report *Manpower requirements to the year 2020.*

232 *Health and personal social services statistics for England.* London: HMSO. Annual.
Prepared by the Government Statistical Service. Tables related to dental staff include analyses of hospital dental staff by grade and sex, grade and age, grade and speciality; of general dental practitioners by age and sex and by regional health authority; of the community dental service by grade and sex, and by grade and number of patients inspected. Information on the number and cost of courses of treatment is taken from the Dental Estimates Board report.

233 **Office of Population, Censuses and Surveys.** 'Children's dental health, 1983'. In: *OPCS monitor*, SS83/2. 11 pp.
The *OPCS monitor* is published regularly but does not normally contain much of

dental interest. This issue publishes the preliminary results of a survey conducted by the OPCS Social Survey Division which is a successor to a previous investigation conducted in 1973; the detailed results are published as **Todd, J. E.** and **Dodd, P.** *Child dental health in the United Kingdom.* London: HMSO, 1985.

Todd, J. E., Walker, A. M. and **Dodd, P.** *Adult dental health, 1978.* (See [645])
This important survey gives figures on caries, periodontal disease and denture provision in England, Scotland and Wales. See the annotation in the 'Public health dentistry' section for further details.

234 Review Body on Doctors' and Dentists' Remuneration. *Reports.* London: HMSO. Annual.
The present Review Body was established in 1971 to advise the prime minister on remuneration to NHS medical and dental staff, but its recommendations are not binding and may not be acted upon. Nevertheless they provide the basis for governmental policy decisions. From the purely statistical point of view, they contain useful tables on recommended and current salary scales, and hours on duty.

235 Scottish Dental Estimates Board. *Report.* Edinburgh: SDEB. Annual.
Tables are similar in scope and content to those for England and Wales.

United States

236 American Dental Association. *Distribution of dentists in the U.S. by state, region, district and county.* Chicago: ADA, 1979. 66 pp.
Tables relate to the numbers of active and inactive dentists, dentist–patient population rate, and give information on household buying income.

American Dental Association. *Survey of dental practice.* (See [581])
The ADA's Bureau of Economic and Behavioral Research conducts this survey regularly from a sample of practitioners. Tables differentiate between 'solo dentists' and 'independent dentists'.

237 National Institute of Dental Research. *Prevalence of dental caries in US children 1979–80: the national caries prevalence survey.* Bethesda, Maryland: National Institute of Dental Research, 1981. 159 pp.
A highly detailed survey, with a greater sample population than previous investigations have had. A sample of 40,000 was evaluated, out of a total population of 48 million, the age range being 5–17 years. Figures are given by region. Although caries surveys had been carried out in 1965 and 1971, the results are not directly comparable because of the size of the population studied and the breakdown by age and social status.

238 *Vital and health statistics.* Data from the National Health Survey, Series 11. 3700 East West Highway, Hyattsville, Maryland 20782: National Center for Health Statistics. Irregular.
Dental reports are issued at irregular intervals. The following are typical examples:

Oral hygiene among youths 12–17 years. 1975.
Prosthodontic care: number and types of denture wearers. 1976.
Assessment of the occlusion of the teeth of youths 12–17 years. 1977.
Diet and dental health. 1982.

Standards *(Chapter 7)*

239 **American Dental Association.** *Specifications.* In: *Guide to dental materials and devices, 1974–75.* 7th ed. Chicago: ADA. 1974.

240 **British Standards Institution.** *Yearbook.* Milton Keynes: BSI. Annual.
Lists standards in numerical order, with a subject index.

241 **United States. National Bureau of Standards.** *Bibliography of publications by the dental medical materials section.* Washington, DC: USNBS, 1979. 51 pp.

242 **United States. National Bureau of Standards.** *Organizations engaged in preparing standards for dental materials and therapeutic agents with a list of standards.* Washington, DC: US Government Printing Office, 1980. 51 pp.

Miscellaneous Sources *(Chapter 7)*

243 *Catalogue of British official publications not published by HMSO.* 1980–. Cambridge: Chadwyck-Healey. Bimonthly. Annual cumulations.
Includes subject, name and author indexes.

244 *Keyword index to British official publications not published by HMSO.* 1984–. Cambridge: Chadwyck-Healey. Bimonthly. Microfiche only.

245 **National Institute of Dental Research.** *Selected list of technical reports in dentistry.* Bethesda, Maryland: National Institute of Dental Research. Annual.
Dental reports received by the National Technical Information Service are listed by NTIS accession number. Entries give the author, title, institution and date. An appendix gives a KWIC index.

Audiovisual Materials: Listings *(Chapter 7)*

246A **BLAT Centre for Health and Medical Education.** *Audiovisual teaching/learning materials for practising dentists or those studying at postgraduate level.* BMA House, Tavistock Square, London WC1H 9JP: BLAT, [1980].
A typescript list of films, tapes, slides and videos.

246B **BLAT/BMA.** *Medical films: selected for their educational value.* London: BLAT/BMA. Irregular.
An annotated subject list of films.

British medicine. (See [24])
Each monthly issue has a subject section for audiovisual materials.

247 British Universities Film and Video Council. *Catalogue.* 55 Greek Street, London W1V 5LR: the Council. Annual.
A microfiche list arranged by subject.

248 Graves Medical Audiovisual Library. *Catalogue of tape and slide programmes.* Chelmsford: Graves Medical Audiovisual Library. Irregular.
A subject list, predominantly of tape–slide programmes.

249 *National Library of Medicine audiovisuals catalog.* 1978–. Bethesda, Maryland: NLM. Quarterly.
The subject sequence is arranged by MESH headings; the file is available online as AVLINE. There are annual cumulations.

250 Oxford Educational Resources. *Title list.* Oxford: OER. Irregular.

Audiovisual Material on Dentistry: British Suppliers

251 **British Dental Health Foundation** (address given in Part III). Slide sets for lay audiences, for dental health education and preventive dentistry.

252 **Camera Talks Ltd**, 31 North Row, London W1R 2EN. Tel. 01–493 2761. Audiovisual course of twenty-three tape–slide programmes to cover the DSAs examination.

253 **CIBA Laboratories**, Horsham, West Sussex RH12 4AB. Collection of medical illustrations includes a set of twenty-nine slides on anatomy of mouth and pharynx, and a set of thirty-nine slides on diseases of the mouth and pharynx. For purchase. Not available for loan.

254 **General Dental Council** (address given in Part III). Slides for lay audiences on oral health, for loan free of charge. Film *Dentistry today* to promote recruitment into the profession and create a wider understanding of the work of dental staff. Available for loan from Central Film Library, Chalfont Grove, Gerrards Cross, Bucks. SL9 8TN.

255 **Gibbs' Oral Hygiene Service** (address given in Part III). Films, videos, pamphlets and slide sets for lay audiences. For hire or purchase.

256 **Graves Medical Audiovisual Library.** Holly House, 220 New London Road, Chelmsford, Essex CM2 9BJ. Tel. (0245) 83351. Tape–slide programmes for dental students and practitioners. For loan or hire.

257 **Health Education Council.** A selection of films and videos on oral health for lay audiences. Loan of films and videos free of charge. Concord Films Council Ltd, 201 Felixstowe Road, Ipswich IP3 9BJ. Tel. (0473) 7612, or Central Film Library, Chalfont Grove, Gerrards Cross, Bucks. SL9 8TN. Sales: Supplies Dept. HEC, 78 New Oxford Street, London WC1A 1AH. Tel. 01–637 1881.

258 Oxford Educational Resources, Botley Road, Oxford OX2 0HE. Tel. (0865) 726625. The largest selection of videos on dentistry, for sale and hire. Programmes are mainly on prosthetics, and are for dentists, students and ancillaries.

Anaesthesia

Dental treatment today is virtually painless, thanks to the developments in anaesthesia and analgesia. Broadly speaking, the major categories are general anaesthesia, local analgesia and conscious sedation, the latter also being called relative analgesia. In the first case the patient is rendered unconscious, while in the latter a sufficient degree of anaesthetic is given so that the patient is relaxed and can tolerate operative procedures, but is still conscious and can hear and respond to questions.

Local anaesthetics are administered by injection, general anaesthesia and relative analgesia induced by inhalation. Intravenous injections may also be used for general anaesthesia.

Current-awareness Lists

259 'Anaesthetic literature'. In: *Anaesthesia.* Monthly.
A subject list compiled from *Current contents life sciences* which includes journal papers, books, and chapters of books of interest to anaesthetists in general. There is a delay of some six to eight months between appearance in *Current contents* and in 'Anaesthetic literature'. The listing is extensive, occupying some eleven pages of the journal.

Books

260 Allen, G. D. *Dental anesthesia and analgesia.* 3rd ed. Baltimore: Williams & Wilkins, 1984. 432 pp.
A standard American text for the clinician, with thorough coverage of techniques used in the United States and Britain.

261 Bennett, C. R. *Conscious sedation in dental practice.* 2nd ed. St. Louis: C. V. Mosby, 1978. 205 pp.
Covers the indications and procedures for relative analgesia.

262 Coplans, M. P. and **Green, R. A.** *Anaesthesia and sedation in dentistry.* Amsterdam: Elsevier, 1983. 421 pp. (Monographs in Anaesthesiology vol. 12.)
This is not a textbook describing standard procedures and techniques, but a discussion of topics of current interest, not all of which are clinical problems. Section I, on basic concepts, is particularly useful for its coverage of aspects rarely treated at length in textbooks, such as training, morbidity and mortality studies, and medico-legal considerations. Sections II and III are on local analgesia, sedation and general anaesthesia.

263 Drummond-Jackson, S. L. *Dental sedation and anaesthesia.* 6th ed. by P. Sykes. London: Society for the Advancement of Anaesthesia in Dentistry, 1979. 393 pp.
The standard British book on intravenous anaesthesia, for reference use and for practical information.

264 Evers, H. and **Haegerstam, G.** *Handbook of dental local anaesthesia.* London: Schulz, 1981. 201 pp.
Almost coming into the category of colour atlas, this profusely illustrated book has comparatively little text, but comprises mainly excellent diagrams and photographs, which deal with anatomical and operative aspects of local anaesthesia.

It is intended for the student and general practitioner. Originally published in Swedish by Schulz; the German edition is published by Springer, the French by MEDSI, and the Italian by Verduci.

265 Jastak, J. T. and **Yagiela, J. A.** *Regional anesthesia of the oral cavity.* St. Louis: C. V. Mosby, 1981. 212 pp.
A well-illustrated text on local anaesthesia for the practitioner.

266 Jorgensen, N. B. and **Hayden, J.** *Premedication, local and general anaesthesia in dentistry.* 3rd ed. Philadelphia: Lea & Febiger, 1980. 299 pp.
Jorgensen's original technique of intravenous anaesthesia is used less frequently today, but the book incorporates modern American practice, with the emphasis on local analgesia.

267 Kaufman, L., Sowray, J. H. and **Rood, J. P.** *General anaesthesia, local analgesia and sedation in dentistry.* Oxford: Blackwell, 1982. 170 pp.
A concise, practical text for the student and general practitioner, well-illustrated with line drawings. There are no references.

268 Langa, H. *Relative analgesia in dental practice: inhalation analgesia and sedation with nitrous oxide.* 2nd ed. Philadelphia: W. B. Saunders, 1976. 419 pp.
This is recognized as the standard text on conscious sedation.

269 Roberts, D. H. and **Sowray, J. H.** *Local analgesia in dentistry.* 2nd ed. Bristol: John Wright, 1979. 155 pp.
A helpful description of techniques for the general practitioner.

270 Smith, W. D. A. *Under the influence: a history of nitrous oxide and oxygen anaesthesia.* London: Macmillan, 1982. 188 pp.
A lavishly illustrated, detailed text. It is compiled from papers originally published in the *British journal of anaesthesia* and other journals, over a fifteen-year period, the collection containing a great deal of unique material.

Journals

271 *Anesthesia progress.* 1954–. Chicago: American Dental Society of Anesthesiology. Bimonthly.

Includes original reports, news, advertisements, book reviews and abstracts from other journals.

272 *Dental anaesthesia and sedation.* 1972–. Sydney: Australian Society for the Advancement of Anaesthesia and Sedation in Dentistry. 3 issues per year.
Publishes clinical papers, news, reviews of recent literature and trade advertisements.

273 *Giornale di anestesia stomatologica.* 1973–. Milan: Masson. Quarterly.
Official organ of the Associazione Italiana per il Progresso del Anestesia in Odontostomatologia. Included are original research reports and translations, practical papers, news and reviews.

274 *SAAD digest.* 1970–. London: Society for the Advancement of Anaesthesia in Dentistry. Quarterly.
One or two original papers per issue are included, plus case reports, correspondence and news items.

General Anaesthesia Journals

Anaesthesia
Anesthesiology
British journal of anaesthesia

Directories

275 *Handbook of British anaesthesia.* Basingstoke: Macmillan. Annual. Issued as a supplement to *British journal of anaesthesia.*
Contents include names and addresses of British and international bodies, specialist societies, regional and local societies, university departments, plus information on manufacturers and their anaesthetic products.

Anatomy, Growth, Histology

These subjects are studied at an elementary level for the undergraduate curriculum, and again for general postgraduate degrees such as the Fellowship in Dental Surgery. Fundamental research at an advanced level continues to be published. Maxillofacial growth has traditionally been studied in relation to orthodontic treatment, and only recently have texts devoted to growth in a wider context been produced.

Although part of the biological sciences, anatomy and growth are treated separately here, because of the number of items to be listed.

Books

276 **Berkovitz, B. K. B., Holland, G. R.** and **Moxham, B. J.** *Colour atlas and textbook of oral anatomy*. London: Wolfe, 1978. 247 pp.
An advanced-level atlas, with macro- and microscopic illustrations of the teeth and oral soft tissues. Of particular interest is the section on comparative anatomy.

277 **Broadbent, B. H. Sr., Broadbent, B. H. Jr.** and **Golden, W. H.** *Bolton standards of dentofacial developmental growth*. St. Louis: C. V. Mosby, 1975. 166 pp. Includes 36 transparencies.
This is an important set of standards of cephalometric normality, developed from a series of averages of individual cases which had optimum facial and dental growth. Measurements from representative male and female Caucasian faces were taken from a database of over 5,000 children, and synthesized to present a norm. The resulting standards can be used for clinical purposes, for diagnostic assessment in oral or maxillofacial surgery or orthodontics; for research, as a baseline for the study of abnormalities; or for education, to demonstrate normal and abnormal growth.
The study is named after Frances Bolton, whose interest in maxillofacial growth was aroused in 1926, and confirmed when her son had orthodontic treatment two years later. The Bolton family has supported this ongoing study since 1929.

278 **Brothwell, D. R.** *Dental anthropology*. Oxford: Pergamon, 1963. 288 pp.
A useful work on the oral structures of primates and primitive man.

279 **Enlow, D. H.** *Handbook of facial growth*. 2nd ed. Philadelphia: W. B. Saunders, 1982. 486 pp.
A standard undergraduate and postgraduate text, with an extensive bibliography.

280 **Goose, D. H.** and **Appleton, J.** *Human dentofacial growth*. Oxford: Pergamon, 1982. 228 pp.
A very detailed book for its size, useful for students.

281 **McMinn, R. M. H., Hutchings, R. T.** and **Logan, B. M.** *Colour atlas of head and neck anatomy*. London: Wolfe, 1981. 240 pp.
Intended to supplement dissection manuals and textbooks, this excellent presentation of the bones and muscles of the face is justifiably popular with students, especially candidates for higher examinations. It is a companion work to Berkovitz, but is the more sought-after of the two.

282 **Orban, B. J.** *Oral histology and embryology*. 9th ed. by S. N. Bhaskar. St. Louis: C. V. Mosby, 1980. 482 pp.
A standard text for undergraduates and for general reference, with comprehensive coverage.

283 Osborn, J. W. and **Ten Cate, A. R.** *Advanced dental histology*. 4th ed. Bristol: John Wright, 1983. 209 pp. (Dental Practitioner Handbooks no. 6)
A useful, detailed book for postgraduate students and practitioners.

284 Peyer, B. *Comparative odontology*. Chicago: University of Chicago, 1968. 347 pp.
The standard work in the field, which currently lacks new texts.

285 Ranly, D. M. *Synopsis of craniofacial growth*. New York: Appleton Century Crofts, 1980. 188 pp.
A concise American introduction

286 Scott, J. H and **Symons, N. B. B.** *Introduction to dental anatomy*. 9th ed. Edinburgh: Churchill Livingstone, 1982. 419 pp.
A traditional student text popular in Britain, with a clear account of the growth and development of the facial bones, periodontium and teeth. The contents are arranged thus: form and arrangement of teeth; development of the face, teeth and jaws; development and histology of dental and oral tissues; functional anatomy; comparative anatomy.

287 Sicher, H. *Oral anatomy*. 7th ed. by E. L. Dubrul. St. Louis: C. V. Mosby, 1980. 572 pp.
A well-established American text, with detailed coverage of the field and its ramifications. The book is divided into two parts. First descriptive and functional anatomy are described, that is, the skull, muscles, temporomandibular joint, viscera, oropharyngeal system, blood vessels, lymphatic system and nerves. The second part, regional and applied anatomy, covers a variety of topics: the structure and relations of the alveolar process, anatomy of local anaesthesia, arterial haemorrhages, the propagation of dental infection, tracheostomy, temporomandibular joint articulation, and the edentulous mouth.

288 University of Michigan. Center for Human Growth and Development. Craniofacial Growth Series. Ann Arbor: the Center, 1972–.
A series of monographs with one or two additions per year, written at research level. Titles include the following:

5. **Moyers, R. E.** *Standards of human occlusal development*. 1976.
6. **McNamara, J. A.** *Factors affecting the growth of the midface*. 1976.
7. **McNamara, J. A.** *Biology of occlusal development*. 1977.
10. **Carlson, D. S.** *Craniofacial biology*. 1981.
14. **McNamara, J. A.** *Clinical alteration of the growing face*. 1983.

289 Van Beek, G. C. *Dental morphology: an illustrated guide*. 2nd ed. Bristol: John Wright, 1983. 135 pp.
A useful revision aid, with brief notes accompanying clear line drawings. The first edition was in the name of G. C. Downer; the author is now naturalized Dutch, hence the name change.

290 Wheeler, R. C. *Pulp cavities of the permanent teeth: an anatomical guide to manipulative endodontics*. Philadelphia: W. B. Saunders, 1976. 211 pp.
A well-illustrated production showing the various forms of the individual teeth, with special reference to root canal therapy, but of wider interest too.

Journals

Acta anatomica
American journal of anatomy
Anatomical record
Archives of oral biology [306]
Journal of anatomy

Biological Sciences in General

Bibliographies and Reviews

For anatomy, see the previous section.

291 *Advances in oral biology*. New York: Academic Press, **1–4** (1964–70).
Four volumes containing state-of-the-art reviews.

292 Catron, A. R. and **Evans, F. G.** *Bibliography on the mechanical and physical properties of teeth*. Ann Arbor: University of Michigan, 1970. 26 pp.
Some 341 references are given covering a period from before 1900 up to 1970, and are arranged by author. Most are in English, but some German and Japanese papers are included. Abstracts and chapters from books are listed.

293 'Current papers in oral biology'. In: *Archives of oral biology*. Monthly.
Some ninety papers are listed in each issue under broad headings such as anatomy, biochemistry and fluorides. Most references are from non-dental journals, and for each one is given the title, author, source and author's address. The time-lag before listing is six to nine months.

Books

294 Adams, D. *Essentials of oral biology*. Edinburgh: Churchill Livingstone, 1981. 132 pp.
A description of physiology and biochemistry for the undergraduate.

295 Cohen, B. and **Kramer, I. R. H.** *Scientific foundations of dentistry*. London: Heinemann, 1976. 688 pp.
A comprehensive work on biology and pathology, containing contributions from eminent specialists, which is mandatory reading for Fellowship in Dental Surgery candidates, and an important general reference text. Chapters cover growth and development, cell structure and function, immunology, microbiology, oncology,

pain and anaesthesia, calcified tissues, periodontal tissues, oral mucosa, salivary glands, bone, masticatory muscles and the temporomandibular joint.

296 *Frontiers of oral physiology.* Basle: Karger, 1974–. Irregular.
A series of monographs for the advanced worker. Titles include the following:
1. Kawamura, Y. *Physiology of mastication.* 1974.
2. Kawamura, Y. *Physiology of oral tissues.* 1976.
3. Ferguson, D. B. *The environment of the teeth.* 1981.
4. Kawamura, Y. *Oral sensory mechanisms.* 1983.

297 Jenkins, G. N. *Physiology of the mouth.* 4th ed. Oxford: Blackwell, 1978. 599 pp.
A standard undergraduate presentation, also useful for general reference.

298 Lavelle, C. L. *Applied physiology of the mouth.* Bristol: John Wright, 1975. 368 pp.
Highlights the aspects of oral physiology that have direct clinical application, which are as follows: metabolism, calcification, bone growth, tooth eruption, plaque, salivary glands, mastication, deglutition, dietary deficiencies, hormone imbalance, blood supply, pain, age changes, wound healing, taste and smell. An invaluable source for undergraduate and advanced students.

299 Miles, A. E. W. *Structural and chemical organization of the teeth.* London: Academic Press, 1967. 2 vols.
The classic work in the field, and a standard reference or bench book for the research worker, with contributions from fourteen eminent authorities in the field. Volume 1 covers the general organization of the teeth and structural organization during development. Volume 2 covers definitive structural organization, physical and chemical organization and organization of the supporting tissues. There are extensive reference lists.

300 'Monographs in Oral Science'. Basle: Karger, 1972–.
A series which includes scholarly reviews, state-of-the-art reports and research papers at an advanced level. Twelve titles had been published up to 1983, of which the following are particularly important:
2. Shannon, I. L. *Saliva: composition and secretion.* 1974.
5. Goodson, J. M. *Analysis of human mandibular movement.* 1975.
7. Myers, H. M. *Fluorides and dental fluorosis.* 1978.
8. Baum, C. L. *The biology of pulp and dentine.* 1980.
12. Cimasoni, L. *The crevicular fluid updated.* 1983.

301 Rowe, A. H. and **Johns, R. B.** *Companion to dental studies.* Oxford: Blackwell, 1982–. 3 vols. in 4 books.
An integrated text of basic and clinical science, for undergraduate and advanced students. Composition of the series is as follows: Volume 1 book 1: Anatomy, biochemistry and physiology; Volume 1 book 2: Dental anatomy and embryology; Volume 2: Clinical methods; Volume 3: Clinical dentistry.

302 Schroeder, H. E. *Orale Strukturbiologie. Entwicklungsgeschichte, Struktur und Funktion normaler Hart- und Weichgewebe der Mundhohle.* 2nd ed. Stuttgart: Thieme, 1982. 368 pp.

303 Shaw, J. H., Sweeney, E. A., Cappuccino, C. C. and **Meller, S. M.** *Textbook of oral biology.* Philadelphia: W. B. Saunders, 1978. 1,178 pp.
An American book with similar scope to that of Cohen and Kramer.

304 Veis, A. *The chemistry and biology of mineralized connective tissues.* Amsterdam: Elsevier, 1982. 680 pp. (Developments in Biochemistry Vol. 22.)
The proceedings of a conference held at Northwestern University Dental School, with an interdisciplinary approach.

305 Williams, R. A. D. and **Elliott, J. C.** *Basic and applied dental biochemistry.* Edinburgh: Churchill Livingstone, 1979. 311 pp.
Approximately half the book is devoted to biochemistry in general, the rest more specifically with the oral cavity.

Journals

306 *Archives of oral biology.* 1959–. Oxford: Pergamon. Monthly.
A prestigious research journal, publishing original reports and short communications on every aspect of oral and dental tissue and bone in vertebrates. These include anatomy, palaeontology, chemistry, physics, pathology, physiology, immunology, bacteriology, epidemiology and genetics. This journal is very highly regarded, and attracts contributions from researchers throughout the world.

307 *Calcified tissue international.* 1967–. New York: Springer. Bimonthly.
This journal covers all aspects of hard tissue research. The present title was assumed in 1979, reflecting the broader readership and source of papers; formerly it was called *Calcified tissue research.*

308 *Journal de biologie buccale.* 1973–. Paris: Société d'Edition de l'Information Dentaire. Quarterly.
Publishes research-level papers on oral biology, mostly in French, but with some in English. Abstracts for all articles are given in English, French and German.

Other Journals

American journal of physical anthropology
Human biology
Journal of biological chemistry
Journal of applied biology

Caries

Tooth decay, caries, is a disease that is known to everyone, and is particularly common in the Western world. It can be studied from various points of view, such as its epidemiology or occurrence, prevention or treatment; dental professionals in all spheres therefore will have an interest in some aspect of the carious process or the affected tooth. Hence relevant material is scattered throughout various sections of this book. For example, surveys on caries prevalence are listed under 'Public health dentistry', while treatment of caries will be discussed under 'Conservative dentistry'. Preventive dentistry is also highly significant.

Bibliographies

309 Bagnall, J. S. *Bibliography on caries research.* Ottawa: National Research Council of Canada, 1950. 557 pp.

Contains brief descriptions of 2,300 English-language items, from the late nineteenth century onwards. Arrangement is under fifteen main headings, with numerous subdivisions, summaries of papers being given in the appropriate section. A bibliography of items described in the main body of the book follows the subject section.

310 Brislin, J. F. and **Cox, G. J.** *Survey of the literature of dental caries; 1948–1960.* Pittsburgh: University of Pittsburgh Press, 1964. 762 pp.

Updates the bibliography by Toverud, and includes over 3,700 abstracts arranged in chronological order. There are author and subject indexes.

311 Toverud, G. and others. *Survey of the literature of dental caries.* Washington, DC: National Academy of Sciences, 1952. 566 pp.

A review of the various aspects of the subject, providing abstracts of papers and critical summaries, followed by a bibliography of cited items, arranged by author.

Books

312 Bibby, B. G. and **Shern, R. J.** *Methods of caries prediction.* London: Information Retrieval, 1978. 326 pp.

A special supplement to *Microbiology abstracts.* A research-level monograph.

313 Lehner, T. *The borderland between caries and periodontal disease.* Vol. I. London: Academic Press, 1977. 288 pp.

Lehner, T. and **Cimasoni, G.** *The borderland between caries and periodontal disease.* Vol. II. London: Academic Press, 1980. 253 pp.

The reports of two important seminars bringing an interdisciplinary approach to the study of oral diseases. They are of interest to the clinician and research worker.

314 Menaker, L. *Biologic basis of dental caries.* Hagerstown: Harper & Row, 1980. 532 pp.

A detailed discussion of all aspects of the carious process, for advanced students and researchers. There are five sections as follows: 'the host' deals with saliva, the salivary glands and tooth composition; 'the disease' with aetiology and epidemiological factors, histopathology and clinical aspects. 'The agents' covers microbial interaction, and 'the environment' deals with caries prevention. 'Research' is the final section.

315 Newbrun, E. *Cariology.* 2nd ed. Baltimore: Williams & Wilkins, 1983. 344 pp.
A comprehensive textbook for students and practitioners. Chapters cover the following topics: historical aspects, aetiology, microflora, diet, sugar and sweeteners, plaque, histopathology, caries activity tests, dentifrices, sealants, prevention and control. There are extensive bibliographies.

316 Schamschula, R. G., Adkins, B. L., Barmes, D. E., Charlton, G. and **Davey, B. G.** *World Health Organization study of dental caries etiology in Papua New Guinea.* Geneva: WHO, 1978. 199 pp.
A key study of a primitive population, of interest to epidemiologists, community dentists and researchers.

317 Silverstone, L. M., Johnson, N. W., Hardie, J. M. and **Williams, R. A. D.** *Dental caries.* London: Macmillan, 1981. 315 pp.
A basic textbook covering aetiology, control and prevention for students and practitioners. One of the most authoritative and helpful texts in the field.

318 Stiles, H. M., Loesch, W. J. and **O'Brien, T. C.** *Microbiological aspects of dental caries.* Washington, DC: Information Retrieval, 1976. 3 vols.
A *Microbiology abstracts* supplement. The proceedings of a workshop attended by dental and medical microbiologists and researchers. The publication is of value to specialists and advanced students in medical and oral microbiology.

319 Tanzer, J. M. *Animal models in cariology.* Washington, DC: Information Retrieval, 1981. 458 pp.
A special supplement to *Microbiology abstracts*, this is the report of a symposium, and of interest to research workers.

320 'Vipeholm dental caries study'. In: *Acta odontologica scandinavica* **11** (1954): 195–388.
The Vipeholm study is a classic research project undertaken in Sweden, which demonstrated conclusively the relationship between diet and dental caries. This was also produced as a separate publication by the journal.

Journals

321 *Caries research.* 1967–. Basle: Karger. Bimonthly.
The official journal of the European Organization for Caries Research (ORCA), and a prestigious research-orientated journal. Supplements have been published as follows:

8 (1974): suppl. 1. *Reports of ORCA on water fluoridation.*
11 (1977): suppl. 1. *Cariostatic mechanisms of fluorides.*

12 (1978): suppl. 1. *Progress in caries prevention.*
17 (1983): suppl. 1. *Monofluorophosphate perspectives.*

Conferences

Proceedings of some of the European Organization for Caries Research congresses, held annually, have been published in various formats, for instance:
9th–12th conferences. *Advances in fluorine research and dental caries prevention* **1–4**. Oxford: Pergamon, 1963–66.
Abstracts of papers:
1976–80 congresses in: *Caries research*
1981 congress in: *Zahn- Mund- und Kieferheilkunde* **69** (1982): 725–49. (Published in English.)
1982 congress in: *Caries research* **17** (1983): 156–92.
1983 congress in: *Caries research* **18** (1984): 153–92.
1984 congress in: *Caries research* **19** (1985): 153–92.

Directories

322 ORCA membership list. In: *Caries research* **12** (1978): 339–52.

Conservative Dentistry

Conservative dentistry is concerned with the preservation of teeth, and the restoration of damaged or diseased parts. Included in the scope of this definition are the removal of carious tooth tissue and the placement of fillings (operative dentistry), and the provision of crowns and bridges (fixed prosthodontics). Endodontics, the study and treatment of diseases affecting the dental pulp, is regarded as part of the speciality.

The term 'restorative dentistry' is often used as a synonym, but has, strictly speaking, a wider context in that it includes dental care for patients with all or some of their natural teeth. It therefore includes, in addition, periodontal and prosthetic aspects, so that the sections on periodontology and prosthetic dentistry will include relevant material. In the former, Schluger, Yuodelis and Page's *Periodontal disease* [561] is a particularly useful text discussing periodontal–restorative aspects, while the *International journal of periodontics and restorative dentistry* [563] will be found to contain relevant case reports.

Bridgework cannot be studied in total without reference to the prosthetic literature as a whole, and a useful source here is the *Glossary of prosthodontic terms* [630].

Occlusion, discussed separately, is of particular relevance to conservative dentistry, for example in relation to the accurate shape of crowns and bridges. The books by Dawson [417], Ramfjord and Ash [423] and Gross [419] are highly recommended.

Reviews

323 'Report of the Committee on Scientific Investigation of the American

Academy of Restorative Dentistry'. An annual review published in the *Journal of prosthetic dentistry* of published papers on all aspects of the field, comprising a narrative section and bibliography of some 250 references. Recent reviews are:
Journal of prosthetic dentistry
43 (1980): 663–86.
45 (1981): 643–89.
47 (1982): 654–80.
50 (1983): 411–36.
51 (1984): 823–46.

Bibliographies

324 *Endodontic references*
This is a listing, arranged by author, of endodontic papers published worldwide, and appears in each issue of the *International endodontic journal*. There is a time-lag of six to nine months between publication of the original paper and its listing, but this delay compares favourably with the *Index to dental literature* for papers published outside the United States.

Textbooks

325 Black, G. V. *Operative dentistry*. 9th ed. Chicago: Medical Dental Publishing Co., 1955. 2 vols.
This classic work on conservative dentistry was first published in 1908, expounding many principles that are still valid today.

326 Cohen, S. and **Burns, R. C.** *Pathways of the pulp*. 3rd ed. St. Louis: C. V. Mosby, 1984. 880 pp.
A comprehensive endodontic text edited by two eminent authorities from the United States. As well as providing standard clinical and technical information there is a useful historical section, and self-assessment quizzes at the end of each chapter.

327 Eccles, J. D. and **Green, R. M.** *The conservation of teeth*. 2nd ed. Oxford: Blackwell, 1983. 254 pp.
A basic undergraduate book, discussing cavity preparation and filling techniques in a clear, easy to read manner.

328 Gerstein, H. *Techniques in clinical endodontics*. Philadelphia: W. B. Saunders, 1983. 394 pp.
This is not a standard textbook, in that it excludes basic science, diagnosis and interdisciplinary relationships. It is devoted to clinical techniques, and is therefore useful for the practising general dentist or specialist.

329 Gilmore, H. W., Lund, M. R. and **Bales, D. J.** *Operative dentistry*. 4th ed. St. Louis: C. V. Mosby, 1982. 379 pp.
An excellent general text for the student and clinician, with wider scope than Eccles or Pickard. Chapters cover cavity preparation, instruments, pulp protec-

tion, and the different kinds of restorations: amalgam, pins, tooth-coloured, cast gold and porcelain.

330 Grossman, L. I. *Endodontic practice.* 10th ed. Philadelphia: Lea & Febiger, 1981. 458 pp.
The classic American book on root canal treatment, first published in 1940 and updated regularly. Unlike many textbooks from the United States it is not filled with superfluous illustrations or excessive description, but has a concise style more akin to the British manner. A minor criticism is that the bibliographies do not include titles of papers cited. Translations of various editions of this important book have been made into Chinese, German, Italian, Japanese, Portuguese and Spanish.

331 Grundy, J. R. *Colour atlas of conservative dentistry.* London: Wolfe, 1980. 152 pp.
An adjunct to standard textbooks illustrating various clinical procedures, but not comprehensive in its coverage.
A French edition has been published by Maloine, and a German edition by Hanser.

332 Harty, F. J. *Endodontics in clinical practice.* 2nd ed. Bristol: John Wright, 1982. 280 pp. (Dental Practitioner Handbook no. 24.)
An invaluable aid for students and practitioners, with a wealth of information succinctly presented. A standard British text.

333 Hess, J. C. *Enseignement d'odontologie conservatrice.* Paris: Maloine, 1983-. 7 vols.
Two volumes are devoted to methods of conservative dentistry in general, the other five to endodontics.

334 McLean, J. W. *Science and art of dental ceramics.* Chicago: Quintessence, 1979–80. 2 vols.
Originally intended for advanced students and researchers, this is also a popular work among clinicians. It is an expansion and update of lectures first published by Louisiana University in 1974. Volume one provides technical information on porcelain, including physical and chemical properties, strengthening and aesthetic aspects. Volume two describes the design and construction of bridges.
German, Italian and Japanese editions are available, all published by Quintessence.

334A Nicholls, E. *Endodontics.* 3rd ed. Bristol: John Wright, 1984. 385 pp.
A popular textbook with students and clinicians, it contains a wealth of information and has good coverage of recent research and developments.

335 Pickard, H. M. *A manual of operative dentistry.* 5th ed. Oxford: Oxford University Press, 1983. 277 pp.
A popular undergraduate text providing a useful introduction to supplement more detailed works.

336 Roberts, D. H. *Fixed bridge prosthesis.* 2nd ed. Bristol: John Wright, 1980. 289 pp.
Describes the basic principles of bridge design for clinicians. Laboratory procedures are generally excluded, except where they are of direct concern to the dentist.

337 Shillingburg, H. T., Hobo, S. and **Whitsett, L. D.** *Fundamentals of fixed prosthodontics.* 2nd ed. Chicago: Quintessence, 1981. 454 pp.
A work originally intended for undergraduates and practitioners, this is widely used also by advanced students. It is a highly practical text; each chapter sets out an armamentarium of equipment or instruments needed for the procedure to be described. Topics covered include mechanical principles and techniques, preparations for veneer crowns, intracoronal cast restorations and extensively damaged teeth. Laboratory procedures are described with the importance of occlusion being stressed throughout. There are no photographs, but excellent line drawings and diagrams. Useful bibliographical references are provided. Quintessence have published editions in French, German, Italian, Japanese, Portuguese and Spanish.

338 Shillingburg, H. T. and **Kessler, J. C.** *Restoration of the endodontically treated tooth.* Chicago: Quintessence, 1982. 382 pp.
Various techniques are described employing dowels or pins to provide a foundation on which crowns can be placed. A practical manual for the clinician, with numerous illustrations and diagrams, but somewhat lacking in critical appraisal. Quintessence also publish a German edition.

339 Simonsen, R., Thomson, V. and **Barrack, G.** *Etched cast restorations.* Chicago: Quintessence, 1983. 180 pp.
A popular text among practitioners, this book covers the relatively new methods of acid-etched retained casting and bridgework, primarily the Rochette technique.

Journals

Most of the general journals regularly carry papers on conservative dentistry, possibly because it is such a broad field, and is practised by the majority of dentists. In consequence there are comparatively few devoted entirely to the speciality, although endodontics is acquiring a sizeable body of literature.

340 *Endodontics and dental traumatology.* 1985–. Copenhagen: Munksgaard. Bimonthly.
Includes original reports and review articles on clinical methods and techniques, and case reports.

341 *International endodontic journal.* 1967–. Oxford: Blackwell. Quarterly.
Formerly the *Journal of the British Endodontic Society*, it assumed its present title in 1980, and is now the official journal of the British and Netherlands societies, the Canadian Academy of Endodontics and the European Society of Endodontics.

Each issue includes original reports, news and information, some twenty-five abstracts from other journals, and a list of endodontic papers published elsewhere.

342 *Japanese journal of conservative dentistry.* 1958–. Koko Hoken Kyokai: 44–2 Komagome, Toshima Ka, Tokyo. 3 issues per year.
In Japanese, with English abstracts.

343 *Journal of endodontics.* 1975–. 424 East Preston Street, Baltimore, Maryland 21202: American Association of Endodontists. Monthly.
Official journal of the society, publishing scientific and clinical papers, case reports, letters and reviews. News items, mostly related to the United States, are included, as is a list of American Association of Endodontists study clubs and related organizations. Trade and classified advertisements are published.

344 *Operative dentistry.* 1976–. School of Dentistry, University of Washington, Seattle, Washington 98195. Quarterly.
Official journal of the American Academy of Gold Foil Operators and the Academy of Operative Dentistry. A little-known but useful journal, with scientific and clinical papers and book reviews.

345 *Revista española de endodoncía.* 1983–. Londres 17, Madrid 28: Editorial Garsi. Irregular.

346 *Revue française d'endodontie.* 1982–. Paris: Prelat. Quarterly.
Official journal of the Société Française d'Endodontie. Original articles have brief English abstracts.

General Dental Journals of Particular Interest

British dental journal [62]
International journal of periodontics and restorative dentistry [563]
Journal of the American Dental Association [74]
Journal of dentistry [78]
Journal of oral rehabilitation [80]
Journal of prosthetic dentistry [81]
Restorative dentistry [88]

Dictionaries

347 American Association of Endodontists. *An annotated glossary of terms used in endodontics.* 4th ed. Chicago: American Association of Endodontists, 1984. 17 pp.
Gives brief definitions of words and phrases used in the speciality.

348 'Verklarende woordenlijst endodontie'. In: *Nederlands tijdschrift voor tandheelkunde* **86** (1979): 41–6.

A glossary of endodontic terms, with explanations, in Dutch. Direct English equivalents are given for most entries.

Academy of Denture Prosthetics. 'Glossary of prosthodontic terms'. (See [630].

History of Dentistry

Medical history is a well-documented area, and many of its sources are useful for dentistry as well. However, this particular branch of medicine does have a sizeable body of literature on its own account, notably general histories of the subject and bibliographies.

Research in this field may also involve searching through early volumes of indexes such as the *Index catalogue of the Library of the Surgeon General's office* [40], the *Index to dental literature* [17] or directories such as the *Dentists register* [193], sources which are standard tools in current or retrospective research.

General Guides

349 Corsi, P. and **Weindling, P.** *Information sources in the history of science and medicine.* London: Butterworth, 1983. 531 pp.

A narrative description of sources covering the historical development of science, research methods, libraries and archives. Dentistry is not specifically discussed, but the book contains much of general interest to the dental historian.

Bibliographies

350 Asbell, M. B. *A bibliography of dentistry in America, 1790–1840.* Cherry Hill, New Jersey: Sussex House Publications, 1973. 107 pp.

Lists in chronological order fifty-nine books published in the United States. Individual entries may include location(s) for the book, bibliographical references to the item, and an annotation. Journal papers, including book reviews, are listed chronologically.

351 Campbell, J. M. *Dental bibliography: British and American, 1682–1880, with an index of authors.* London: Low, 1949. 63 pp.

Entries are arranged into two groups, British and American, and then listed chronologically. This bibliography is widely used by historians and collectors.

352 Crowley, C. G. *Dental bibliography: a standard reference list of books on dentistry published throughout the world from 1536 to 1885.* Philadelphia: S. S. White, 1885. 180 pp.

Lists over 2,000 books chronologically, giving for each item the author, title, size, place of publication and date. There is an author index.

353 David, T. *Bibliographie française de l'art dentaire.* Paris: Germer-Baillière, 1889. (Reprinted by Liberac, Nieuwe Herengracht 31, Amsterdam, 1970.) 307 pp.

After a list of twenty-two journals, the main body of the book is a list of books, pamphlets and theses arranged by author. Details for each entry include title in the original language and in French, place of publication, publisher, size, number of pages, edition, date, and name of translator. The subject section is divided into broad groups, some with subheadings, and lists authors.

354 Morton, L. T. *A medical bibliography (Garrison and Morton)*. 4th ed. Aldershot: Gower, 1983. 1,000 pp.
Subtitled *Annotated checklist of texts illustrating the history of medicine.* Included are forty dental entries, including English- and foreign-language titles, and significant journal papers.

355 Poletti, I. B. *De re dentaria apud veteres*. 2nd ed. by L. Diotallevi. Milan: Mediolani, 1951. 214 pp.
A list of dental books, and medical books of dental interest, published before 1900. Arrangement is by author, and details include title, date, size, pagination and edition. Occasional annotations, in Italian, are given.

356 Stromgren, H. L. *Index of dental and adjacent topics in medical and surgical works before 1800*. Copenhagen: Munksgaard, 1955. 255 pp. (Library Research Monographs vol. 4.)
The main sequence is arranged by author, and gives title, date, place of publication and publisher. Most entries have annotations giving the relevant pages in the book listed. A subject sequence lists authors.

357 Weinberger, B. W. *Dental bibliography*. New York: First District Dental Society. Part 1: 1929; Part 2: 1932.
Compiled from Weinberger's own library and that of the New York Academy of Medicine, this is one of the most useful historical bibliographies. It includes foreign-language material, and reprints from journals. Part 1 is arranged by author, and entries give the title, in the original language, place of publication, date, number of pages, and size. Also in Part 1 is a list, arranged geographically, of dental periodicals held by the New York Academy of Medicine. Part 2 lists additional material, from all periods, and contains a subject index to both volumes.

358 Werner, E. *Entwicklungsgeschichte und Bibliographie der zahnheilkundlichen Bibliographien*. Frankfurt am Main: University, 1957. 108 pp.
Notes are given on bibliographies published from 1793 to 1956. There is a bibliography of bibliographies, and a list of useful twentieth-century references.

Library Catalogues

359 British Dental Association. Robert and Lilian Lindsay Library. *Catalogue of the rare book room*. London: BDA, 1964. 28 pp.
A chronological listing of some 600 items, from the sixteenth to the twentieth century. Bibliographical details given are author, title, edition, place of

publication and date. Typescript supplements are available listing new additions to the collection up to 1983.

360 Northwestern University Dental School Library. *Catalogue of the rare book collection.* [Chicago]: NUDS, 1976. 136 pp.
Includes almost 1,400 volumes, of which about three-quarters were published before 1865. Forty-five percent of titles are in English, 35 percent in French. Arrangement is by author; other details listed are title, place, publisher, year and pages. Occasional annotations are given.

Indexing Services

361 *Bibliography on the history of dentistry.* 1976–. In: Lindsay Club Occasional Newsletter (See [382]).
A list of articles from journals received in the British Dental Association's library, arranged in three groupings: general articles, people and places, equipment and techniques. Foreign titles are translated into English, and the existence of English abstracts is noted.

362 *Bibliography of the history of medicine.* 1965–. Bethesda, Maryland: National Library of Medicine. Annual, with five-year cumulations.
Entries are arranged under broad headings.

363 *Current work in the history of medicine.* 1954–. 183 Euston Road, London NW1 2BP: Wellcome Institute for the History of Medicine. Quarterly.
This important source has international coverage. It is based on a Medline printout, to which other material, such as papers from non-medical journals, is added. Arrangement is by subject headings; most dental references are indexed under 'dentistry', but multiple entry is common. There is an interval of about twelve to eighteen months between publication of the original paper and its inclusion in *Current work.* Regrettably, there are no cumulations.

364 *Histline.* 1970–. Bethesda, Maryland: National Library of Medicine.
This is an online database now used as the basis for the *Bibliography of the history of medicine*, and it is updated quarterly. It includes articles, monographs and symposia, with a total of over 50,000 citations. Unlike Medline, it is not routinely offered by many host systems.

Books

365 British Dental Association. *Advance of the dental profession: a centenary history, 1880–1980.* London: BDA, 1979. 289 pp.
A description of the early years, and the growth of the various groups, branches and administrative sections, compiled by members of the Lindsay Club. To compile the history, extensive use was made of minute books held in the BDA archives.

366 British Dental Association. *Jubilee book.* London: John Bale, Sons & Danielsson, 1930. 145 pp.
A summary of the BDA's history for the period 1880–1930, with numerous portraits.

367 Campbell, J. M. *Dentistry then and now.* 3rd ed. of *From a trade to a profession.* Edinburgh, privately printed (available via the British Dental Association), 1981. 395 pp.
An anthology of some of Campbell's papers originally published in journals. Topics include dental advertisements, toothbrushes, reminiscences of early days in training and practice, and biographical sketches. There is a bibliography of his other writings.

368 Colyer, F. *Old instruments used for extracting teeth.* London: Staples, 1952. 245 pp.
An authoritative, much used text, describing instruments according to groups: pelicans, elevators, keys, screws, and forceps.

369 Cope, Z. *Sir John Tomes: a pioneer of British dentistry.* London: Dawson, 1961. 108 pp.
John Tomes (1815–95) was prominent in the formation of the Odontological Society and in its early work, and was the first president of the British Dental Association. He published *A course of lectures on dental physiology* in 1848 and the classic *System of dental surgery* in 1859.

370 Guerini, V. *History of dentistry.* Philadelphia: Lea & Febiger, 1909. 355 pp.
This is the most accurate of the older histories, and covers the period 4000 BC to the early 1800s. It is an eminently readable book, with useful illustrations. Arrangement is chronological. There is no bibliography, but footnotes are provided.

371 Hill, A. *History of the reform movement in the dental profession in Britain during the last twenty years.* London: Trubner, 1877. 400 pp.
This important publication documents events and describes important personalities during the years leading to the introduction of Britain's first Dentists Act in 1878.

372 Hoffmann-Axthelm, W. *History of dentistry.* Chicago: Quintessence, 1981. 435 pp.
A revision of the original German edition, which was published in 1973, but with the sections for the nineteenth and twentieth centuries considerably expanded. This is a scholarly text, for the specialist and research worker, not the layman. There are numerous footnotes and extensive reference lists, and the book is profusely illustrated with black and white photographs. The scope of the subject is from earliest times to the mid twentieth century, at first discussed chronologically and then with chapters devoted to different specialities. This major textbook is the modern successor to Guerini.

373 Lässig, H. E. and **Muller, R. A.** *Die Zahnheilkunde in Kunst und Kulturgeschichte.* Cologne: Dumont Buchverlag, 1983. 219 pp.
A lavish pictorial history of dentistry from 2000 BC to the present day, with photographs of equipment and instruments, and reproductions of paintings, many not previously reproduced. The illustrations are of high quality, and there is a useful bibliography.

374 Lindsay, L. *Short history of dentistry.* London: John Bale, Sons & Danielsson, 1933. 88 pp.
A concise, easy-to-read account, particularly for the non-specialist. There is no bibliography.

375 Lufkin, A. W. *History of dentistry.* 2nd ed. London: Kimpton, 1948. 367 pp.
A description of early history, and dental development in different countries, chiefly educational and legislative aspects. Chapters on different specialities are included.

376 Pindborg, J. J. and **Marvitz, L.** *The dentist in art.* Copenhagen: Munksgaard, 1960. 144 pp.
A depiction of works of art with dental features; dentists at work, the patient, and humour. A classic collection of paintings, drawings and cartoons each with a short description, and the location of the original.

377 Prinz, H. *Dental chronology: a record of the more important events in the evolution of dentistry.* London: Kimpton, 1945. 189 pp.
A listing by date of noteworthy occasions, from 5000 BC to 1944.

378 Proskauer, C. and **Witt, F. H.** *Bildgeschichte der Zahnheilkunde.* Cologne: Dumont Schauberg, 1962. 220 pp.
A chronological history of dentistry as illustrated by drawings and paintings. The text comprises a foreword, introduction and notes on each illustration, and is given in German, English, French, Italian and Spanish.

379 Weinberger, B. W. *Introduction to the history of dentistry.* St. Louis: C. V. Mosby, 1948. 2 vols.
Volume 1 covers the period from prehistoric times up to the eighteenth century, and includes useful bibliographical information. There is a bibliography of important books up to 1800, a bibliography of bibliographies on medicine and dentistry and a bibliography on the history of dentistry. Volume 2 describes the history of dentistry in America from 1620 to 1800.

Histories of particular branches of dentistry are described in the appropriate subject chapters, for instance Woodforde's *Strange story of false teeth* [626] under prosthetics, and Weinberger's *Orthodontics: a historical review of its origin and evolution* [516] in the orthodontic section.

Journals

380 *Bulletin of the history of dentistry.* 1953–. Division of Behavioral Sciences, School of Dentistry, University of Oregon Health Sciences Center, 611 SW Campus Drive, Portland, Oregon 97201. Twice yearly.

The official journal of the American Academy of the History of Dentistry, the *Bulletin* includes original articles and numerous snippets of information from early books and journals.

381 *Bulletin of the Society for Social History in Medicine.* 1970–. The Society. Twice yearly.

Mainly publishes shortened versions of papers presented at meetings of the Society, which from time to time include dental topics. Editor: M. Pelling, Wellcome Unit for the History of Medicine, 47 Banbury Road, Oxford OX2 6PE, England.

382 *Dental historian.* 1975–. British Dental Association. Annual.

A typescript publication from the British Dental Association's History of Dentistry group, the Lindsay Club. Contents vary from year to year, but a regular feature is a bibliography on history, compiled in the BDA library. Available from the BDA Librarian. Current title adopted in 1985, formerly called the *Lindsay Club occasional newsletter.*

383 *Medical history.* 1975–. 183 Euston Road, London NW1 2BP: Wellcome Institute for the History of Medicine. Quarterly.

A scholarly journal publishing papers on all aspects of medical history. There is a lengthy book review section, which includes foreign-language as well as English titles.

Lists of Theses

384 Konrad, M. *Die Hochschulschriften zur Geschichte der Zahnmedizin 1919–1969. Ein Bibliographie.* Tecklenburg: Burg Verlag, 1982. 181 pp. (Medical dissertation, Berlin University, 1981.)

A list of 963 theses accepted in German institutions, arranged by author, giving the title, institution and date for each thesis. There are indexes of personal names (people who are the subjects of theses), places studied, and a general subject index.

Museum Catalogue

385 Campbell, J. M. *Catalogue of the Menzies Campbell collection of dental instruments, pictures, appliances, ornaments. etc.* Edinburgh: Royal College of Surgeons of Edinburgh, 1966. 137pp.

This collection was one of the most comprehensive in private hands. The catalogue is arranged in groups according to objects, which are mostly instruments: pelicans, elevators, keys, forceps, etc. There is a list of instrument makers at the end of the catalogue.

Laboratory Technology

The dentist relies considerably on technicians working in laboratories, notably for the fabrication of crowns, bridges and dentures. The dentist will take study models, and the laboratory then makes the prosthesis or appliance to the dentist's specifications. With the advances made in materials and techniques, and the importance of accuracy and aesthetics, close collaboration between dentist and technician is essential, and an understanding of each other's work is invaluable.

Books

386 Eissmann, H. F., Rudd, K. D. and **Morrow, R. M.** *Dental laboratory procedures*; vol. 2, *Fixed partial dentures*. St. Louis: C. V. Mosby, 1980. 367 pp.

An exhaustive presentation of the subject, of interest to dentists and laboratory staff. The three volumes by these authors give detailed descriptions of laboratory techniques accompanied by numerous black and white photographs. At the beginning of each chapter are given definitions of new terms that will be encountered in the pages which follow.

387 Martinelli, N. and **Spinella, S. C.** *Dental laboratory technology*. 3rd ed. St. Louis: C. V. Mosby, 1981. 502 pp.

A standard American book for technicians, covering the construction of dentures, bridges, porcelain fused to metal restorations and wrought wires and bars.

388 Morrow, R. M., Rudd, K. D. and **Eissmann, H. F.** *Dental laboratory procedures*; vol. 1, *Complete dentures*. St. Louis: C. V Mosby, 1980. 541 pp.

A companion volume to [386].

389 Osborne, J., Wilson, H. J. and **Mansfield, M. A.** *Dental technology and materials for students*. 7th ed. Oxford: Blackwell, 1979. 391 pp.

A well-established British text for technicians and dental students, which describes laboratory procedures in relation to prosthetic work. Previous editions were entitled *Dental mechanics for students*.

390 Rudd, K. D., Morrow, R. M. and **Eissmann, H. F.** *Dental laboratory procedures*: vol. 3, *Removable partial dentures*. St. Louis: C. V. Mosby, 1981. 675 pp.

A companion volume to [386] and [388].

391 Stananought, D. *Laboratory procedures for full and partial dentures*. Oxford: Blackwell, 1978. 226 pp.

A practical manual for dental students and trainee technicians. It is well illustrated with numerous line drawings.

392 Stananought, D. *Laboratory procedures for inlays, crowns and bridges.* Oxford: Blackwell, 1975. 132 pp.
A companion volume to [391].

Journals

393 *Dental echo.* 1950–. Turnerstrasse 20, D-6900 Heidelberg: Helmut Haase Verlag. Monthly.
Describes itself as an 'international journal for product development and information'. It is published in German, but each issue has substantial sections in English, French, Spanish and Italian.

394 *Dental laboratory.* 1975–. Nottingham: Dental Laboratories Association. Bimonthly.
For laboratory owners and managers.

395 *Dental laboratory world.* 1973–. San Antonio, Texas: Huthig Esco. Monthly.
The present title was adopted in 1980; it was formerly called *Dental laboratory age.*

396 *Dental technician.* 1948–. Epsom: A. E. Morgan. Monthly.
In newspaper format, this useful publication has articles on new products and techniques, plus advertisements, book reviews and correspondence.

396A Institute of Maxillofacial Technology. *Proceedings.* 1975–. Annual.
Contains original reports.

397 *Quintessence of dental technology.* 1976–. Chicago: Quintessence. Monthly.
Includes original papers, often accompanied by colour photographs, information on new products, and advertisements. German and Japanese editions of the journal are also published.

398 *Zahntechnik.* 1942–. Badenerstrasse 41, CH-8004 Zürich: Landesverband freier Schweizer Arbeitnehmer Zentralsekretariat. Bimonthly.
Official organ of the Schweizerischen Zahntechniker Vereinigung. Includes original articles, news, announcements, and advertisements. Predominantly in German, but some papers are in French or Italian.

Directories

Dental technician yearbook and directory. (See [204])
Includes information relating to British organizations, a product directory, a list of manufacturers and traders, and directory of commercial laboratories.

Materials

All clinicians use a wide range of materials in their daily practice, and new products are continually under development. Not only dentists are involved in research and development, but materials scientists, such as metallurgists and polymer chemists, who make large contributions to the published literature.

Information on dental materials science is therefore spread among a wide range of clinical and technical sources. Patents and standards in the dental field relate primarily to materials; therefore *see also* Chapter 7 and [239]–[242] for information on these special kinds of material.

Bibliographies

399 'Dental materials: literature review'. A narrative report and accompanying bibliography is published in the *Journal of dentistry*. This covers the literature for a given year, from 1973 onwards. It is compiled by the Panel for Dental Materials Studies in the United Kingdom, various contributors having a separate section. A core list of thirty-seven journals is scanned, but other sources are included if considered appropriate. Some 400 papers are listed, the majority being in English.

Literature review for:	*Journal of dentistry*
1976	**6** (1978): 1–22; 95–119
1977	**7** (1979): 275–303; **8** (1980): 43–67
1978	**8** (1980): 189–248
1979	**9** (1981): 177–209; 271–298
1980	**11** (1983): 1–34; 95–132
1981	**12** (1984): 1–28; 95–121

Books

American Dental Association. *Dentists' desk reference: materials, instruments and equipment.* (See [215])
A practical guide to the selection and use of materials for the American clinician, but also useful in other countries. The book supersedes *Guide to dental materials and devices*, which included ADA specifications; unfortunately these are excluded from this new format.

400 Anderson, J. N. *Applied dental materials.* 6th ed. by J. F. McCabe. Oxford: Blackwell, 1985. 178 pp.
A guide to the manipulation of materials, notably those for prosthetic use. A useful text for dental students and practitioners, but especially for technicians.

401 Combe, E. C. *Notes on dental materials.* 4th ed. Edinburgh: Churchill Livingstone, 1981. 333 pp.
Concise data on clinical and technical aspects, for dental practitioners.

402 Craig, R. G. *Restorative dental materials.* 6th ed. St. Louis: C. V. Mosby, 1980. 478 pp.
An excellent undergraduate text with thorough coverage.

403 Skinner, E. W. *Science of dental materials.* 8th ed. by R. W. Phillips. Philadelphia: W. B. Saunders, 1982. 646 pp.
The most exhaustive book on the technical aspects of materials. Emphasis is placed on the reasons for selecting and choosing particular materials, and descriptions of clinical procedures are also given. The whole range of intra-oral materials is included—resins, metals and porcelain—as are impression materials. Chemistry, composition and manipulative techniques are described. The bibliographies are up to date, and there is an extensive subject index.

404 Smith, D. C. and **Williams, D. F.** *Bicompatibility of dental materials.* Boca Raton, Florida: CRC, 1982. 4 vols.
A series of monographs for researchers. Volume 1 deals with characteristics of dental tissues and their response to dental materials; volume 2 deals with preventive materials and bonding agents; volume 3 with restorative materials, volume 4 with prosthodontic materials.

405 Stecher, P. G. *New dental materials.* Park Ridge: Noyes Data Group, 1980. 353 pp.
Comprises summaries of relevant U.S. patents issued since 1970, arranged by type of material: alloys, composites, cements, adhesives and sealants, artificial teeth and crowns, denture materials, impression materials. The author and patent number are given for each item, and chemical formulae where appropriate.

406 Williams, D. F. and **Cunningham, J.** *Materials in clinical dentistry.* Oxford: Oxford University Press. 376 pp.
A description of the application of materials for undergraduates and practising dentists. The authors emphasize the relationship between science and the clinical uses of materials, but the scientific content is of a level to promote the understanding of the clinical properties, and is not the primary focus of the text. Endodontics, preventive dentistry, orthodontics, periodontology and oral surgery are briefly covered. There are no references.
There is a Spanish edition by Editorial Mundi.

Journals

407 *Biomaterials.* 1980–. Guildford: Butterworth. 6 issues per year.
Published in association with the Biological Engineering Society, this journal regularly includes papers of interest to the postgraduate student or researcher in dentistry.

408 *Journal of biomedical materials research.* 1967–. New York: John Wiley. 6 issues per year.
The comparable American equivalent to *Biomaterials.*

409 *Journal of the Japanese Society for Dental Materials and Devices.* 1983–. Koku Hoken Kyokai: 44–2 Komagone, Toshima Ku, Tokyo. Bimonthly.
Japanese, with English abstracts. Succeeds *Journal of the Japanese Society for Dental Apparatus and Materials.*

410 *Dental materials.* 1985–. Copenhagen: Munksgaard. Bimonthly.
Includes papers on clinical and laboratory, basic and applied research, related to the properties or performance of materials, or the reaction of host tissues. Laboratory technology may also be relevant.

Other Journals

Most general journals include papers on materials, but the following are particularly useful:

Journal of dentistry [78]
Journal of dental research [77]
Journal of oral rehabilitation [80]
Journal of prosthetic dentistry [81]

Microbiology and Immunology

Microbiology developed following Anton van Leeuwenhoek's discovery of the microscope as long ago as the 1680s, when he was able to identify tiny organisms that could not be seen with the naked eye. It has long been recognized that bacteria are involved in caries and periodontal disease, and are responsible for other dental infections as well; the classic treatise on the aetiology of caries, W. D. Miller's *Microbiology of the human mouth*, was published in 1882.

Immunology is currently a growth area in medicine generally and hence in dentistry too, and evidence is being acquired on the role of immunological processes in the pathogenesis of oral disease. Although basic texts are available, much of the journal literature on oral immunology is written at an advanced level, and frequently in specialized immunological, rather than dental journals. The microbiology of caries and periodontal disease specifically are, however, also covered in texts and journals related to those particular diseases.

Books

411 McCracken, A. W. and **Cawson, R. A.** *Clinical and oral microbiology.* Washington, DC: Hemisphere, 1983. 629 pp.
Most of the book deals with general medical microbiology; bacteria, fungi, viruses, treatment and prevention of infections, and immunity. Approximately 150 pages are devoted to oral microbiology, and discuss caries, periodontal diseases, and infections. This text is easier to read and assimilate than some others, but still contains a wealth of detail.

412 Melville, T. H. and **Russell, C.** *Microbiology for dental students.* London: Heinemann, 1981. 394 pp.
A popular book with British undergraduates and practitioners. Part 1 discusses fundamentals of microbiology, part 2 has chapters on different groups of bacteria, and part 3 is devoted to microorganisms of the mouth.

413 Newman, H. N. *Dental plaque: the ecology of the flora on human teeth.* Springfield: Thomas, 1980. 102 pp.
A simplified outline is provided for students and clinicians. Chapters describe plaque microorganisms, plaque formation, structure and biology, plaque-associated diseases and plaque control.

414 Nolte, W. A. *Oral microbiology.* 3rd ed. St. Louis: C. V. Mosby, 1977. 683pp.
A well-established American text, with more detail and a wider scope than other books listed in this section. Two-thirds of the contents relate to general microbiological principles and the various varieties of microorganisms; dental topics covered are periodontal disease, caries, the pulp, hypersensitivity of dentine and focal infection.

415 Roitt, I. M. and **Lehner, T.** *Immunology of oral diseases.* 2nd ed. Oxford: Blackwell, 1983. 448 pp.
Approximately half the book is a modification of Roitt's short but classic *Essential immunology*, the rest is devoted to immunological aspects of caries and periodontal disease. The work is intended for undergraduate and postgraduate students.

Journals

There are no serials specifically devoted to oral microbiology or immunology, but the following regularly carry papers of interest:

Archives of oral biology [306]
Caries research [321]
Immunology
Infection and immunity
Journal de biologie buccale [308]
Journal of hospital infection
Journal of clinical periodontology [565]
Journal of immunology
Journal of periodontal research [566]
Journal of periodontology [567]

Occlusion

The definition one finds of the phrase 'dental occlusion' will vary according to the source consulted, which, in its turn, is influenced by its country of origin. The British Standards Institution's *Glossary of dental terms*, for instance, defines occlusion as 'any contact between the teeth of opposing dental arches, usually referring to contact between the occlusal surfaces'. A much broader area is, however, covered by the definition in Jablonski's *Illustrated dictionary of dentistry*: 'the relationship between all the components of the masticatory system in normal function, dysfunction and parafunction. This includes the contact of opposing teeth and restorations, occlusal trauma and dysfunction, neuromuscular physiology, temporomandibular and muscle dysfunction, swallowing and mastication, psychophysiological status, diagnosis, prevention and treatment of functional disorders of the masticatory system.'

Whichever definition is chosen, it is evident that occlusion impinges on a wide range of physiological and clinical aspects of dentistry. In Britain its teaching is fragmented, but in the main it is studied as a part of the syllabus of conservative dentistry, periodontology and prosthetics. In the United States, by contrast, dental schools have departments of occlusion, hence Jablonski's all-embracing definition.

This publication takes a middle course, listing important sources relating to occlusion in the more specific sense, but also including within its scope the temporomandibular joint. Mastication is discussed in the context of the biological sciences, and is covered by [291]–[308].

Malocclusion, the abnormal meeting of the cusps of the upper and lower teeth, falls into the province of orthodontics.

Books

416 Arnold, N. R. and **Frumker, S. C.** *Occlusal treatment.* Philadelphia: Lea & Febiger, 1976. 163 pp.

A practical handbook of procedures for the general practitioner. It includes many useful diagrams, but there is no index.

417 Dawson, P. E. *Evaluation, diagnosis and treatment of occlusal problems.* St. Louis: C. V. Mosby, 1974. 407 pp.

This is accepted as the most comprehensive book on the subject in Britain and North America, and is popular with advanced students and serious practitioners. It is an authoritative text with a well-deserved reputation. French edition published by Prelat, German by Zahnärztlich-medizinisches Schrifttum.

418 Gelb, H. *Clinical management of head, neck and temporomandibular joint pain and dysfunction: a multidisciplinary approach to diagnosis and treatment.* 2nd ed. Philadelphia: W. B. Saunders, 1985. 635 pp.

The management of temporomandibular joint problems remains a controversial subject. This book presents a variety of treatments, and is of interest to general practitioners and specialists.

419 Gross, M. D. *Occlusion in restorative dentistry.* Edinburgh: Churchill Livingstone, 1982. 194 pp.

An introduction for general practitioners and undergraduates. There are numerous diagrams, and a helpful glossary.

420 Morgan, D. H., House, L. R., Hall, W. P. and **Vamvass, S. J.** *Diseases of*

the temporomandibular joint: a multidisciplinary approach. 2nd ed. St. Louis: C. V. Mosby, 1982. 695 pp.
A companion volume to [418], covering growth and development, diagnosis, and the various treatment options.

421 **Ogus, H. D.** and **Toller, P. A.** *Common disorders of the temporomandibular joint.* Bristol: John Wright, 1981. 105 pp. (Dental Practitioner Handbook no. 26.)
A practical introduction to the subject, with an emphasis on nonsurgical treatment. A German edition is published by Quintessence.

422 **Posselt, U.** *Physiology of occlusion and rehabilitation.* 2nd ed. Oxford: Blackwell, 1968. 331 pp.
Now superseded by Dawson [417] in popularity, but still regarded as an authoritative work, and valuable for its explanation of theoretical and practical points. A French edition is published by Prelat.

423 **Ramfjord, S.** and **Ash, M. M.** *Occlusion.* 3rd ed. Philadelphia: W. B. Saunders, 1983. 544 pp.
A classic text for advanced students, covering the subject in its widest context, as defined by Jablonski. The scope includes the anatomy and physiology of the masticatory system, epidemiology and aetiology of occlusal problems (which includes bruxism, trauma from occlusion and the temporomandibular joint syndrome), diagnosis and treatment. This last aspect deals with therapy for bruxism and temporomandibular joint problems, occlusal adjustment, orthodontics, restorative dentistry and splints. With Dawson [417], one of the most comprehensive books on occlusion. A French edition is published by Prelat, an Italian one by Piccin.

424 **Thomson, H.** *Occlusion in clinical practice.* Bristol: John Wright, 1981. 188 pp. (Dental Practitioner Handbook no. 30.)
A presentation of a complex subject in a highly readable style. The approach is practical rather than theoretical, and intended for clinicians.

425 **Watt, D. M.** *Gnathosonic diagnosis and occlusal dynamics.* Eastbourne: Praeger, 1981. 218 pp.
Describes the sounds made by the masticatory mechanism, that is, the occlusion and temporomandibular joint (TMJ), and how these sounds can be used to diagnose and assist treatment of TMJ dysfunction. The book is accompanied by a cassette tape of occlusal and TMJ sounds. Intended users are clinicians and occlusion specialists.

426 **Zarb, G. A.** and **Carlsson, C. E.** *Temporomandibular joint function and dysfunction.* Copenhagen: Munksgaard, 1979. 467 pp.
A collection of papers by acknowledged experts, on all aspects of the subject, originally published in *Oral sciences reviews*, which is a series of review monographs. Topics covered include the anatomy, physiology and epidemiology of dysfunction, neurophysiological studies, psychological implications, radiology, therapy and surgery. Each section has an extensive bibliography.

Journals

427 *Journal of craniomandibular practice.* 1983–. 5323 Brainerd Road, Chattanooga, Tennessee 37411: Chroma. Quarterly.
Includes original papers, advertisements and announcements, and a listing of relevant subject entries from *Index medicus*, this last feature occupying some eight pages per issue.

428 *Journal of gnathology.* 1982–. PO Box 1085, La Mesa, California: International Academy of Gnathology. Twice yearly.

Other Journals

Journal of oral rehabilitation [80]
Journal of prosthetic dentistry [81]

Oral Medicine

The sources listed under this heading are few. It is difficult to define precise boundaries between oral medicine and various other disciplines, such as oral surgery, pathology and pharmacology, and published works commonly discuss several aspects of the condition being described. Other sections, therefore, will also contain relevant material.

Books

429 Astley-Hope, H. D. and **Hellier, M. D.** *Disease, drugs and the dentist.* Chichester: John Wiley, 1983. 254 pp.
A pocket-sized handbook for the clinician. The first half of the book is devoted to medical conditions, the second half comprises notes on drugs.

430 Burket, L. W. *Oral medicine.* 8th ed. by M. A. Lynch. Philadelphia: J. B. Lippincott, 1984. 958 pp.
Burket is accepted as one of the most authoritative and comprehensive titles in the field. The contents are divided into three sections: principles of diagnosis, oral disease and systemic disease.

431 Gayford, J. J. and **Haskell, R.** *Clinical oral medicine.* Bristol: John Wright, 1979. 285 pp.
A book intended for students and clinicians, which is popular in Britain.

432 Gorlin, R.J., Pindborg, J. J. and **Cohen, M. M.** *Syndromes of the head and neck.* 2nd ed. New York: McGraw-Hill, 1976. 812 pp.
An important reference book for all workers concerned with congenital abnormalities. For each syndrome, the oral manifestations are described, and differential diagnoses discussed. Important references are listed, and there are ample black and white illustrations.

433 Jones, J. H. and **Mason, D. K.** *Oral manifestations of systemic disease.* London: W. B. Saunders, 1980. 559 pp.
Discusses diseases of the whole body, or specific parts of it, that affect the mouth. A significant book for clinicians in both medicine and dentistry.

434 Kennedy, A. C. and **Blumgart, L. H.** *Essentials of medicine and surgery for dental students.* 4th ed. Edinburgh: Churchill Livingstone, 1982. 355 pp.
Simplified accounts are given of various disorders, omitting details that are not relevant to the dentist. There is greater coverage of facial problems.

435 Little, J. W. and **Falace, D. A.** *Dental management of the medically compromised patient.* 2nd ed. St. Louis: C. V. Mosby, 1984. 320 pp.
This was the first book to approach its subject material in this way, filling an important gap in the literature. Clinicians may find the summary section, printed on blue paper for ease of identification, particularly useful for quick reference.

436 McCarthy, P. L. and **Shklar, G.** *Diseases of the oral mucosa.* 2nd ed. Philadelphia: Lea & Febiger, 1980. 579 pp.
A well-illustrated book covering clinical and pathological aspects of the subject.

437 Malamed, S. F. *Handbook of medical emergencies in the dental office.* 2nd ed. St. Louis: C. V. Mosby, 1982. 408 pp.
Chapters are arranged according to clinical signs and symptoms, such as respiratory difficulty, altered consciousness, seizures, and drug-related emergencies.

438 Mumford, J. M. *Orofacial pain: aetiology, diagnosis and treatment.* 3rd ed. Edinburgh: Churchill Livingstone, 1982.
There are preliminary chapters on pain in general, but most of the book is devoted to specific causes, such as pulp diseases, or soft tissue lesions. The main emphasis is on the cause of pain and its diagnosis; treatment is discussed only briefly.

439 Pindborg, J. J. *Atlas of diseases of the oral mucosa.* Copenhagen: Munksgaard, 1980. 316 pp.
This colour atlas is devoted primarily to clinical diagnosis.

440 Scully, C. and **Cawson, R. A.** *Medical problems in dentistry.* Bristol: John Wright, 1982. 514 pp.
A popular British equivalent to Little and Falace [435], which is of immense value to students and practitioners.

441 Tyldesley, W. *Colour atlas of oral medicine.* London: Wolfe, 1978. 111 pp.
A diagnostic aid, comprising over 250 colour photographs, predominantly of lesions of the mouth mucosa. There are brief accompanying notes for each illustration.

442 Wood, N. K. and **Goaz, P. W.** *Differential diagnosis of oral lesions*. 2nd ed. St. Louis: C. V. Mosby, 1980. 662 pp.
Diseases are described according to the oral symptoms.

Journals

443 *Journal of oral medicine*. 1946–. New York: Academy of Oral Medicine. Quarterly.
Official publication of the American Academy of Oral Medicine. Until 1965 entitled *Journal of dental medicine*.

Oral surgery, oral medicine, oral pathology. (See [486])
This core journal is described in the oral surgery section. It is the official journal of the Organization of Teachers of Oral Diagnosis, and has a section each month devoted to oral medicine.

Oral Pathology

Pathology is concerned with the structural and functional changes caused by disease, and is therefore part of a triad with medicine and surgery. It is common for clinical and pathological aspects of a disease to be discussed together, especially in diagnosis, thus much material on oral medicine and surgery will also be relevant to oral pathology. Also important are sources in general pathology, since the techniques used, such as histology and microscopy, are universal, and diseases manifested in the mouth may be linked to other disorders elsewhere in the body.

Books

444 Banoczy, J. *Oral leukoplakia*. Hague: Martinus Nijhoff, 1982. (Developments in Oncology vol. 8.) 231 pp.
A specialist review by a world authority on precancerous lesions, for researchers in the field.

445 Batsakis, J. G. *Tumors of the head and neck: clinical and pathological considerations*. 2nd ed. Baltimore: Williams & Wilkins, 1979. 573 pp.
Comprehensive coverage of neoplasms and non-neoplastic lesions. Tissue types and diseases are preferred to anatomical sites for many chapter headings.

446 Cawson, R. A. *Aids to oral pathology and diagnosis*. Edinburgh: Churchill Livingstone, 1981. 126 pp.
Brief notes for undergraduate revision.

447 Cawson, R. A. *Essentials of dental surgery and pathology*. 4th ed. Edinburgh: Churchill Livingstone, 1984. 454 pp.
A clear presentation for students and practitioners, with the emphasis on pathology and oral medicine. A German edition is published by Hanser.

448 Colby, R. A., Kerr, D. A. and **Robinson, H. B. G.** *Color atlas of oral pathology*. 4th ed. by H. B. G. Robinson and A. S. Miller. Philadelphia: J. B. Lippincott, 1983. 192 pp.
For students and practitioners.

449 Dolby, A. E. *Oral mucosa in health and disease*. Oxford: Blackwell, 1975. 512 pp.
A review of current knowledge for clinicians and researchers. The topics covered are the structure, function and physiology of the oral mucosa; its significance in systemic diseases; and mucosal diseases.

450 Lucas, R. B. *Pathology of tumours of the oral tissues*. 4th ed. Edinburgh: Churchill Livingstone, 1984. 427 pp.
An excellent British textbook, for practising pathologists and advanced students. The scope is narrower than Batsakis [445]; diagnostic aspects are emphasized.

451 Mackenzie, I. C., Dabelsteen, E. and **Squier, C. A.** *Oral premalignancy*. Iowa City: University of Iowa Press, 1980. 353 pp.
This monograph comprises the edited proceedings of a symposium bringing together oral and general pathologists and basic scientists, resulting in an interdisciplinary approach to precancerous lesions. Sections cover clinical and histopathological concepts, aetiology, models, cell behaviour patterns, and diagnosis, offering substantial reviews by international authorities.

452 Marsland, E. A. and **Browne, R. M.** *Colour atlas of oral histopathology*. Aylesbury: HM&M, 1975. 95 pp.
Intended to supplement textbooks, and aid laboratory studies and diagnosis, this text has over 400 photomicrographs, arranged by tissue type. The largest section is devoted to the oral mucosa.

453 Pindborg, J. J. *Oral cancer and precancer*. Bristol: John Wright, 1980. 177 pp.
A concise review for postgraduate students. In contrast to traditional approaches, cancerous and premalignant lesions are discussed together, in chapters devoted to anatomical sites. Four chapters at the end of the book deal with oral leukoplakia. A selected list of references, with a cut-off date of 1978, occupies some sixteen pages. A German edition is published by Quintessenz.

454 Pindborg, J. J. *Pathology of the dental hard tissues*. Copenhagen: Munksgaard, 1970. 443 pp.
Excellent general coverage, not confined to enamel lesions. Subjects covered include abnormalities of tooth morphology, disturbances of tooth formation, eruption problems, caries, fractures, mechanical, physical and chemical injuries, resorption, ankylosis, and odontogenic tumours. An important reference work, despite its publication date.

455 Pindborg, J. J. and **Kramer, I. R. H.** *Histological typing of odontogenic tumours, jaw cysts and allied lesions*. Geneva: WHO, 1971. 44 pp. (International Histological Classification of Tumours no. 5.)

One of a series of reference manuals for practising pathologists, valuable also for postgraduate students.

456 Schroeder, H. E. *Pathobiologie orale Strukturen: Zahn, Pulpa, Paradont.* Basle: Karger, 1983. 210 pp.

457 Shafer, W. G., Hine, M. K. and **Levy, B. M.** *Textbook of oral pathology.* 4th ed. Philadelphia: W. B. Saunders, 1983. 917 pp.
An authoritative textbook and work of reference for students and practitioners, emphasizing the diseases and processes encountered most frequently in general practice. It is recognized as a standard source, of high reputation, on both sides of the Atlantic. There is a Spanish edition by Nueva Editorial Interamericana and a Portuguese one by Editôra Interamericana.

458 Shear, M. *Cysts of the oral regions.* 2nd ed. Bristol: John Wright, 1983. 218 pp.
Occurrence, pathology and treatment are described for the clinician.

459 Stewart, R. E. and **Prescott, G. H.** *Oral facial genetics.* St. Louis: C. V. Mosby, 1976. 680 pp.
A review of the diseases of the mouth and face that are directly or indirectly affected by genetic influences, intended for students and practitioners of dentistry and medicine, and for geneticists. It is not a textbook of genetics. Information is provided on the factors and mechanisms which influence disturbances in craniofacial development; on disturbances in the various parts of the tooth and in the soft tissues; on immunological disorders, errors of metabolism, blood disorders, cytogenetic anomalies and cleft lip and palate.

460 Thoma, K. H. *Oral pathology.* 6th ed. by R. J. Gorlin and H. M. Goldman. St. Louis: C. V. Mosby, 1970. 2 vols.
Still the most comprehensive general text in the field, despite its publication date.

461 Walter, J. B., Hamilton, M. C. and **Israel, M. S.** *Principles of pathology for dental students.* 4th ed. Edinburgh: Churchill Livingstone, 1981. 668 pp.
Two-thirds of the book is devoted to the general concepts and principles of the field; the smaller second section covers individual systems and organs. As its title indicates, it is a book about pathology in general, not specifically oral pathology. It is a standard undergraduate text, but also popular for revision purposes for higher examinations.

Important Books Described in Other Sections

Cohen, B. and **Kramer, I. R. H.** *Scientific foundations of dentistry.* [295].

Gorlin, R. J., Pindborg, J. J. and **Cohen, M. M.** *Syndromes of the head and neck* [432].

Jones, J. H. and **Mason, D. K.** *Oral manifestations of systemic disease.* [433].

Pindborg, J. J. *Atlas of diseases of the oral mucosa* [439].

Journals

462 *Journal of head and neck pathology.* 1982–. Avenue de Duc Jean 71–73, B-1080 Brussels: Centre Tête et Cou. Quarterly.
Succeeds *Postgraduate journal for mouth, head and neck pathology.* Papers in English, Dutch or French, with English abstracts.

Oral surgery, oral medicine, oral pathology. (See [486]). Monthly.
The official organ of three American oral pathology societies, publishing four to six papers or case reports in each issue.

463 *Journal of oral pathology.* 1972–. Munksgaard: Copenhagen. 10 issues per year.
The core journal, and official organ of the International Association of Oral Pathologists. Includes scientific papers, case reports, review articles, and book reviews.

Medical and Scientific Journals

Papers of interest to workers in the field of oral pathology are scattered widely. As well as the general dental journals, the following titles are a selection of the most important serials which may include useful case reports or descriptions of techniques.

Acta pathologica microbiologica immunologica scandinavica. Section A
American journal of clinical pathology
Archives of dermatology
Archives of pathology and laboratory medicine
British journal of cancer
British journal of dermatology
Calcified tissue international
Cancer
Journal of clinical pathology
Journal of histochemistry and cytochemistry
Journal of investigative dermatology
Journal of pathology
Journal of ultrastructure research

Dictionary

464 Courtois, J. *Lexique des termes de pathologie dentaire.* Paris: Prelat, 1972. 71 pp.

Oral Surgery

Surgery is closely linked with the disciplines of pathology and medicine. In the literature too they are often discussed together, for instance in case reports published in journals, and in textbooks. This section therefore cannot stand alone, but must be regarded as part of a triad with those on oral medicine and oral pathology. In a wider context, oral surgery has close links with plastic surgery, the two disciplines having developed in conjunction with each other as a result of the need for treatment of casualties with serious maxillofacial injuries during the Second World War. Today there is an increasing trend towards the performance of jaw surgery for aesthetic reasons, often coordinated with orthodontic treatment.

Books

465 Bell, W. H., Proffit, W. R. and **White, R. P.** *Surgical correction of dentofacial deformities*. Philadelphia: W. B. Saunders, 1980–85. 3 vols.
Diagnostic and clinical guidelines for surgery are given; orthodontic and surgical procedures are described and illustrated.

466 Epker, B. N. and **Wolford, L. M.** *Dentofacial deformities: surgical orthodontic correction*. St. Louis: C. V. Mosby, 1980. 477 pp.
An atlas of line drawings demonstrating techniques, accompanied by brief descriptions. There is no index.

467 Haunfelder, D. and **Lehnert, S.** *Zahnärztliche Mundchirurgie*. 3rd ed. Heidelberg: Huthig, 1981. 200 pp.

468 Howe, G. L. *Minor oral surgery*. 2nd ed. Bristol: John Wright, 1971. 335 pp.
Essential reading for undergraduates and graduates, on basic principles and techniques.

469 Killey, H. C. *Fractures of the mandible*. 3rd ed. by P. Banks. Bristol: John Wright, 1983. 118 pp. (Dental Practitioner Handbook no. 5.)
A concise summary for the student and practitioner. Aspects covered include surgical anatomy, the edentulous mandible, and fractures in children.

470 Killey, H. C. *Fractures of the middle third of the facial skeleton*. 3rd ed. Bristol: John Wright, 1977. 87 pp. (Dental Practitioner Handbook no. 3.)
Summarizes the surgical anatomy, clinical findings and management of these fractures.

471 Killey, H. C. and **Kay, L. W.** *The prevention of complications in oral surgery*. 2nd ed. Edinburgh: Churchill Livingstone, 1977. 210 pp.
A practical guide of value to any clinician.

472 Killey, H. C., Kay, L. W. and **Seward, G. R.** *Benign cystic lesions of the jaws*. 3rd ed. Edinburgh: Churchill Livingstone, 1977. 175 pp.
A succinct coverage of diagnosis and treatment.

473 Killey, H. C., Seward, G. R. and **Kay, L. W.** *Outline of oral surgery*. Bristol: John Wright, 1975. 2 vols. (Dental Practitioner Handbook no. 11.)
A popular text with British clinicians. Volume 1 discusses the practical aspects of

minor oral surgery, of interest to all practitioners. Volume 2 covers diagnosis and treatment of conditions encountered by surgeons in a hospital setting.

474 Moore, J. R. and **Gillbe, G. V.** *Principles of oral surgery*. 3rd ed. Manchester: Manchester University Press, 1981. 256 pp.
An introductory work for undergraduate students.

475 Oringer, M. J. *Electrosurgery in dentistry*. 2nd ed. Philadelphia: W. B. Saunders, 1975. 1,134 pp.
A comprehensive description of the principles and clinical applications of this specialized technique.

476 Rowe, N. L. and **Williams, J. Ll.** *Maxillofacial injuries*. Edinburgh: Churchill Livingstone, 1985. 2 vols.
The long-awaited successor to N. L. Rowe and H. C. Killey's *Fractures of the facial skeleton*, a classic text long out of print, this is a valuable work for students and practitioners. Chapters are contributed by eminent authorities in the field, predominantly from Great Britain.

477 Starshak, T. J. and **Saunders, B.** *Preprosthetic oral and maxillofacial surgery*. St. Louis: C. V. Mosby, 1980. 189 pp.
Discusses surgical techniques to recontour the mouth and jaws in order that dentures can be satisfactorily retained.

Reviews

478 *Current advances in oral surgery*. 1974–. Edited by W. B. Irby. St. Louis: C. V. Mosby. Every three years.
Volumes 1, 2 and 4 are general in coverage; volume 3 is devoted to the temporomandibular joint.

479 *Fortschritte der Kiefer- und Gesichtschirurgie*. 1955–. Stuttgart: Thieme. Annual.
Each volume is dedicated to a particular topic. Papers are predominantly in German, but with an occasional contribution in English.

Journals

480 *British journal of oral and maxillofacial surgery*. 1963–. Edinburgh: Churchill Livingstone. 6 issues per year.
Official journal of the British Association of Oral and Maxillofacial Surgeons, and the major British journal in the speciality. The title changed in 1984; it was formerly called *British journal of oral surgery*. Includes original papers, with an emphasis on case reports, book reviews and topical information.

481 *Deutsche Zeitschrift für Mund-, Kiefer- und Gesichtschirurgie*. 1977–. Munich: Hanser. 6 issues per year.
Official journal of the Deutsche Gesellschaft für Mund-, Kiefer- und Gesichtschirurgie and the Bundesverband Deutsche Ärzte für Mund-, Kiefer- und Gesichtschirurgie.

482 *Head and neck surgery*. 1978–. New York: John Wiley. 6 issues per year.
A commercially produced journal which is becoming an important title, and has published some significant review articles. It includes original reports, advertisements for products and situations vacant, and abstracts from other journals.

483 *International journal of oral surgery*. 1972–. Copenhagen: Munksgaard. 6 issues per year.
The official journal of the International Association of Oral Surgeons, and a major title. It publishes original research, review articles, case reports and book reviews, and has included papers presented at the 5th, 6th and 7th conferences on oral surgery. All papers are published in English, but with French and German abstracts.

484 *Journal of maxillofacial surgery*. 1981–. Stuttgart: Thieme. 6 issues per year.
Published for the European Association for Maxillofacial Surgery, and includes original research, book reviews and advertisements. Papers are predominantly in English.

485 *Journal of oral and maxillofacial surgery*. 1943–. Philadelphia: W. B. Saunders. Monthly.
Official organ of the American Association of Oral and Maxillofacial Surgeons. The title changed in 1982; it was formerly called *Journal of oral surgery*. One of the core journals in the field, it publishes scientific and clinical papers, case reports, abstracts from other journals, book reviews, correspondence and advertisements.

486 *Oral surgery, oral medicine, oral pathology*. 1948–. St. Louis: C. V. Mosby. Monthly.
Although the organ of several societies in related disciplines, it is not the journal of an oral surgery association. It.is, however, one of the most widely read serials in the field. Sections cover surgery, medicine and pathology, also endodontics and radiology, publishing scientific and clinical research, and case reports. Advertisements are included, for appropriate products and for books. From 1919 to 1947 the journal was a part of the *International journal of orthodontia and oral surgery*.

487 *Revue de stomatologie et de chirurgie maxillofaciale*. 1894–. Paris: Masson. Bimonthly.
Journal of the Société de Stomatologie et de Chirurgie Maxillofaciale de France. The title changed in 1969; it was formerly called *Revue de stomatologie*. It publishes original reports, and abstracts from other journals, not necessarily French. It includes a title page in English, and gives English abstracts for its papers.

General Surgery Journals of Particular Interest

488 *Annals of the Royal College of Surgeons of England*. 1947–. Lincoln's Inn Fields, London WC2A 3PN: Royal College of Surgeons of England. Bimonthly.
Includes papers by members of the RCS Faculty of Dental Surgery.

489 *British journal of plastic surgery.* 1948–. Edinburgh: Churchill Livingstone. Quarterly.
Official journal of the British Association of Plastic Surgeons.

490 *Plastic and reconstructive surgery.* 1946–. Baltimore: Williams & Wilkins.
Organ of four American plastic or maxillofacial surgeons' societies.

491 *Scandinavian journal of plastic and reconstructive surgery.* 1967–. Stockholm: Almqvist & Wiksell.

Lexicons

492 American Society of Oral Surgeons. *Oral and maxillofacial surgery procedural terminology with glossary.* Chicago: American Society of Oral Surgeons, 1975. 203 pp.

Directories

493 *Oral and maxillofacial surgery directory of the world.* Edited by W. H. Archer. 5th ed. 71 Osage Drive, Pittsburgh 15243: the author, 1976.
Despite the title, useful mainly for information on American surgeons. Lists are included of diplomates of the American Board of Oral Surgeons and members of the American Society of Oral Surgeons. Biographical information is given on oral surgeons in America, arranged by state; there are brief details for surgeons in other countries. An interesting section describes the history of the speciality in the USA.

Conferences

494 The International Association of Oral Surgeons holds a conference every three years, and the *Transactions* have appeared in a variety of formats:

2nd conference, 1965. Edited by E. Husted and E. Hjørting-Hansen. Copenhagen: Munksgaard, 1967.
3rd conference, 1968. Edited by R. V. Walker. Edinburgh: Churchill Livingstone, 1970.
4th conference, 1971. Edited by L. W. Kay. Copenhagen: Munksgaard, 1973.
5th conference, 1974. Published in the *International journal of oral surgery* **3** (1974): 213–361.
6th conference, 1977. Published in the *International journal of oral surgery* **7** (1978): 234–425.
7th conference, 1980. Published in the *International journal of oral surgery* **10** (1981): supplement 1.
8th conference, 1983. Edited by E. Hjørting-Hansen. Chicago: Quintessence, 1985.

Orthodontics

Orthodontics deals with the cause, prevention and treatment of irregularities of jaw shape, and of the position of the teeth. Most work is on children, although an increasing number of adults are now seeking treatment for aesthetic reasons. Many children have jaws that are too small to allow all the teeth to erupt into their correct positions. Sometimes teeth are rotated, misplaced or crooked. The jaws may be in an unsatisfactory relationship to each other. These conditions are treated by the orthodontist, normally by appliances either fixed to the teeth or capable of being removed by the patient. Occasionally surgery is performed on the jaws.

Oral hygiene is important for the orthodontic patient, to prevent tooth decay in hard-to-clean areas of the mouth, so the orthodontist must be aware of the importance of preventive and conservative dentistry. There may also be periodontal implications in rotating teeth, or in forcing the eruption of submerged teeth.

Since orthodontic treatment is undertaken on healthy teeth, usually for the sake of appearance, it is a field of dentistry that is practised in developed countries, rather than in the Third World, where treatment of caries and periodontal disease take priority.

Books

495 Angle, E. H. *Treatment of malocclusion of the teeth.* 7th ed. Philadelphia: S. S. White, 1907. 628 pp.

Angle is regarded as the founder of modern orthodontics, and this is his classic work.

496 Bassigny, F. *Manuel d'orthopédie dentofaciale.* Paris, Masson: 1983. 210 pp.

497 Begg, P. R. and **Kesling, P. C.** *Begg orthodontic theory and technique.* 3rd ed. Philadelphia: W B. Saunders, 1977. 705 pp.

Describes a standard fixed appliance mode of treatment, which is based on a differential force technique. The authoritative text on the subject, discussing concepts of occlusion, diagnosis and practical treatment, in general terms and for specific kinds of malocclusion.

French edition published by Prelat, Italian by Edizione Odontologiche.

498 Bernlau, K. and **Bertzbach, K.** *Geschichte der deutschen Gesellschaft für Kieferorthopädie, 1907–1978.* Munich: Urban & Schwarzenberg, 1981. 200 pp.

Broadbent, B. H. Sr., Broadbent, B. H. Jr. and **Golden, W. H.** *Bolton standards of dentofacial developmental growth.* (See [277])

An important collection of cephalometric studies, described fully in the Anatomy section.

499 Foster, T. D. *Textbook of orthodontics.* 2nd ed. Oxford: Blackwell, 1982. 374 pp.

A detailed review of orthodontics and related topics: growth; the classification, diagnosis and treatment of malocclusion; orthodontic and preventive relationships. A useful book for students and clinicians.

500 **Graber, T. M.** and **Neumann, B.** *Removable orthodontic appliances.* 2nd edition. Philadelphia: W. B. Saunders, 1984. 631 pp.
An authoritative review by an American and a Czech. Chapters devoted to specific appliances describe the activator and the Bimler, Kinetor and Fränkel appliances. The uses, advantages and disadvantages of each are given, and diagnostic factors are emphasized. This is a standard text for practitioners, and often the most convenient source for information on specific appliances.

501 **Graber, T. M.** and **Swain, B. F.** *Orthodontics. Current principles and techniques.* St. Louis: C. V. Mosby, 1985. 915 pp.
This is the successor to the authoritative two-volume work by the same authors entitled *Current orthodontic concepts and techniques*, published ten years previously by W. B. Saunders. Diagnosis and treatment planning, techniques and treatment are covered, including functional, edgewise and straightwire appliances, bonding, adult orthodontics and retention.

502 **Harvold, E. P.** *The activator in interceptive orthodontics.* St. Louis: C. V. Mosby, 1974. 229 pp.
The classic text on this Scandinavian appliance, which is the subject of many journal articles but not textbooks.

503 **Houston, W. J. B.** *Orthodontic diagnosis.* 3rd ed. Bristol: John Wright, 1982. 123 pp. (Dental Practitioner Handbook no. 4.)
A concise but detailed account for students and practitioners, covering occlusion, records, relationship of the jaws, and treatment planning. Treatment methods are not discussed.
An Italian edition is published by Piccin.

504 **Houston, W. J. B.** and **Isaacson, K. G.** *Orthodontic treatment with removable appliances.* 2nd ed. Bristol: John Wright, 1980. 189 pp. (Dental Practitioner Handbook no. 25.)
Concentrates on the practical aspects of appliance design and case management, without examining specific appliances in detail.

505 **Isaacson, K. G.** and **Williams, J. K.** *Introduction to fixed appliances.* 3rd ed. Bristol: John Wright, 1984. 173 pp. (Dental Practitioner Handbook no. 17.)
Explains the basic principles common to all techniques, rather than emphasizing a particular system.
These three handbooks are a useful trio for the British practitioner or student.

506 **Mayoral, J., Mayoral, G.** and **Mayoral, P.** *Ortodoncia; principios fundamentales y practica.* 4th ed. Barcelona: Editorial Labor, 1983. 659 pp.
Acknowledged as an outstanding Spanish textbook.

507 Mills, J. R. E. *Principles and practice of orthodontics.* Edinburgh: Churchill Livingstone, 1982. 251 pp.

Designed as a basis for advanced students, but also of interest to undergraduates and clinicians. Discusses maxillofacial growth, aetiology, diagnosis and treatment of various kinds of malocclusion, cephalometry, and surgical orthodontics.

508 Muir, J. D. and **Reed, R. T.** *Tooth movement with removable appliances.* London: Pitman, 1979. 167 pp.

A practical bench manual for the general practitioner, with numerous line drawings. The emphasis is on space assessment, anchorage control and measurement of progress; functional appliance therapy is deliberately excluded. There are no bibliographical references.

509 Rakosi, T. *Atlas and manual of cephalometric radiology.* London: Wolfe, 1982. 228 pp.

Covers the general principles of cephalometry: facial landmarks, lines and angles, the significance of various skeletal, dental and soft tissue assessments, interpretation of results, and growth. Demonstrates treatment planning for class II malocclusion. A translation of the original German edition, published by Hanser.

510 Shankland, W. M. *The American Association of Orthodontists: the biography of a specialty organization.* St. Louis: American Association of Orthodontists, 1971. 843 pp.

The Association was founded in 1901, with E. H. Angle as its first president. This book chronicles its history up to 1967.

511 Thurow, R. C. *Edgewise orthodontics.* 4th ed. St. Louis: C. V. Mosby, 1982. 361 pp.

Covers the bioengineering aspects of the technique, followed by a description of the clinical procedures involved.

A German edition is published by Verlag Zahnärztlich-medizinisches Schrifttum.

512 Timms, D. J. *Rapid maxillary expansion.* Chicago: Quintessence, 1981. 140 pp.

A description of the palatal expansion technique of correcting a narrow dental arch, which uses lateral force to separate the maxillary bones and move the teeth. Topics covered include anatomy, a description of the appliance, its clinical use, prevention of relapse, and medical and surgical aspects.

513 United States. National Center for Health Statistics. *Orthodontic treatment priority index.* By R. M. Grainger. Washington, DC: Public Health Service, 1967. 49 pp.

An important document for orthodontists and planners in community dentistry, which describes the development and use of a system for studying malocclusion in population groups. It provides a means of ranking individuals according to the severity of malocclusion, degree of handicap or priority for treatment. Sixteen tables of distribution of various malocclusions are given. Findings from field examinations are weighted and summed on a ten-point scale of severity through the use of multiple regression analysis.

514 University of Michigan. Center for Human Growth and Development. *Monographs.* Craniofacial Growth Series. Ann Arbor: the Center, 1972–.

Over fifteen monographs on growth in relation to orthodontic treatment have been published, for the use of the advanced student or researcher (See also [288].) Of particular interest are:

No. 5 *Standards of human occlusal development.* 1976.
No. 6. *Factors affecting the growth of the midface.* 1976.
No. 14. *Clinical alteration of the growing face.* 1983.

515 Walther, D. P. *Orthodontic notes.* 4th ed. by W. J. B. Houston. Bristol: John Wright, 1983. 218 pp.

A short undergraduate text that provides a basis for more extensive reading. Also useful for clinicians, for quick reference or for revision. A French edition is published by Saccardin.

516 Weinberger, B. W. *Orthodontics: a historical review of its origin and evolution.* St. Louis: C. V. Mosby, 1926. 2 vols.

Volume 1 has some 200 pages on the history of dentistry in general, and a further 250 on early orthodontics up to 1870. Volume 2, also comprising some 500 pages, covers 1870–1900. Extensive quotations and illustrations from original papers are notable features of the book, and there is an extensive fifty-page bibliography.

Journals

517 *American journal of orthodontics.* 1915–. St. Louis: C. V. Mosby. Monthly.

The official journal of the American Association of Orthodontists (AAO), its constituent societies and the American Board for Orthodontics (ABO). Until 1937 it was entitled the *International journal of orthodontia and oral surgery* and was divided into two appropriate sections. In 1938 it became the *American journal of orthodontics and oral surgery*, and adopted its present title in 1948. It is one of the major journals in the speciality. Each issue includes original reports, advertisements, reviews of books and other papers, situations vacant, news, and directories of AAO and ABO officers.

518 *Angle orthodontist.* 1931–. 103 West College Avenue, Appleton, Wisconsin 54911: Angle Orthodontists Research and Education Foundation. Quarterly.

Established by the co-workers of E. H. Angle, in his memory, and an important journal in the field.

519 *British journal of orthodontics.* 1973–. Edinburgh: Churchill Livingstone. Quarterly.

Official journal of the British Society for the Study of Orthodontics. It succeeds the *Transactions of the BSSO*, which were published annually from 1908 to 1971. It is primarily devoted to original papers and case reports.

520 *European journal of orthodontics*. 1979–. Edinburgh: Churchill Livingstone. Quarterly.
Succeeds the *Transactions of the EOS*, published annually from 1909 to 1977. Published in English, but with numerous contributions by European authors.

521 *Fortschritte der Kieferorthopädie*. 1940–. Munich: Urban & Schwarzenburg. 6 issues per year.
Journal of the Deutschen Gesellschaft für Kieferorthopädie, publishing original reports, book reviews, advertisements and announcements. In German, with English and French abstracts.

522 *Information aus Orthodontie und Kieferorthopädie mit Beiträgen aus der internationalen Literatur*. 1969–. Munich: Zahnärtzlich-medizinisches Schrifttum. Quarterly.

523 *International journal of orthodontics*. 1962–. 1408 North Meade Street, Appleton, Wisconsin 54911: Federation of Orthodontic Associations. Quarterly.
An American journal, despite its title, being the organ of five organizations from the USA. Each issue lists their respective officers, and includes original papers and case reports.

524 *Journal of clinical orthodontics*. 1967–. 1828 Pearl Street, Boulder, Colorado 80302: JCO Inc. Monthly.
A popular serial among practitioners both sides of the Atlantic, with clinical papers, product news and advertisements. The current title was adopted in 1970; it was previously called *Journal of practical orthodontics*.

525 *Mondo ortodontico*. 1976–. Milan: Masson Italia Editori. 6 issues per year.
The official organ of the Società Italiana di Ortodonzia. Original papers are accompanied by English abstracts; the journal also carries news items and trade advertisements.

526 *Orthodontie française*. 1921–. Paris: Prelat. Annual.
Proceedings of the Société Française d'Orthopédie Dentofaciale. Each volume includes a list of members.

527 *Revue d'orthopédie dentofaciale*. 1969–. Paris: Association de la Revue d'Orthopédie Dentofaciale. Quarterly.

Dictionaries

528 American Association of Orthodontists. *Glossary of dentofacial orthopedic terms: orthodontic glossary*. St. Louis: AAO, 1981. 19 pp.
A simple and practical listing of common terms used in the speciality, for workers in the field, and for insurance or third pary use.

529 **Kurlyandskii, V. Y.** *Dictionary of orthopaedic stomatology.* Tashkent: Medit-sina, 1977. 428 pp.
In Russian.

Directories

530 **British Association of Orthodontists.** *Yearbook.* BAO. Annual. Available from the Honorary Secretary.
Lists members alphabetically, and gives a geographic list. Addresses of dental traders and laboratories are also given.

531 **British Society for the Study of Orthodontics.** *Membership list.* BSSO. Issued at approximately two-year intervals. Available from the Honorary Secretary.

532 **Consultant Orthodontists Group.** *Directory of consultant orthodontists.* COG, 1984. 16 pp. Available from P. H. Morse, Booth Hall Hospital, Manchester M9 2AA, England.
Lists consultants in the British hospital service.

533 *Orthodontic directory of the world.* 31st ed. Nashville: Orthodontic Directory of the World, 1982. 413 pp. plus supplement.
Lists orthodontic societies throughout the world. Gives a list of names and addresses of orthodontists, arranged by country, and has a name index.

534 **Indian Orthodontic Society.** *Directory.* IOS, 1980. 20 pp. Secretary: Dr. R. Godiawala, 5KB Community Centre, Ahmedabad.

Paedodontics

The emphasis in children's dentistry today is primarily on the prevention of dental caries and gingivitis. Because the oral structures of the child are still growing, development of the jaws and eruption of the permanent teeth have to be taken into account when planning treatment, a situation not applicable for the adult patient. Children's behaviour may give rise to problems; a child's fear or lack of cooperation have to be overcome before treatment can be carried out. The disease pattern varies between children and adults; the former are more likely to suffer from caries and to break or damage teeth, whereas adults are more prone to periodontal disease. It is apparent, therefore, that sources on anatomy and growth, preventive dentistry and orthodontics will be related items of particular interest.

Textbooks

535 **Andlaw, R. J.** and **Rock, W. P.** *Manual of paedodontics.* Edinburgh: Churchill Livingstone, 1982. 209 pp.
A useful manual for students and practitioners, describing treatment procedures

for caries, soft tissue lesions, abnormalities and traumatic injuries. Excluded are other aspects such as aetiology, clinical features, histopathology and surgery.

536 **Andreasen, J. O.** *Traumatic injuries of the teeth.* 2nd ed. Copenhagen: Munksgaard, 1981. 462 pp.
Although not restricted to the treatment of children, the emphasis is inevitably on children's teeth. The aetiology and incidence of the various kinds of injury are discussed, and treatment of fractured, dislocated and knocked-out teeth described. This is a standard reference work for all clinicians. An Italian edition is published by Edition Labor.

537 **Braham, R. L.** and **Morris, M. E.** *Textbook of pediatric dentistry.* Baltimore: Williams & Wilkins, 1980. 556 pp.
Provides a general overview of the field for practitioners and advanced students but with more detail than many other texts. Discusses growth and development, aetiology of dental disease, diagnosis and treatment, behavioural aspects and public dental health.

538 **Davis, J. M., Law, D. B.** and **Lewis, T. M.** *Atlas of pedodontics.* 2nd ed. Philadelphia: W. B. Saunders, 1981.
A volume predominantly of black and white photographs accompanied by brief descriptions, of clinical conditions and methods of treatment. Intended for practising dentists.

539 **Holloway, P. J.** and **Swallow, J. N.** *Child dental health.* 3rd ed. Bristol: John Wright, 1982. 225 pp.
A useful introduction for students or practitioners wanting a concise general introduction to the subject.

540 **Kennedy, D. B.** *Paediatric operative dentistry.* 2nd ed. Bristol: John Wright, 1979. 275 pp. (Dental Practitioner Handbook series no. 21.)
A practical manual describing conservative procedures in relation to the deciduous teeth. Topics include anatomy, radiography, treatment of carious lesions according to site, crowns and root canal treatment.

541 **McDonald, R. E.** and **Avery, D. R.** *Dentistry for the child and adolescent.* 4th ed. St. Louis: C. V. Mosby, 1983. 845 pp.
This is a standard American work on paedodontics for workers or students at all levels.

542 **Magnusson, B. O.** *Pedodontics: a systematic approach.* Copenhagen: Munksgaard, 1981. 386 pp.
A presentation of Scandinavian philosophy and practice.

543 **Rapp, R.** and **Winter, G. B.** *Colour atlas of clinical conditions in paedodontics.* London: Wolfe, 1979. 142 pp.
A collection of photographs, accompanied by brief descriptions, this is a useful adjunct to diagnosis for students and clinicians, and a supplement to conven-

tional textbooks. A French edition is published by Maloine, a German one by Hanser.

544 Sanders, B. *Pediatric oral and maxillofacial surgery.* St. Louis: C. V. Mosby, 1979. 606 pp.
A range of subjects relating to surgery are discussed, including techniques, infections, pathology, and congenital abnormalities. A useful text for general practitioners, orthodontists and paediatricians as well as paedodontists.

545 Wright, G. Z., Starkey, P. E. and **Gardner, D. E.** *Managing children's behavior in the dental office.* St. Louis: C. V. Mosby, 1983. 337 pp.
A case-orientated approach on a range of topics which include anaesthesia, gagging, restorative procedures and communication. For each theme the same format is used: case presentation, case analysis and discussion. Individual chapters do not have reading lists, but a bibliography of over 300 references is appended at the end of the book.

Journals

546 *Acta odontologica pediatrica.* 1980–. Centro de Odontología Pediatrica, Jose Joaquin Perez 101, Zona 1, Aptdo Postal 2753, Santo Domingo, Dominica. Semi-annual.
Original articles are published in English or Spanish; other features such as book reviews, abstracts from other journals and advertisements are in Spanish.

547 *Journal of dentistry for children.* 1940–. 211 East Chicago Avenue, Chicago, Illinois 60611: American Society of Dentistry for Children. Monthly.
The longest-established journal in the field with original papers, abstracts, letters and reviews. It also carries extensive advertising for products and situations vacant.

548 *Journal of the International Association of Dentistry for Children.* 1970–. International Association of Dentistry for Children. Semi-annual.
Includes original papers, reviews and advertisements. Further information from the secretary of the Association, Prof. J. J. Murray, University of Newcastle, Framlington Place, Newcastle NE2 4BW.

549 *Journal of pedodontics.* 1976–. Boston: Warren, Gorham & Lamont. Quarterly.
A publication restricted to scientific and clinical papers.

550 *Pediatric dentistry.* 1979–. 211 East Chicago Avenue, Chicago, Illinois 60611: American Academy of Pedodontics. Quarterly.
Predominantly containing scientific and clinical papers, it also includes abstracts, book reviews and advertisements.

551 *Proceedings of the British Paedodontic Society.* 1971–1984. Annual.

Published some four to six papers. From 1985, succeeded by *Journal of paediatric dentistry*. Oxford: Blackwell. Twice-yearly.

Periodontology

Periodontology comprises the study of supporting tissues of the teeth; that is, the gums and underlying bone, and the linking periodontal ligament. As far as the literature is concerned, it is a relatively self-sufficient speciality, with three core journals as the main documentary sources. In recent years, however, research on the aetiology of periodontal disease, particularly chronic inflammatory periodontal disease, has drawn on work in the fields of microbiology and immunology, which is now being reflected in citations. Entries [411]–[415] will therefore also be of interest.

Abstracting services

552 *Journal of the Western Society of Periodontology/Periodontal abstracts.* 1952–. 2626 Highland Avenue, Santa Monica, California 90405: Western Society of Periodontology. Quarterly.

Editorial policy is to present abstracts from as wide a range of journals as possible, but inevitably there is a bias towards journals in the speciality. Each issue contains approximately sixty informative, signed abstracts, equally divided into two groups, laboratory studies and clinical studies, plus an important review article. There is an interval of approximately nine months between publication of original and abstract.

Textbooks

553 **Berkovitz, B. K. B., Moxham, B. J.** and **Newman, H. N.** *The periodontal ligament in health and disease.* Oxford: Pergamon, 1982. 470 pp.

A scholarly description of current knowledge on biology and pathology, but not treatment. Intended for postgraduate students and research workers.

554 **Cimasoni, G.** *Crevicular fluid updated.* Basle: Karger, 1983. 152 pp (Monographs in Oral Science vol. 12.)

A follow-up to Cimasoni's earlier title *The crevicular fluid*, on the structure and function of the gingival fluid. For advanced workers.

555 **Fourel, J.** and **Falabregues, R.** *Parodontologie pratique.* 2nd ed. Paris: Prelat, 1980. 200 pp.

Standard French textbook.

556 **Glickman, I.** *Clinical periodontology.* 6th ed. by F. A. Carranza. Philadelphia: W. B. Saunders, 1984. 979 pp.

A comprehensive textbook for students and practitioners. It covers the periodontal tissues, the aetiology and pathology of periodontal diseases, and their treatment. Extensive reference lists are included. A useful innovation is the highlighting of key sentences by printing them in bold type. There is a French edition by Prelat, an Italian one by Editrice Scientifica, a Portuguese one by Interamericana and a Spanish by Nueva Editorial.

557 Goldman, H. M. and **Cohen, D. W.** *Periodontal therapy*. 6th ed. St. Louis: C. V. Mosby, 1980. 1,217 pp.
A standard American work for students and clinicians.

558 Lindhe, J. *Textbook of clinical periodontology*. Copenhagen: Munksgaard, 1983. 544 pp.
Contributions from eminent Scandinavian periodontologists have been coordinated by the editor of *Journal of clinical periodontology*. Half the book is devoted to the disease state itself; especially emphasized are the role of plaque as an aetiological factor, and the pathogenesis of plaque-associated periodontal disorders.

559 MacPhee, T. and **Cowley, G.** *Essentials of periodontology and periodontics*. 3rd ed. Oxford: Blackwell, 1981. 328 pp.

560 Manson, J. D. *Periodontics*. 3rd ed. London: Kimpton, 1980. 291 pp.
MacPhee [559] and this work are standard British undergraduate texts.

561 Schluger, S., Yuodelis, R. A. and **Page, R. C.** *Periodontal disease: basic phenomena, clinical management and occlusal and restorative relations*. Philadelphia: Lea & Febiger, 1977. 737 pp.
An important work for postgraduate students and clinicians in the field. The sections on occlusion and restoration are also useful for a wider readership.

562 Strahan, J. D. and **Waite, I. M.** *Colour atlas of periodontology*. London: Wolfe, 1978. 144 pp.
A useful adjunct to textbooks for students and practitioners. A French edition is published by Maloine and a German one by Hanser.

Journals

563 *International journal of periodontics and restorative dentistry*. 1981–. Chicago, Berlin, Tokyo: Quintessence. 6 issues per year.
Chiefly case reports involving periodontal and operative techniques, profusely illustrated with colour photographs and diagrams. Japanese, German, French and Italian editions are also available.

564 *Journal de parodontologie*. 1982–. Paris: Société d'Edition de l'Information Dentaire. Quarterly.
Journal of the Société Française de Parodontologie.

565 *Journal of clinical periodontology*. 1974–. Copenhagen: Munksgaard. Monthly.
Official organ of the periodontal societies of Belgium, Great Britain, France,

Holland, Germany, Greece, Ireland, Italy, Scandinavia, Spain and Switzerland. A very important title. Lengthy abstracts of each paper are given in French and German.

566 *Journal of periodontal research*. 1966–. Copenhagen: Munksgaard. 6 issues per year.
The international forum for research workers. Supplements are published irregularly, comprising abstracts or papers from the International Association for Dental Research periodontal research group conferences, and other appropriate topics.

567 *Journal of periodontology*. 1930–. Chicago: American Academy of Periodontology. Monthly.
The oldest-established extant title and the most widely read journal in the field. Includes abstracts from other journals.

568 *Journal of the New Zealand Society of Periodontology*. 1956–. Dunedin: The Society. Twice yearly.
Includes scientific papers and news.

569 *Periodontal case reports*. 1979–. New York: NE Society of Periodontologists. Twice yearly.

570 *Periodontology*. 1980–. Australian Society of Periodontology. Irregular.

SSO Schweizerische Monatsschrift für Zahnmedizin. (See [132])
Four times a year includes *Acta parodontologica*, on behalf of the Schweizerische Gesellschaft für Parodontologie. Papers are in German or French, accompanied by English, French and German abstracts. Summaries of papers in other journals are given.

Dictionaries

571 American Academy of Periodontology. *Current procedural terminology for periodontics, and insurance reporting manual*. 4th ed. American Academy of Periodontology. 1977. 52 pp.
Facilitates the reporting of periodontal services to third parties who have no specialist knowledge. Includes non-technical descriptions of periodontal procedures, and a glossary of simplified definitions.

572 American Academy of Periodontology. Committee on Nomenclature. 'Glossary of terms used in periodontology' In: *Journal of periodontology* **48** (1977): supplement 1. 31 pp.
A listing suitable for use by all dental staff.

573 Baume, L. J. 'L'adaptation de la terminologie parodontale uniformisée aux acquisitions récentes'. *Schweizerische Monatsschrift für Zahnheilkunde* **93** (1983): 649–64.

A discussion of terminology, with a lexicon of English, French and German equivalents. A modified English version is 'The adaptation in various languages of standardized periodontal terminology to recent acquisitions.' *International dental journal* **34** (1984): 135–40.

Directories

574 American Academy of Periodontology. *Directory of members of the American Academy of Periodontology.* Chicago: the Academy, 1980. 117 pp.

Pharmacology

Drugs are used in dentistry, as in medicine generally for anaesthetic, prophylactic and therapeutic purposes. It may also be significant for the dentist to know if a patient is taking any medicaments prescribed by his doctor, in case these are likely to interact with other drugs, affect dental treatment in some way, or even be responsible for oral problems. For example, phenytoin, prescribed for epileptic patients, is known to cause enlargement of the gums, while patients taking anticoagulants would obviously need special treatment if dental extractions were necessary. A precautionary course of penicillin is sometimes given to patients undergoing minor oral surgery, so the dentist will need to be notified of any allergy to this drug and be ready to substitute an alternative.

Books

575 American Dental Association. *Accepted dental therapeutics.* 39th ed. Chicago: ADA, 1982. 424 pp. Published every two years.

An invaluable handbook designed to assist the American dentist in selecting appropriate drugs and procedures for the prevention and treatment of oral disease. Includes therapeutic agents, such as anaesthetics, antimicrobial agents and antiseptics, and preventive agents, for instance fluoride compounds, dentifrices and mouthwashes. For individual drugs the actions and indications are described, as are adverse reactions, contraindications and dosage. Indexes cover distributors and brand names. Until the 32nd edition in 1967, the book was entitled *Accepted dental remedies.* Although intended for American dentists, and obviously only including drugs and brand names used in the United States, this is a valuable text for dentists in other countries as well.

Astley-Hope, H. D. and **Hellier, M. D.** *Disease, drugs and the dentist.* (See [429])
A pocket-sized *aide-mémoire* for the practitioner, intended to assist the dentist when a patient is receiving a particular drug, or has a medical condition. There are two sections: an alphabetical list of conditions, and an alphabetical list of drugs, which includes pharmacological and proprietary names.

Pharmacopoeias and Formularies

Each country will have its own pharmacopoeia, so these are not listed. The titles below relate to Britain, but are typical of publications that may be found in other countries.

576 **Association of the British Pharmaceutical Industry.** *Data sheet compendium.* London: Datapharm. Annual.
A collection of data sheets compiled and supplied by manufacturers. It is arranged alphabetically by manufacturer, and has an index of products. For each drug is given information on presentation, uses, doses and administration, contraindications, and package quantities. A useful adjunct to the *British national formulary.*

577 'Dental practitioners' formulary, 1984–1986'. In: *British national formulary.* No. 8 1984. London: British Medical Association and the Pharmaceutical Press, 1984. 33 pp.
The *British national formulary* is published quarterly, but it is envisaged that the accompanying formulary for dentists will be issued every two years. It lists preparations that dentists can prescribe for patients receiving treatment under the National Health Service; other drugs that can be prescribed to patients being treated privately are not included. As well as notes on specific preparations, there is information on prescribing for patients with systemic disease and on medical emergencies.

578 *Martindale: the extra pharmacopoeia.* 28th ed. London: Pharmaceutical Press, for the Pharmaceutical Society, 1982. 2,025 pp.
This famous publication provides a summary of the properties, actions and uses of drugs and medicines mainly for the pharmacist and medical practitioner, but will also be valuable in the dental field. The bulk of the volume contains monographs on 3,990 substances, arranged in 105 chapters, bringing together drugs of similar uses or actions. There is also information on new drugs and obsolescent ones. Over-the-counter proprietary medicines are listed. There are several indexes as follows: manufacturers' names and addresses with worldwide coverage, clinical uses, Martindale identity numbers, and of course the general index, which includes 50,000 entries to drugs, listing generic and proprietary names. For each drug, references in national pharmacopoeias and trade names used throughout the world are given. *Martindale* is available online via Data-Star.

Journals

579 *MIMS: monthly index of medical specialties.* London: Haymarket Publications. Monthly.
Issued free of charge to doctors. A valuable source for ascertaining the possible interactions or side-effects of drugs prescribed by general medical practitioners.

580 *Pharmacology and therapeutics in dentistry.* 1970–. PO Box 1452, Grand Central Post Office, New York, NY 10017: Cadmus Publishers. Quarterly.

Other Journals

Drug and therapeutics bulletin
Journal of oral medicine [443]
Oral surgery, oral medicine, oral pathology [486]

Practice Management

Included in this section are sources relevant to the administration and business side of dentistry, as opposed to the clinical aspects, which take up most of the book. Dentists wishing to practise in other countries need information on the legislation and current situation in those countries. The importance of a well-run practice is being increasingly recognized, with the present decline in caries and likelihood of overmanning in the profession. In the United States particularly, advertising, marketing and the threat of litigation are areas of current concern.

Books

581 American Dental Association. Bureau of Economic and Behavioral Research. *1982 survey of dental practice.* Chicago: ADA, [1982]. 77 pp.
The latest in a series of surveys which are conducted every two or three years, sampling dentists in private practice. There are two parts: solo dentists and independent dentists. Tables cover a wide range of topics, including the number of appointments and patient visits per week, staff, income and expenditure.

582 Barnard, P. D. *Australian dental practice surveys.* Sydney: Australian Dental Association. Annual.
Similar in scope to the American surveys, and useful for planners, administrators and practitioners.

583 Crosthwaite, D. W. *Handbook of dental practice management.* Edinburgh: Churchill Livingstone, 1982. 117 pp.
An introduction to the subject for the dentist in Britain new to general practice.

584 Department of Health and Social Security. *Dental manpower: report of the departmental study group.* Stanmore: DHSS, 1983. 109 pp.
A research document predicting future manpower requirements in Britain, but containing a considerable amount of useful statistical data. Also included is a British Dental Association report entitled *Manpower requirements to the year 2020.*

585 Domer, L. R., Snyder, T. L. and **Heid, D. W.** *Dental practice management: concepts and application.* St. Louis: C. V. Mosby, 1980. 381 pp.
More detail is given on running a practice than in Crosthwaite's book [583], but the intended readership is American, and much information is applicable only to the United States.

586 Farthing, P. *Diary of a squat; all about starting a dental practice.* Holly Tree House, 1 Blacksmiths Lane, Welby, Lincolnshire: Easicast Publications, 1982. 187 pp.

A spiral-bound, typescript publication, which is a case study of one practitioner's experience in starting a practice. The only practical book of its kind in Britain, giving facts and figures, graphs and financial data not available elsewhere.

Fédération Dentaire Internationale. *Basic fact sheets.* (See [217])

A loose-leaf publication which gives brief details on manpower, education, specialization and practice in about 100 countries.

587 Fédération Dentaire Internationale. *Handbook of regulations of dental practice.* 2nd ed. London: FDI, 1976.

A loose-leaf booklet with brief notes on legislation and regulations in some 100 countries, of particular interest to dentists wishing to practise abroad.

588 Forrest, J. O. *A guide to successful dental practice.* Bristol: John Wright, 1984. 132 pp.

Intended for the same readership as Crosthwaite [583], but with somewhat more detail.

589 Gehrman, R. E. *Dental photography: today's camera and the growing practice.* Tulsa: Penwell Books, 1982. 182 pp.

Describes techniques and equipment for the general practitioner.

590 Kilpatrick, H. C. *Work simplification in dental practice.* 3rd ed. Philadelphia: W. B. Saunders, 1974. 804 pp.

This important book is subtitled *Applied time and motion studies* but has a wider scope. Topics covered include surgery layout and design, administrative procedures, selection and use of equipment, and physical fitness. Much material is not readily accessible elsewhere. A French edition is published by Prelat.

591 Parkin, S. F. and **Oakley, J. R.** *A textbook for dental surgery assistants.* 2nd ed. London: Faber, 1983. 247 pp.

Gives an overview of professional practice in Britain, and covers anatomy, physiology and clinical dentistry in nontechnical language. Intended for student dental surgery assistants, but useful for qualified assistants too, and all non-specialists.

592 Paul, J. E. *Manual of four-handed dentistry.* Chicago: Quintessence, 1980. 155 pp.

The standard work on close support dentistry, that is, the optimum use of the dental surgery assistant in clinical dentistry. A lavishly illustrated, practical manual for clinicians in all specialities.

593 Seear, J. *Law and ethics in dentistry.* 2nd ed. Bristol: John Wright, 1981. 251 pp. (Dental Practitioner Handbooks no. 19.)

A thorough description of the professional code and legislative situation in Britain.

Journals

594 *Dental economics.* 1911–. Tulsa: Penwell Publications. Monthly.
A controlled-circulation journal, distributed in the USA.

595 *Dental management.* 1961–. New York: Harcourt Brace Jovanovich. Monthly.

Dental practice. (See [68])
A newspaper-format publication, which includes clinical articles as well as practice management. However, it is the most detailed source of features relating to the administration of a British general practice.

596 *Dentalpractice.* 1980–. 3700 West Waco Drive, Waco, Texas 76710: Stevens Publishing Corporation. Monthly.

597 *Journal of dental practice management.* 1984–. Philadelphia: J. B. Lippincott. Quarterly.
This journal and [594], [595] and [596] relate to practice in the United States. General articles are of interest to dentists outside the USA, but much material will not be relevant to practice outside North America on account of different administrative and legislative systems.

Classification

598 American Dental Association. 'Code on dental procedures and nomenclature'. 3rd ed. In: *Journal of the American Dental Association* **104** (1982): 351–6.
Designed for computer use, to facilitate payment of insurance claims. Arranges procedures and services into ten categories.

Preventive Dentistry

Although the literature of preventive dentistry relates predominantly to the prevention of dental caries, especially in children, there is today a growing awareness of the need to promote good oral hygiene in adults as well. Because caries, gingivitis and periodontal disease are related particularly to individual life style, dental health education is seen as an essential part of preventive care. In the case of caries, dietary advice plays a prominent role, whereas plaque control is essential to the prevention of periodontal disease. (Microbiological aspects of plaque are discussed elsewhere.)

Dental health education is provided by dentists on an individual basis, and also by charitable, medical or government-sponsored organizations concerned with health. To a smaller extent it is also provided by other health professionals and by manufacturers of dental products. As well as promoting appropriate attitudes and practices among the public, preventive dentistry is concerned with the actual methods the dentist can use or advocate. These include the use of fluoride in various forms, and the application of fissure sealants to children's teeth.

Books

599 Fejerskov, O. *Fluorid i tandplejen.* Copenhagen: Munksgaard, 1981. 131 pp.

600 Forrest, J. O. *The good teeth guide.* London: Granada, 1981. 192 pp.
An excellent, easy to read introduction to oral health written for the layman.

601 Forrest, J. O. *Preventive dentistry.* Bristol: John Wright, 1981. 128 pp. (Dental Practitioner Handbook no. 22.)
Discusses the chemical, irrigation and mechanical methods of plaque control, and the use of fluorides. Material also covers mother and child aspects, and prevention in relation to conservative dentistry and sports injuries.

602 Holzinger, W. *Prophylaxefibel.* 3rd ed. Munich: Hanser, 1982. 160 pp.

603 Johansen, E., Taves, D. R. and **Olsen, T. U.** *Continuing evaluation of the use of fluorides.* Boulder, Colorado: Westview Press, 1979. 321 pp. (American Association for the Advancement of Science Selected Symposia no. 11.)
Publications in this series are designed for rapid dissemination, and are therefore reproduced from camera-ready copy. This book gives a reasonably balanced view of an emotive subject. Topics covered are historical perspectives, water fluoridation, topical applications, treatment for osteoporosis, fluoride in the blood, its distribution in the body, toxicity and safety.

604 Murray, J. J. *The prevention of dental disease.* Oxford: Oxford University Press, 1983. 362 pp.
Summarizes current clinical and epidemiological knowledge on the prevention of caries and periodontal disease, with chapters written by British authorities. Chapters cover the following aspects: diet and caries, fluorides, oral cleanliness, fissure sealants, the early carious lesion, immunology and vaccines for caries, periodontal disease, orthodontics and social factors. There are extensive reference lists. The book is particularly valuable for clinicians, students at all levels and community dentists.

605 Murray, J. J. and **Rugg-Gunn, A. J.** *Fluorides in caries prevention.* 2nd ed. Bristol: John Wright, 1982. 263 pp. (Dental Practitioner Handbook no. 20.)
A description of the various uses of fluoride, including water fluoridation, tablets and drops, toothpaste and mouthwashes. Physiological aspects, fluoride toxicity and the chemical's mode of action are also covered.

606 Randolph, P. M. and **Dennison, C. I.** *Diet, nutrition and dentistry.* St. Louis: C. V. Mosby, 1981. 358 pp.
A third of the book is devoted to the principles of nutrition in general. The chapters relating to dentistry cover diet counselling, nutritional requirements for oral growth, the effect of diet on caries and periodontal disease, and the special needs of particular classes of patient: the pregnant, the aged, cancer patients and children. A text of interest to the clinician, dental health educator and dietitian, but with some controversial ideas.

607 Royal College of Physicians. *Fluoride, teeth and health.* London: Pitman, 1976. 84 pp.
Discusses the physiology and toxicology of fluoride, and the various disorders which it has been said to cause or aggravate. The report, regarded as an authoritative document by the medical communities, vindicates the safety of fluoride used for caries prevention, and recommends its addition to water supplies where appropriate levels are not already present.

608 Stallard, R. E. *Textbook of preventive dentistry.* 2nd ed. Philadelphia: W. B. Saunders, 1982. 403 pp.
An important American textbook for student and practitioner, with a wider scope than the British books. As well as covering caries and periodontology, it covers the epidemiology of oral cancer, nutrition, radiological aspects, preventive orthodontics, and the marketing of preventive dentistry.

Journals

Caries research. (See [321])
Includes academic studies on the inhibition of plaque and prevention of caries.

609 *Clinical preventive dentistry.* 1974–. Philadelphia: J. B. Lippincott. Bimonthly.
Includes original articles, product news and book reviews, and is of particular interest to the practising dentist rather than the researcher. Each issue has separate pagination. This journal succeeds the *Journal of preventive dentistry*, which was published from 1974 to 1978.

610 *Oralprophylaxe.* 1979–. Schichaustrasse 3–5, D-6000 Frankfurt am Main: W. Gerhards & Co. Quarterly.
Journal of the Deutscher Medizinischer Informationsdienst and the Verein für Zahnhygiene. The title changed in 1984; it was formerly called *Kariesprophylaxe.*

611 *Prevenzione Stomatologica.* 1973–. Milan: Masson. Bimonthly.
Includes original papers and some translations. Most articles have English summaries.

Audiovisual Material

Most countries have organizations responsible for the promotion of dental health, and many of these produce material suitable for distribution or demonstration to patients. Important British sources are as follows:

British Dental Health Foundation. (See [251]) Slide sets available for purchase.
General Dental Council. (See [254]) Slide sets available for free loan.
Gibbs' Oral Hygiene Service. (See [255]) Films, videos, pamphlets and slide sets for hire or purchase.
Health Education Council. (See [257]) Films and videos available for hire or purchase.

In the United States, the American Dental Association produces an extensive range of material, and issues a catalogue.

Prosthetic Dentistry

Prosthetics, or prosthodontics to use the American term, deals with the replacement of natural human substance which for some reason is no longer present in the body. Dental prosthetics, therefore, is concerned with the replacement of missing teeth and the associated dentoalveolar tissues, most commonly by the provision of full or partial dentures, following the loss of some or all of the natural teeth. Crowns and bridges (fixed prosthodontics) may be regarded in this category, but for the purposes of this book are treated with conservative dentistry. On a broader basis, prostheses for parts of the face itself, such as jaw implants which may be inserted following cancer operations, are included in this speciality.

Since the materials used for prostheses are of interest to all working in this field, entries [399]–[410], which deal with materials, may be of relevance. Dentists who design and fit prosthetic appliances work closely with technicians, who make the actual appliances; entries [386]–[398], on laboratory technology, may therefore also be of interest.

Books

612 Anderson, J. N. and **Storer, R.** *Immediate and replacement dentures*. 3rd ed. Oxford: Blackwell, 1981. 351 pp.

A realistic approach to complete denture prosthetics, covering the provision of temporary dentures immediately after extraction, and the modification or replacement of existing dentures. This is a practical book of value to students and clinicians.

613 Basker, R. M., Davenport, J. C. and **Tomlin, H. R.** *Prosthetic treatment of the edentulous patient*. 2nd ed. London: Macmillan, 1983. 234 pp.

A concise description of the theoretical background and clinical practice for undergraduates and practising dentists. Excluded is background information on materials, preprosthetic surgery, and laboratory techniques.

614 Boucher, C. O. *Prosthodontic treatment for edentulous patients*. 8th ed. by J. C. Hickey and G. A. Zarb. St. Louis: C. V. Mosby, 1980. 630 pp.

A standard American textbook which was known for its first six editions as *Swenson's complete dentures*. Technical and clinical procedures are described in detail, and there is a useful bibliography.

615 Brewer, A. A. and **Morrow, R. M.** *Overdentures*. 2nd ed. St. Louis: C. V. Mosby, 1980. 426 pp.

This is the most useful of several books on this specialized kind of denture, providing good descriptions of the rationale and technique for using retained roots to support a prosthesis.

616 Grant, A. A. and **Johnson, W.** *Introduction to removable denture prosthetics.* Edinburgh: Churchill Livingstone, 1983. 230 pp.
An undergraduate text for British students.

617 Heimke, G. *Dental implants, materials and systems.* Munich: Hanser, 1980. 132 pp.
Papers presented at a symposium of the European Society for Biomaterials, 1979, covering the compatibility of different materials, results of experimental studies and clinical results. Published in English, but most contributors are German.

618 Hoffmann, M. *Totale Prothesen nach dem All-Oral Verfahren.* 3rd ed. Munich: Hanser, 1981. 236 pp.

619 Lejoyeux, J. *Prothèse complète.* 3 vols. Paris: Maloine, 1976–79.

620 McCracken, W. L. *Removable partial prosthodontics.* 7th ed. by D. Henderson, G. P. McGivney and D. J. Castleberry. St. Louis: C. V. Mosby, 1981. 498 pp.
An authoritative American textbook for students and clinicians.

621 Neill, D. J. and **Nairn, R. I.** *Complete denture prosthetics: a clinical and laboratory manual.* 2nd ed. Bristol: John Wright, 1983. 172 pp.
A practical manual for undergraduate dental students and trainee or qualified technicians. Principles and procedures are explained in a simple style, and the significance of various laboratory procedures described.

622 Neill, D. J. and **Walter, J. B.** *Partial dentures.* 2nd ed. Oxford: Blackwell, 1983. 119 pp.
A companion to Neill and Nairn [621], enumerating the clinical and laboratory stages of partial denture construction, for students and clinicians.

623 Preiskel, H. W. *Precision attachments in dentistry.* 3rd ed. London: Kimpton, 1979. 292 pp.
The standard work on this specialized aspect of denture retention. Particularly useful are the descriptions of the many commercially available devices. The book is helpfully illustrated with photographs and diagrams.

624 Schnitman, P. A. and **Schulman, L. B.** *Dental implants: benefit and risk.* Bethesda, Maryland: National Institutes of Health, 1980. 351 pp. (Proceedings of a National Institutes of Health–Harvard Development Conference, 1978.)
A significant contribution to the literature on the effects of biomaterials on the body, for researchers and practising implantologists.

625 Watt, D. M. and **MacGregor, A. R.** *Designing complete dentures.* Philadelphia: W. B. Saunders, 1976. 414 pp.
Principles of design are described for students and practitioners, topics including muscle balance, support, occlusal balance, and appearance. The actual tech-

niques used are discussed in appendices, which occupy a quarter of the book. Immediate and partial dentures are excluded.

626 Woodforde, J. *The strange story of false teeth.* London: Routledge & Kegan Paul, 1968. 141 pp.
A nontechnical history of prosthetics, especially useful for the nonspecialist or lay reader. There are few references for further reading.

Journals

627 *Cahiers de prothèse.* 1973–. Paris: Prelat. Quarterly.
Papers in French, with English abstracts.

Journal of prosthetic dentistry (See [81])
The official journal of twenty-one American societies, and one of the most widely read journals in dentistry. Includes scientific and clinical papers, case reports, advertisements, news and correspondence.

628 *Proceedings of the British Society for the Study of Prosthetic Dentistry.* 1953–. Annual.
Available from the honorary secretary.

629 *Proceedings of the European Prosthodontic Association.* 1977–. Annual.
Includes abstracts or edited papers from the EPA annual conference. Copies of the *Proceedings* are usually obtainable from the honorary secretary (W. M. Murphy, Department of Restorative Dentistry, Dental School, Heath Park, Cardiff CF4 4XY, Wales).

Other Journals

Journal of dentistry [78]
Journal of oral rehabilitation [80]

Glossaries

630 Academy of Denture Prosthetics. 'Glossary of prosthodontic terms'. In: *Journal of prosthetic dentistry* **38** (1977): 70–109. Available as a separate publication from the Education and Research Foundation of Prosthodontics (c/o T. Curtis, University of California School of Dentistry, San Francisco, California 94143).
Comprises brief definitions, usually single sentences, for clinicians.

631 Batarec, E. *Lexique des termes de prothèse dentaire.* 2nd ed. Paris: Prelat, 1980. 90 pp.
Includes some English-language terms, and proper names. Provides short definitions, and often an English translation.

Public Health Dentistry

Community dentistry, as public health dentistry is also called, deals with the planning and provision of oral health services for populations rather than individuals. Groups of patients may be national (for instance, the entire population of a country), local (such as in a district health authority), or may comprise particular kinds of patient, such as children, old people or the handicapped.

The study of dental diseases, notably caries and periodontal disease, and in particular their occurrence, control and prevention is central to community dentistry. Entries [309]–[322] and [552]–[574] will therefore be relevant in this context, as will Chapter 7 and entries [229]–[238], which deal with statistical matters and surveys of dental health not described here.

Note that uniformly presented oral health data for many countries can be provided by the World Health Organization's Oral Health Unit Global Data Bank, which is described in Chapter 1, section 1.4.2.

General Sources

632 Young, A. and others. *Sources of data relating to dentistry: a catalog*. Hyattsville; Bureau of Health Manpower, 1980. 119 pp.

Available from the US National Technical Information Service, or its agencies outside the United States.

A document reproduced from typescript, for planners and administrators wanting information on the United States. Arrangement of data is by subject groups, on such topics as manpower, education, services, facilities, economics and epidemiology. For each source is given details of the data available and variables, the year they were collected and an address to contact for obtaining information.

Current-awareness Sources

633 'Current titles in community dentistry and oral epidemiology'. 1973–. In: *Community dentistry and oral epidemiology*.

About ninety papers listed in each issue, in seven subject groups, from Scandinavian, English- and German-language journals. There is a delay of some twelve months between original publication and listing.

Bibliographies

634 Hine, M. K. *Epidemiology of selected dental conditions*. Fédération Dentaire Internationale, 1963. 124 pp.

Sections are devoted to caries (the largest section), periodontal diseases, malocclusion, and cleft lip and palate, and cover studies published during the years 1950–63. Within each section papers are arranged by country studied. Only prevalence or incidence studies are listed, aetiology and treatment are excluded.

Books

635 Cormier, P. P. and **Levy, J. I.** *Community oral health: a systems approach for the dental health professional.* New York: Appleton Century Crofts, 1981. 237 pp.
Emphasizes the situation in the United States.

636 Cowell, C. R. and **Sheiham, A.** *Promoting dental health.* London: King Edward's Hospital Fund for London, 1981. 129 pp.
Discusses the causes and prevalence of dental diseases, methods of prevention and the promotion of dental health. An international comparison of dental delivery systems is made, but the provision and effectiveness of the system in the United Kingdom is the main topic under consideration.

637 Dunning, J. M. *Principles of dental public health.* 3rd ed. Cambridge, Massachusetts: Harvard University Press, 1979. 654 pp.
The standard American book on public health dentistry, this is a comprehensive text covering all aspects of the field including statistical and epidemiological methods. There is inevitably greater coverage of the delivery system in the United States than of those in other countries.

638 Frandsen, A. *Dental health care in Scandinavia.* Chicago: Quintessence, 1982. 259 pp.
A description of dental care delivery systems, dental disease, evaluation of preventive programmes, also behavioural and environmental factors and economics. There is a Spanish edition, also published by Quintessence.

639 Ingle, J. I. and **Blair, P.** *International dental care delivery systems: issues in dental health policies.* Cambridge, Massachusetts: Ballinger, 1978. 263 pp. (The proceedings of a conference sponsored by the Panamerican Health Organization.)
Chapters describe the national systems for providing dental care in thirteen countries, ranging from the United States to China, Australia and Norway. Manpower, finance and private practice in each country are discussed as appropriate. Also included are useful statistical information and many tables.

640 Kostlan, J. *Oral health in Europe.* Copenhagen: WHO Regional Office for Europe, 1979. 141 pp.
A general review of the different patterns of care, including dental health insurance, private practice and public health services. The systems in the twenty-eight individual countries in the Region are briefly described, under the following headings: historical introduction, management of oral health services, provision of these services, delivery of oral care, current problems and future plans.

641 Rhodes, J. R. and **Haire, T. H.** *Adult dental survey Northern Ireland 1979.* Belfast: HMSO, 1981. 172 pp.
A report with scope and arrangement similar to those of the more widely known survey by Todd [645].

642 Slack, G. L. *Dental public health: an introduction to community dentistry.* 2nd ed. Bristol: John Wright, 1981. 343 pp.

A standard British book and essential reading for students or practitioners in the United Kingdom. Chapters are contributed by acknowledged authorities in the field, and cover a wide range of topics: preventive dentistry, epidemiology, statistical methods, use of computers, the British dental system, planning national services, manpower needs, ancillaries, dental health education and dental education.

643 Striffler, D. F., Young, W. O. and **Burt, B. A.** *Dentistry, dental practice and the community.* 3rd ed. Philadelphia: W. B. Saunders, 1983. 512 pp.

Less biased towards the United States than some titles, it includes coverage of the sociology of dental practice, evaluation of scientific information, and epidemiology, as well as the standard topics.

644 Tiemann, B. and **Herber, R.** *System der zahnärztlichen Versorgung in der Bundesrepublik Deutschland.* Cologne: Deutsche Artzte-Verlag, 1980. 196 pp.

A valuable description of the system of dental care in West Germany; historical development, professional representation, sick funds, the panel dentist system, the benefit and contract system of dental care. This covers some seventy pages; English and French translations occupy the rest of the book.

645 Todd, J. E., Walker, A. M. and **Dodd, P.** *Adult dental health, 1978.* London: HMSO, 1980, 1982. 2 vols.

An important survey on the prevalence of dental disease, the state of teeth, and attitudes of the general public in Britain, based on a sample of some 7,200 people. The survey was undertaken by the Office of Population, Censuses and Surveys in collaboration with the University of Birmingham, and is the successor to the 1968 investigation in England and Wales, and the 1972 Scottish survey. Volume 1, *England and Wales 1968–1978*, compares the findings with those of the previous survey, describes the methodology, and covers tooth loss, sound, decayed, missing and filled teeth, and changes in dental attitudes. Volume 2, *United Kingdom 1978*, gives further analyses of the 1978 results, and tables for Scotland. Also in this volume are chapters on orthodontic–periodontal conditions, dental visits, treatment received and prosthetics.

646 World Health Organization. *Oral health surveys: basic methods.* Geneva: WHO, 1977. 68 pp.

A description of the general principles for planning, organizing and conducting surveys, the procedures for collecting basic data, for estimating treatment needs and oral health status, and for preparing survey reports.

647 World Health Organization. *Planning oral health services.* Geneva: WHO, 1980. 49 pp. (WHO Offset Publication no. 49.)

Primarily for administrators and planners in developing countries, this document describes the steps to be followed in organizing the provision of dental services, and gives examples of oral health plans. Useful facts and figures are given, many in tabular form.

Journals

648 *Community dental health.* 1984–. London: Libbey. Quarterly.
Published in collaboration with the British Association for the Study of Community Dentistry, this is especially relevant to the British situation.

649 *Community dentistry and oral epidemiology.* 1973–. Copenhagen: Munksgaard. 6 issues per year.
A commercially produced journal with international scope, which attracts authors and readers from countries all over the world. Papers are grouped into subject sections: public health dentistry, treatment needs, behavioural dental sciences, health hazards, methodology and oral epidemiology. No advertisements are carried.

650 *Journal of public health dentistry.* 1941–. Raleigh, North Carolina: American Association of Public Health Dentists. Quarterly.
Most papers relate to North America, but there is nevertheless much of interest to readers in other countries. Original reports, advertisements and book reviews are included.

Other Journals of Interest

American journal of public health
Community medicine
International journal of epidemiology
Journal of epidemiology and community health
Public health reports
Royal Society of Health journal

Dictionaries

651 Petterson, E., Loader, D. and **Nystrom, G. P.** 'Glossary of Swedish dental terms: translation of Swedish expressions to British and American English'. *Tandlakartidningen* **71** (1979): 23–9.
A listing of predominantly administrative terms used in community dentistry.

Directories

652 British Association for the Study of Community Dentistry. *Register of research projects in community dentistry* No. 2. BASCOD, 1981. 32 pp. Available from the Secretary.
Lists research in progress in Britain.

Radiography

An integral part of the diagnostic process, radiography is used by clinicians as a matter of routine. It is a tool applicable to all disciplines.

Books

653 Barr, J. H. and **Stevens, R. G.** *Dental radiology: pertinent basic concepts and their application in clinical practice.* Philadelphia: W. B. Saunders, 1980. 439 pp.
An informative, well-presented book for students and practitioners.

654 Langeland, O. E., Langlais, R. P. and **Morris, C. R.** *Principles and practice of panoramic radiology.* Philadelphia: W. B. Saunders, 1982. 458 pp.
Although early work on whole-mouth radiography was done in the late 1940s, the procedure was not widely adopted until the 1970s. This comprehensive text covers theories and techniques, but places particular emphasis on interpretation.

655 Mason, R. A. *Guide to dental radiography.* 2nd ed. Bristol: John Wright, 1982. 165 pp. (Dental Practitioner Handbook no. 27.)
A practical manual of radiographical techniques for the clinician.

656 Poyton, H. G. *Oral radiology.* Baltimore: Williams & Wilkins, 1982. 403 pp.
Primarily devoted to the interpretation of radiographs, and therefore predominantly comprising photographs with short textual accompaniments.

657 Smith, N. J. D. *Dental radiography.* Oxford: Blackwell, 1980. 132 pp.
A selective text describing techniques and use of equipment for students. Interpretation is not discussed. A useful book, but not as detailed as Mason [655].

658 Wuehrmann, A. H. and **Manson-Hing, L. R.** *Dental radiology.* 5th ed. St. Louis: C. V. Mosby, 1981. 508 pp.
An important American text, covering all aspects of the subject.

Journals

659 British Society of Dental and Maxillofacial Radiology. *Newsletter.* 1977–. Irregular.
Includes news, information and technical notes. A library list gives references to papers in other journals from the previous year; selected abstracts and book reviews are included. Available from the secretary.

660 *Dental radiography and photography.* 1928–. Rochester, New York: Eastman-Kodak. 3 or 4 issues per year.
Publishes case reports and original articles, plus some news items.

661 *Dentomaxillofacial radiology.* 1972–. International Association of Dentomaxillofacial Radiology. Twice yearly.
A highly specialized title with technical papers and case reports. Occasional supplements are published. Editor: Professor U. Welander, School of Dentistry, University of Umea, S-901 87 Umea, Sweden.

Oral surgery, oral medicine, oral pathology (See [486]).
Has a section on dental radiology each month, with two or three papers or case reports. The journal is the official publication of the American Academy of Dental Radiology.

Glossaries

662 **American Academy of Dental Roentgenology**. *Glossary of terms used in dental radiology*. Chapel Hill, North Carolina: the Academy, 1978. 64 pp.

Miscellaneous Subjects

663 **Cameron, J. M.** and **Sims, B. G.** *Forensic dentistry*. Edinburgh: Livingstone, 1974. 158 pp.

664 **Dworkin, S. F., Ference, T. P.** and **Giddon, D. B.** *Behavioral science and dental practice*. St. Louis: C. V. Mosby, 1978. 291 pp.

665 **Bates, J. F., Adams, D.** and **Stafford, G. D.** *Dental treatment of the elderly*. Bristol: John Wright, 1984. 158 pp.

666 **Nowak, A. J.** *Dentistry for the handicapped patient*. St. Louis: C. V. Mosby, 1976. 419 pp.

PART III

Directory of Organizations

Directory of Organizations

Selected List of Dental Libraries

Australia

667 Dentistry Library, University of Sydney, 2 Chalmers Street, Surry Hills, New South Wales 2010

Brazil

668 Dental Library, Faculty of Dentistry, University of São Paulo, Cidade Universitaria Armando de Salles Oliveira, 05508 São Paulo

Canada

669 Dental Library, University of Manitoba, 780 Bannatyne Avenue, Winnipeg, Manitoba R3E 0W3

Denmark

670 Royal Dental College Library, Vennelyst Boulevard, DK-8000 Arhus C

Finland

671 Dental Library, University of Helsinki, Kytosuontie 9–11, SF-00280 Helsinki 28

France

672 Centre Française de Documentation Odontostomatologique, 45 rue de la Tour d'Auvergne, F-75009 Paris

German Federal Republic

673 Bundesverband der Deutschen Zahnärzte, Universitätstrasse 73, D-5000 Cologne 41

Hong Kong

674 University of Hong Kong Dental Library, Prince Philip Dental Hospital, Hospital Road, Hong Kong

Italy

675 Universita degli Studi–Bari, Clinica Odontoiatrica e Stomatologia e Scuola de Specializzazione, Bari

Japan

676 Tokyo Dental College, 2–9–18 Misakicho, Chiyoda-Ku, Tokyo

Netherlands

677 Dental Library, Subfaculty of Dentistry, University of Nijmegen, Philips van Leijdenlaan 25, NL-6500 HB Nijmegen

Norway

678 Universitetsbiblioteket i Oslo, Odontologiske Facultet, Bibliotekjenesten, Getmyrsveien 69, Oslo 4

South Africa

679 Dental Library, University of Pretoria, PO Box 3034, Pretoria 0001

Sweden

680 University of Lund, Faculty of Odontology Library, School of Dentistry, Karl Gustafs väg 34, S-214 21 Malmö

Switzerland

681 Zahnärztliches Institut der Universität Zurich, Bibliothek, Zurich

United Kingdom

682 Library, British Dental Association, 64 Wimpole Street, London W1M 8AL

United States of America

683 Bureau of Library Services, American Dental Association, 211 East Chicago Avenue, Chicago, Illinois 60611

684 Northwestern University, Dental School Library, 311 East Chicago Avenue, Chicago, Illinois 60611

National Dental Associations

An asterisk indicates a member of the Fédération Dentaire Internationale.

Argentina

685 Asociación Odontológica Argentina, Junin 959 CP (1113), 1025 Buenos Aires

***686** Confederación Odontológica de la Republica Argentina, Rio Bamba 373–2° piso 'D', 1025 Buenos Aires

Aruba

687 Dental Association of Aruba, PO Box 230, Oranjestad, Aruba, Netherlands Antilles, W.I.

Australia

***688** Australian Dental Association, 116 Pacific Highway, North Sydney, New South Wales 2060

Austria

***689** Bundesfachgruppe für Zahnheilkunde der Österreichischen Ärztekammer, Weihburggasse 10–12, A-1011 Vienna

***690** Österreichische Gesellschaft für Zahn-, Mund- und Kieferheilkunde, Verein Österreichischer Zahnärzte, Weihburggasse 10–12, A-1011 Vienna

Bahama Islands

***691** Bahama Islands Dental Association, PO Box N-8186, Nassau, NP

Bangladesh

692 Bangladesh Dental Association, 60 Bangabandhu Avenue, Ashraf Chamber (1st Floor), Dacca

Barbados

***693** Barbados Dental Association, PO Box 95, Bridgetown, Barbados, W.I.

Belgium

694 Fédération Nationale des Chambres Syndicales Dentaires, Weggevoerdenlaan, 2 Bus Cl, B-8500 Kortrijk

***695** Société Royal Belge de Médecine Dentaire, Maison des Dentistes, Avenue de Jette 165, B-1090 Brussels

696 Société Royal Belge de Stomatologie, 16 Koningstraat, B-9000 Gent

697 Société Scientifique de Stomatologie, Maison des Médecins, 54 Boulevard de Waterloo, Brussels 1.

Bermuda

698 Bermuda Dental Association, PO Box 380, Hamilton 5

Bolivia

***699** Colegio de Odontólogos de Bolivia, Casilla 2203, La Paz

Brazil

***700** Associação Brasileira de Odontologia, Rua Alvaro de Alvim 33/37, Salas 514, Rio de Janeiro, Guanabara

Bulgaria

***701** Association Médicale Scientifique Républicaine de Stomatologie, 1, G. Sofiisky, Sofia

Burma

***702** Burma Dental Association, PO Box 1299, Rangoon

Canada

***703** Canadian Dental Association, 1815 Alta Vista Drive, Ottawa, Ontario K1G 3Y6

Chile

***704** Colegio de Dentistas de Chile, Avenida Santa Maria 1990, Castilla de Correos 252-V, Santiago

Colombia

***705** Federación Odontológica Colombiana, Calle 71 #11–10, Of. 1101, Apartado Aereo 52925, Bogotá, DE

Costa Rica

706 Colegio de Cirujanos Dentistas de Costa Rica, Ap. 698, Calle 21, avenidas 2–6 No 229, San José

Cuba

***707** Sociedad Cubana de Estomatología, 23 Y N-Vedado, Havana

Cyprus

***708** Pancyprian Dental Association, Princess Zina De Tyras Building, PO Box 2063, Nicosia

Czechoslovakia

***709** Ceskoslovenská Stomatologická Spolecnost, Karlovo nám 32, 121 11 Praha 2

Denmark

***710** Dansk Tandlaegeforening, Amaliegade 17, PO Box 143, DK-1004 Copenhagen K

Dominican Republic

***711** Asociación Odontológica Dominicana, El Conde No. 256, Apto. 202, Apartado 1002, Santo Domingo

Ecuador

***712** Federación Odontológica Ecuatoriana, PO Box 2046, Quito

Egypt

***713** Egyptian Dental Association, 42 Kasr-El-Aini Street, Cairo

El Salvador

714 Sociedad Dental de El Salvador, Av. Olimpica 4620, Col. Flor Bianca, San Salvador

Fiji

715 Fiji Dental Association, GPO Box 115, Suva

Finland

***716** Odontologiska Samfundet i Finland (Swedish-Speaking Dentists' Society), Järnvägsmannag 6, SF-00520 Helsinki 52

***717** Suomen Hammaslääkäiseura-Finska Tanlakarsallskapet (Finnish Dental Society), Akavatalo, Rautatieläisenkatu 6, SF-00520 Helsinki 52

***718** Suomen Hammaslääkäriliito-Finlands Tanläkarförbund r.y. (Finnish Dental Association), Rautatieläisenkatu 6, SF-00520 Helsinki 52.

719 Suomen Naishammaslääkärit r.y. (Finnish Women Dentists' Association), Akavatalo, Rautatieläisenkatu 6, SF-00520 Helsinki 52.

France

***720** Association Dentaire Française, 92 Avenue de Wagram, F-75017 Paris

German Democratic Republic

***721** Gesellschaft für Stomatologie der DDR, Nordhäuser Strasse 74, 50 Erfurt

German Federal Republic

***722** Bundesverband der Deutschen Zahnärzte, e.v., Universitätsstrasse 73, D-5000 Köln 41

Greece

***723** Hellenic Dental Association, 38 Themistocleous Street, Athens 142.

***724** Stomatological Society of Greece, 17 Kallirroes Street, Athens TT 410.

Guam

***725** Guam Dental Society, PO Box 2679, Agana, Guam 96910, Mariana Islands

Guatemala

726 Sociedad Dental de Guatemala, 17 Calle 14–40, Zone 13, Apartado Postal 1579, Guatemala City

Haiti

***727** Association Dentaire Haïtienne, BP 2410, 74 rue Capois, Port-au-Prince

Honduras

728 Asociación Estomatológica Honduren, Apartado Postal 274, Tegucigalpa, DC

729 Colegio Estomatológico de Honduras, Apartado Postal 555, Tegucigalpa, DC

Hong Kong

***730** Hong Kong Dental Association, Duke of Windsor Social Services Building, 8th Floor, 15 Hennessy Road, Hong Kong

Hungary

***731** Hungarian Dental Association, POB 258, H-1428 Budapest

Iceland

***732** Icelandic Dental Association, Sidúmula 35, PO Box 788, Reykjavik

India

***733** Indian Dental Association, M-75 Connaught Circus, New Delhi 110 001

Indonesia

***734** Indonesian Dental Association, Jl Salemba Raya No. 4, Jakarta Pusat

Iran

***735** Iranian Dental Association, 469 Hafez Avenue, Tehran

Iraq

***736** Iraqi Dental Association, PO Box 6040, Mansour-Ma-ari Street, Baghdad

Ireland

***737** Irish Dental Association, 29 Kenilworth Square, Dublin 6.

Israel

***738** Israeli Dental Association, 49 Bar-Kochba Street, 73427 Tel Aviv

Italy

***739** Associazione Medici Dentisti Italiani, Via Savoia No. 78, I-00198 Rome

Jamaica

***740** Jamaica Dental Association, PO Box 19, Kingston 5, Jamaica, WI

Japan

***741** Japan Dental Association, 3–16 Hayabusa cho, Chiyoda-ku, Tokyo 102

Jordan

***742** Jordan Dental Association, PO Box 1326, Amman

Kenya

***743** Kenya Dental Association, PO Box 20059, Nairobi

Korea

***744** Korean Dental Association, PO Box 41, Yung-Deung-Po, Seoul

Kuwait

***745** Kuwait Dental Association, PO Box 11066 Salaibikhat

Lebanon

***746** Ordre du Corps Dentaire du Liban, Station Nazareth, Rue Sodeco, BP 2266, Beirut

Luxembourg

***747** Association des Médecins et Médecins-Dentistes du Grand-Duché de Luxembourg, 29 rue de Vianden, Luxembourg

Malaysia

***748** Malaysian Dental Association, PO Box 237, 28 Jalan Sultan 52/4, Petaling Jaya, Selangor

Malta

***749** Dental Association of Malta, Center of the Federation of Professional Bodies, 1 Wilga Street, Paceville

Mauritius

750 Mauritius Dental Association, St. Paul Road, Vacoas

Mexico

***751** Asociación Dental Mexicana, a.c., Ezequiel Montes No. 92, Mexico 4, DF

Morocco

***752** Conseil Supérieur de l'Ordre des Chirurgiens-Dentistes du Maroc, 17 rue d'Assafi, Rabat

The Netherlands

***753** Nederlandsche Maatschappij tot Bevordering der Tandheelkunde, Beneluxlaan 31–33, PO Box 2000, NL-3430 CA Nieuwegein

754 Nederlandsch Tandheelkundig Genootschap, c/o T.G. J. Kuiperes, Valklaan 19, Maartensdijk

755 Nederlandse Vereniging van Tandartsen, Margrietlaan 21, Utrecht

New Zealand

***756** New Zealand Dental Association, 238 Remuera Road, PO Box 28–084, Remuera, Auckland 5

Nicaragua

757 Asociación Dental de Nicaragua, Apartado Postal 2606, Managua, DN

Nigeria

***758** Nigerian Dental Association, Division of Dentistry, College of Medicine, PMB 12003, Lagos

Norway

***759** Den Norske Tannlaegeforening, Kronprinsensgt. 9, Oslo 2

Pakistan

760 Pakistan Dental Association, 65 Shahrah-e-Quaid-i-Azam, Lahore

Panama

761 Asociación Odontológica Panamena, Apartado Postal 6777, Panama 5

Paraguay

***762** Circulo de Odontólogos del Paraguay, Gral. Diaz No. 980, Casilla de Correos 565, Asunción

Peru

***763** Colegio Odontológico de Perú, Los Proceres 261, Santa Constanza-Monterrico, Zona 33, Lima

***764** Academia de Estomatología del Peru, Jiron Chota No. 760, Casilla 2467, Lima

Philippines

***765** Philippines Dental Association, Cor. Kamagong and Ayala Ave., Makati, Metro Manila

Poland

***766** Polish Stomatological Society, 43/45 Kuznicza Street, 50–138 Wrocław

Portugal

***767** Associação Portuguesa de Odontologia, Rua do Barao de Sabrosa, 91–1° dito, Lisboa 1

***768** Sociedade Portuguesa de Estomatologia, Avenida Rainha da Amélia, 36 R/C dito, Lisboa 5

Romania

***769** Société de Stomatologie de l'Union des Sociétés Médicales de la République Socialiste de Roumanie, 8 rue Progresului, Bucharest 45

Senegal

***770** Association Nationale des Chirurgiens Dentistes Sénégalais, IOS/Faculté de Médecine, Dakar-Fann

Sierra Leone

***771** Sierra Leone Association of Dental Surgeons, c/o Dental Department, Connaught Hospital, Freetown

Singapore

***772** Singapore Dental Association, Alumni Medical Centre, 4A College Road, Singapore 3

South Africa

***773** Dental Association of South Africa, Private Bag 1, Houghton 2041, Transvaal

Spain

***774** Consejo General de Colegios de Odontólogos y Estomatólogos de España, Villanueva 11, Madrid 1

Sri Lanka

775 Sri Lanka Dental Association, Professional Centre, 275/5 Bauddhaloka Mawatha, Colombo 7

Sweden

***776** Swedish Dental Association, Box 5843, S-102 48 Stockholm

Switzerland

***777** Société Suisse d'Odonto-Stomatologie, Münzgraben 2, CH-3011 Bern

Syria

***778** Syrian Dental Association, Jisser Al Abiad Raiss, Egypt Street bld, No. 52, PO Box 11104, Damascus

Taiwan

779 Dental Association of the Republic of China, 199 Dung-hwa North Road, Taipei

Tanzania

***780** Tanzania Dental Association, Muhimbili Medical Centre, Dental Department, PO Box 65014, Dar es Salaam

Thailand

***781** Dental Association of Thailand, 12 Soi Prasarnmit, Sukumvit 23, Bangkok

Trinidad and Tobago

782 Dental Association of Trinidad and Tobago, 115 Abercromby Street, Port-of-Spain, Trinidad, WI

Turkey

***783** Türk Dis Tabipleri Cemiyeti, Mesrutiyet Caddesi 182, Sishane-Istanbul

Union of Soviet Socialist Republics

***784** Vsesoiuznoe Nauchno Meditsinskoe Obschestvo Stomatology (All Union Medical Society of Stomatologists), Timur Frunze Street 16, CSP Moscow 3

United Arab Emirates

***785** Emirates Medical Association, Dubai, PO Box 6600, Sh. Rashid Building, Flat 305, Zabil Street

United Kingdom

***786** British Dental Association, 64 Wimpole Street, London W1M 8AL

United States of America

***787** American Dental Association, 211 East Chicago Avenue, Chicago, Illinois 60611

Uruguay

***788** Asociación Odontológica Uruguaya, Avda. del Libertador Brig. Gal. Juan A. Lavalleja, 1464-Piso 13, Montevideo

Venezuela

***789** Colegio de Odontólogos de Venezuela, Apartado de Correos 1341, Caracas

Vietnam

790 Vietnam Dental Association, 1 Hung-Vuong Street, Ho Chi Minh City 5

Yugoslavia

***791** Stomatoloska Sekcija Szd, Komenskega 4, 61000 Ljubljana

792 Association of Yugoslav Stomatologists, Bjelave 64, Sarajevo

Zambia

***793** Zambia Dental Association, PO Box RW50 363, Lusaka

Zimbabwe

***794** Dental Association of Zimbabwe, Department of Community Medicine, Godfrey Huggins School of Medicine, PO Box A 178, Avondale, Harare

Dental Associations and Societies

795 Academy of Dentistry for the Handicapped, 4100 McEwen, Suite 101, Dallas, Texas 75234, USA
Contact point: Executive Secretary
Publication: *Special care in dentistry*

796 Academy of Operative Dentistry, PO Box 177, Menomonie, Wisconsin 54751, USA
Tel. (715) 235 7566
Contact point: Secretary-Treasurer
Publication: *Operative dentistry*

797 American Academy of Gold Foil Operators, 2514 Watts Road, Houston, Texas 77030, USA
Tel. (713) 664 3537
Contact point: Secretary
Publication: *Operative dentistry*

798 American Academy of the History of Dentistry, 3804 Hadley Square East, Baltimore, Maryland 21218, USA
Tel. (301) 243 5744 Telex 1M 301 243 5744 2
Contact point: Secretary
Publication: *Bulletin of the history of dentistry*

799 American Academy of Periodontology, 211 East Chicago Avenue, Room 924, Chicago, Illinois 60611, USA
Tel. (312) 787 5518
Contact point: Executive Secretary
Publications: *Journal of periodontology*; specialist newsletters

800 American Association of Dental Schools, 1619 Massachusetts Avenue NW, Washington, DC 20036, USA
Tel. (301) 667 9433
Contact point: Director of Business Administration
Publications: *Journal of dental education*; *Bulletin of dental education*; *Admission requirements of US and Canadian dental schools*; *Directory of dental educators*; a selection of career guidance material

801 American Association of Oral and Maxillofacial Surgeons, 211 East Chicago Avenue, Chicago, Illinois 60611, USA
Tel. (312) 642 6446
Contact point: Secretary
Publication: *Journal of oral and maxillofacial surgery*

802 American Association of Orthodontists, 460 North Lindbergh Boulevard, St. Louis, Missouri 63141, USA
Tel. (314) 993 1700
Contact point: Executive Director
Publication: *American journal of orthodontics*

803 American Association of Public Health Dentistry, 10619 Jousting Lane, Richmond, Virginia 23235, USA
Tel. (804) 786 3556
Contact point: Secretary/Treasurer
Publication: *Journal of public health dentistry*

804 American Dental Trade Association, 4222 King Street, Alexandria, Virginia 22302, USA
Contact point: Executive Secretary
Publication: *Directory*

805 American Society of Dentistry for Children, 211 East Chicago Avenue, Suite 920, Chicago, Illinois 60611, USA
Tel. (312) 943 1244
Contact point: Secretary
Publication: *Journal of dentistry for children*

806 Association of British Dental Surgery Assistants, DSA House, 29 London Street, Fleetwood, Lancashire FY7 6JY, England
Tel. (03917) 78631
Contact point: Secretary
Publication: *British dental surgery assistant*

806A Association of Dental Anaesthetists, Corbett Hospital, c/o Department of Anaesthesia, Stourbridge, West Midlands DY9 4JB, England
Contact point: Honorary Secretary

806B Association of Industrial Dental Surgeons, c/o Health Services, Marks & Spencer Plc, 47 Baker Street, London W1A 1DN, England
Contact point: Honorary Secretary

807 Australian Society for the Advancement of Anaesthesia and Sedation in Dentistry, 127 Malabar Road, South Cougee, New South Wales 2034, Australia
Tel. (02) 349 7940
Contact point: Secretary
Publication: *Dental anaesthesia and sedation*

808 British Association for Forensic Odontology, c/o 14 South Street, Romford, Essex, England
Tel. (0708) 40063
Contact point: Honorary Secretary

809 British Association for the Study of Community Dentistry, c/o Tameside and Glossop Health Authority, Greenfield Street, Hyde, Greater Manchester SK14 1DB, England
Tel. 061–368 4242
Contact point: Honorary Secretary
Publication: *Community dental health*

810 British Association of Orthodontists, c/o 6 Park Terrace, Stirling, Scotland
Contact point: Honorary Secretary
Publications: Codes of practice; Newsletter

811 British Dental Health Foundation, 88 Gurnard's Avenue, Fishermead, Milton Keynes MK6 2BL, England
Tel. (0908) 667063
Contact point: Executive Director
Publication: Newsletter; dental health education materials

812 British Dental Trade Association, 64 Wimpole Street, London W1M 8AL, England
Tel. 01–486 4856
Contact point: Secretary
Publication: *Dental trader*

813 British Endodontic Society, c/o 35 Harley Street, London W1N 1HA, England
Tel. 01–580 2710
Contact point: Honorary Secretary
Publication: *International endodontic journal*

814 British Postgraduate Medical Federation, Dental Department, 33 Millman Street, London WC1N 3EJ, England
Tel. 01–831 6222
Contact point: Postgraduate Dental Dean
Publications: *Postgraduate courses in the four Thames regions*; plus a variety of reports on postgraduate education and vocational training

815 British Society for Dental Research (incorporating the British Division of the IADR), c/o Department of Oral Biology, Dental School, Heath Park, Cardiff CF4 4XY, Wales
Tel. (0222) 755944
Contact point: Honorary Secretary

816 British Society for Restorative Dentistry, c/o Floor 27, Guy's Hospital Dental School, London SE1 9RT, England
Tel. 01–407 7600 ext. 3013
Contact point: Secretary
Publication: *Restorative dentistry*

817 British Society for the Study of Orthodontics, c/o Orthodontic Department, Eastman Dental Hospital, Gray's Inn Road, London WC1X 8LD, England
Tel. 01–837 3646
Contact point: Honorary Secretary
Publication: *British journal of orthodontics*

818 British Society for the Study of Prosthetic Dentistry, c/o Department of Prosthetic Dentistry, London Hospital Medical College Dental School, Turner Street, London E1 2AD, England
Tel. 01–247 5454 ext. 202
Contact point: Honorary Secretary
Publication: *Annual proceedings*

819 British Society of Dental and Maxillofacial Radiology, c/o Dental Hospital, Clarendon Way, Leeds LS2 9LU, England
Tel. (0532) 440111 ext. 247
Contact point: Honorary Secretary
Publication: Newsletter

820 British Society of Dentistry for the Handicapped, c/o Dental Office, Frimley Children's Centre, Camberley, Surrey GU16 5AD
Tel. 0276 681 636 ext. 227
Contact point: Secretary

821 British Society of Periodontology, c/o King's College Hospital Dental School, Denmark Hill, London SE5 8RY, England
Tel. 01–274 6222
Contact point: Honorary Secretary

822 Dental Laboratories Association, Chapel House, Noel Street, Nottingham NG7 6AS, England
Tel. (0602) 704321
Contact point: Secretary
Publication: *Dental laboratory*

823 European Dental Society, 12 Flag Walk, Eastcote, Pinner, Middlesex HA5 2EP, England
Contact point: Secretary
Publication: Newsletter

European Organization for Caries Research, (see [843])

824 European Orthodontic Society, 64 Wimpole Street, London W1M 8AL, England
Tel. 01–935 2795
Contact point: Honorary Secretary
Publication: *European journal of orthodontics*

825 European Prosthodontic Association, c/o Department of Prosthetic Dentistry, Dental Hospital and School, Heath Park, Cardiff CF4 4XY, Wales
Tel. (0222) 755944 ext. 2510
Contact point: Secretary
Publication: *Proceedings of the European Prosthodontic Association*

826 Fédération Dentaire Internationale, 64 Wimpole Street, London W1M 8AL, England
Tel. 01–935 7852 Telex 21879 IND
Contact point: Executive Director
Publications: *International dental journal*; *FDI newsletter*; *Basic fact sheets*; *Regulations of dental practice*; *Dental lexicon*; Technical reports

827 General Dental Council, 37 Wimpole Street, London W1M 8DQ, England
Tel. 01–487 2171
Contact point: Registrar
Publication: *Dentists register*

828 General Dental Practitioners' Association, 49 Cromwell Grove, Levenshulme, Manchester M19 3QD, England
Tel. 061–224 7442
Contact point: Secretary
Publication: *Probe*

829 Gibbs Oral Hygiene Service, Hesketh House, Portman Square, London W1A 1DY, England
Tel. 01–409 6445 Telex 261815 ELIGB G
Contact point: Administrator
Publication: Health education literature in various formats

830 Groupement International pour la Recherche Scientifique en Stomatologie et Odontologie, Hôpital Université St. Pierre, 322 rue Haute, B-1000 Brussels, Belgium
Publication: *Bulletin*

831 Health Education Council, 78 New Oxford Street, London WC1A 1AH, England
Tel. 01–637 1881
Contact point: Information Section
Publications: A variety of material relating to health education

832 Institute of Maxillofacial Technology, c/o West Midlands Regional Plastic and Jaw Surgery Unit, Wordsley Hospital, Stream Road, Wordsley, West Midlands DY8 5QX, England
Tel. Kingswinford (0384) 288778 ext. 259
Contact point: Honorary Secretary
Publication: *Proceedings of the Institute of Maxillofacial Technology*

833 International Academy of Gnathology, c/o 4323 Palm Avenue, La Mesa, California 92041, USA
Tel. (619) 462 9933
Contact point: President
Publication: *Journal of gnathology*

834 International Association for Dental Research, 734 15th Street NW, Suite 809, Washington, DC 20005, USA
Tel. (202) 638 1515
Contact point: Executive Director
Publication: *Journal of dental research*

835 International Association of Dentistry for the Handicapped, c/o Tandvårdsnämnden, S-172 86 Sundbyberg, Sweden
Tel. (8) 987170
Contact point: Secretary-Treasurer
Publication: Newsletter; Congress proceedings

836 International Association of Dentomaxillofacial Radiology, c/o Department of Radiology, School of Dentistry, Box 33070, S-400 33 Göteborg, Sweden
Tel. (031) 85 31 66
Contact point: Secretary General
Publication: *Journal of dentomaxillofacial radiology*

837 International Association of Oral and Maxillofacial Surgeons, c/o Department of Oral and Maxillofacial Surgery, Guy's Hospital, London SE1 9RT, England
Tel. 01–839 1758
Contact point: Secretary General
Publication: *International journal of oral surgery*

838 International Association of Oral Pathologists, c/o Faculty of Dentistry, University of Toronto, 124 Edward Street, Toronto, Ontario M5S 1G6, Canada.
Tel. (416) 978 6332
Contact point: Secretary

838A International Federation of Dental Anaesthesiology Societies, 53 Wimpole Street, London W1M 7DF, England
Tel. 01–935 1727
Contact point: Honorary Secretary

839 Lindsay Club [history of dentistry society], c/o Library, British Dental Association, 64 Wimpole Street, London W1M 8AL, England
Tel. 01–935 0875 ext. 207
Contact point: Honorary Secretary
Publication: Newsletter

840 National Advice Centre for Postgraduate Medical and Dental Education and Training, 7 Marylebone Road, London NW1 5HH, England
Tel. 01–637 5766
Contact point: Secretary to the Dental Adviser
Publications: *Careers in dentistry*; *Guide to postgraduate degrees, diplomas and courses in dentistry*

841 National Institute for Dental Research, National Institutes of Health, Bethesda, Maryland 20205, USA
Tel (301) 496 4261
Contact point: Office of Scientific and Health Reports
Publications: *NIR abstracts*; *NIDR research news; Journal of dental research*

842 Nordisk Institutt for Odontologisk Materialprøvning (Scandinavian Institute of Dental Materials), Forskningsveien 1, N-0371 Oslo 3, Norway
Tel. (02) 45 24 01
Contact point: Administrative Secretary
Publication: Annual report

843 ORCA (European Organization for Caries Research), c/o 4 Stanley Avenue, Bebington, Wirral, Merseyside, England
Tel. 051–645 2000 ext. 8837
Contact point: Secretary General
Publication: *Caries research*

844 Royal Australasian College of Dental Surgeons, 229 Macquarie Street, Sydney, New South Wales 2000, Australia.
Tel. (232) 3059
Contact point: Honorary Secretary/Registrar
Publication: *Annals of the Royal Australasian College of Dental Surgeons*

845 Société Française d'Orthopédie Dentofaciale, 9 rue de l'Arc de Triomphe, F-75017 Paris, France
Tel. (380) 72 26
Contact point: Secretary
Publication: *Orthodontie française*

846 Society for the Advancement of Anaesthesia in Dentistry, 53 Wimpole Street, London W1M 7DF, England
Tel. 01–935 1727
Contact point: Secretary
Publication: *SAAD digest*

847 Society for the Social History of Medicine, c/o 45–47 Banbury Road, Oxford OX2 6PE, England
Tel. (0865) 511730
Contact point: Secretary
Publication: Bulletin

848 World Health Organization, Avenue Appia, CH-1211 Geneva 27, Switzerland
Tel. (022) 91 3453
Contact point: Scientific Technical Officer, Oral Health
Publications: Extensive range of books, journals, reports and monographs; consult WHO catalogue for details

Schools and University Departments

Afghanistan

849 Kabul Dental Clinic and Dental School, Kabul

Algeria

850 Institut Odontologique, Institut des Sciences Médicales, Hôpital de Mustapha, Alger

~~Iraq~~
Jordan
Saudi Arabia
Ghana
~~[illegible]~~
Libya
Zaire
Sudan
Malawi
Mozambique
~~Sri Lanka~~
~~Fiji~~
Zimbabwe
Bahrain

Marmara
– Turkey

Argentina

851 Facultad de Odontología, Universidad de Buenos Aires, Marcelo T. de Alvear 2142, (1122) Buenos Aires

852 Facultad de Odontología, Universidad Nacional de la Plata, Calle 51 e/1 y 115, (1900) La Plata – prov. de Buenos Aires

853 Facultad de Odontología, Universidad Nacional de Córdoba, Estafeta No. 32 – Ciudad Universitaria, Pabellon Argentina (5000) Córdoba.

854 Facultad de Odontología, Universidad Nacional del Nordeste, Córdoba 794, (3400) Corrientes.

855 Escuela de Odontología, Universidad Nacional de Cuyo, Casilla de Correo 378, (5500) Mendoza

856 Facultad de Odontología, Universidad Nacional de Rosario, Santa Fe 3160, (2000) Rosario – Prov. de Santa Fe

857 Facultad de Odontología, Universidad Nacional de Tucuman, Av. Benjamin Araoz – 8a. cuadra, (4000) San Miguel de Tucumán

Australia

858 Dental School, University of Adelaide, Frome Road, Adelaide, South Australia 5000

859 Dental School, University of Queensland, Turbot Street, Brisbane, Queensland 4000.

860 Faculty of Dental Science, University of Melbourne, 711 Elizabeth Street, Melbourne, Victoria 3000

861 Dental School, University of Western Australia, 179 Wellington Street, Perth, Western Australia 6000

862 Faculty of Dentistry, University of Sydney, 2 Chalmers Street, Surry Hills, New South Wales 2010

863 Westmead Dental Clinical School, Old Windsor Road, Westmead, New South Wales 2145

Austria

864 Universitätsklinik für Zahn-, Mund- und Kieferheilkunde, Landeskrankhaus, A-8063 Graz

865 Universitätsklinik für Zahn-, Mund- und Kieferheilkunde, Annichstrasse 35, A-6020 Innsbruck

866 Klinik für Kiefer und Gesichtschirurgie der Universität Wien, Alser Strasse 4, A-1090 Wien

867 Universitätsklinik für Zahn-, Mund- und Kieferheilkunde, Wahringer Strasse 25a, A-1090 Wien

Bangladesh

868 Dacca Dental College, University of Dacca, Ramna, Dacca

Belgium

869 Vrije Universiteit te Brussel, AZ Dienst Tandheelkunde, Larbeeklaan 101, B-1090 Brussel

870 Université Libre de Bruxelles, Clinique Stomatologique, Hôpital Universitaire Saint Pierre, rue Haute 322, B-1000 Bruxelles

871 Rijksuniversiteit te Gent, Akademisch Ziekenhuis, Klinik voor Tand-Mond- en Kaakziekten, De Pintelaan 135, B-9000 Gent

872 Université de Liège, Institut de Stomatologie, Hôpital de Bavière, Boulevard de la Constitution 66, B-4000 Liège

873 Katholieke Universiteit te Leuven, Akademisch Ziekenhuis 'Sint Raphael' Stomatologie en Tandheelkunde, Capucijnenvoer 7, B-3000 Leuven

874 Université Catholique de Louvain, Ecole de Médecine Dentaire et de Stomatologie, Avenue Hippocrate 15, B-1200 Bruxelles

Bolivia

875 Colegio Departamental de Cochabamba, Casilla No. 1409, Cochabamba.

876 Facultad de Odontología, Universidad Mayor de San Andres, Avenida de Saavedra No. 2244, La Paz

877 Colegio Departamental de la Paz, Casilla No. 2203, La Paz

878 Escuela de Odontología de Bolivia, Colegio Departamental de Odontólogos de La Paz, La Paz

879 Colegio Departamental de Oruro, Casilla No. 329, Oruro

880 Colegio Departamental de Postosi, Hospital Unificada, Casilla No. 30, Postosi

881 Colegio Departamental de Santa Cruz, Casilla no. 4114, Santa Cruz

882 Colegio Departamental de Sucre, Casilla No. 452, Sucre

883 Facultad de Odontología, Universidad de San Francisco Xavier, Casilla Postal 266, Sucre

884 Colegio Departamental de Tarija, Casilla no. 1240, Tarija

885 Facultad de Odontología, Universidad Autonoma 'Juan Misael Saracho', Ave. Domingo Paz No. 428, Tarija

Brazil

886 Faculdade de Farmacia e de Odontologia, Universidade do Amazonas, Rua Simao Bolivar 245, Manaus, Amazonas

887 Faculdade de Odontologia, Universidade Federal do Ceará, Praca Jose de Alencar, Fortaleza, Ceará

888 Faculdade de Odontologia, Universidade Federal do Espirito Santo, Ladeira de Sao Bento 66, Vitória, Espirito Santo

889 Faculdade de Odontologia, Universidade Federal de Goias, Av. Universitaria s/n, Caixa Postal 125, Goiânia, Goiás

890 Faculdade de Odontologia, Universidade do Estado da Guanabara, Av. Pasteur, 438 – ZC82 Urca, Rio de Janeiro, Guanabara

891 Faculdade de Odontologia, Universidade do Estado de Guanabara, Avenida 28 Setembre, 87 fundos, Vila Izabel – ZC11, Rio de Janeiro, Guanabara

892 Faculdade de Odontologia, Fundação Universidade do Maranhão, Rua 13 de Maio 506, São Luís, Maranhão

893 Faculdade de Odontologia, Universidade Federal de Minas Gerais, Rua Conde de Linhares 141, Belo Horizonte, Minas Gerais

894 Faculdade de Farmácia e Odontologia, Universidade Federal de Juiz de Fora, Rua Espirito Santo 1023, Juiz de Fora, Minas Gerais

895 Escola de Farmácia e Odontologia de Alfenas, Praca de Bandeira 46, Alfenas, Minas Gerais

896 Faculdade de Odontologia de Diamantina, Rua da Gloria 201, Diamantina, Minas Gerais

897 Faculdade de Odontologia do Triângulo Mineiro, Av. Guilherme Ferreira 217, Uberaba, Minas Gerais

898 Faculdade de Odontologia, Autarquia Educacional de Uberlândia, Bairro Jardim Umuarama, Caixa Postal 564, Uberlândia, Minas Gerais

899 Faculdade de Odontologia, Universidade Federal do Pará, Praca Batista Campos 17, Belem, Pará

900 Faculdade de Odontologia, Universidade Federal da Paraíba, Rua das Trincheiras 275, João Pessoa, Paraíba

901 Faculdade de Odontologia, Universidade Federal do Paraná, Praca Santos Andrade, s/n, Caixa Postal 2558, Curitiba, Paraná

902 Faculdade Estadual de Odontologia de Londrina, Rua Pernambuco, s/n C.P.M., Londrina, Paraná

903 Faculdade Estadual de Odontologia de Ponta Grossa, Praca Santos Andrade, Edeficio das Faculdades, Terreo, Punta Grossa, Paraná

904 Faculdade de Odontologia de Pernambuco, Rua do Hospicio 949, Boa Vista, Recife, Pernambuco

905 Faculdade de Odontologia, Universidade Federal de Pernambuco, Rua Amauri de Medeiros 200, Derby, Recife, Pernambuco.

906 Faculdade de Odontologia do Piauí, Rua Benjamon Constant 1706, Terezina, Piauí

907 Faculdade de Odontologia, Universidade Federal Fluminense, Rua Visconde de Morais 101, Niteroi, Rio de Janeiro

908 Faculdade de Odontologia de Valenca, Rua Carneiro de Mendonca 139, Valenca, Rio de Janeiro

909 Escola de Odontologia de Volta Redonda, Rua Richard Nixon 76, Aterrado, Volta Redonda, Rio de Janeiro

910 Faculdade de Odontologia, Universidade Federal de Rio Grande do Norte, Av. Salgado Filho 1787, Bairro Boa Sorte, Caixa Postal 336, Natal, Rio Grande do Norte

911 Faculdade de Odontologia do Porto Alegre, Universidade Federal do Rio Grande do Sul, Rua Ramiro Barcelos 2492, Caixa Postal 1118, 90000 Porto Alegre, Rio Grande do Sul

912 Faculdade de Odontologia, Pontifacia Universidade Catolica do Rio Grande do Sul, Av. Ipiranga 6681, Bairro Partenon, Porto Alegre, Rio Grande do Sul

913 Faculdade de Odontologia de Passo Fundo, Rua Paissandu 743, Passo Fundo, Rio Grande do Sul

914 Faculdade de Odontologia de Pelotas, Universidade Federal do Rio Grande do Sul, Rua Goncalvez Chavez, s/n, Pelotas, Rio Grande do Sul

915 Faculdade de Odontologia, Universidade Federal de Santa Maria, Rua Floriano Peixoto 1184, Santa Maria, Rio Grande do Sul

916 Faculdade de Odontologia, Universidade de Santa Catarina, Rua São Francisco No. 9, Centro Florianopolis, Santa Catarina

917 Faculdade de Odontologia, Universidade de São Paulo, Rua Tres Rios 363, Caixa Postal 8216, São Paulo

918 Faculdade de Farmacia e Odontologia de Aracatuba, Rua Jose Bonifacio 1126, Aracatuba, São Paulo

919 Faculdade de Farmacia e Odontologia de Araraquara, Rua Expedicionarios do Brasil 1621, Araraquara, São Paulo

920 Faculdade de Odontologia de Bauru, Universidade de São Paulo, Alameda Universitaria 9/75, Caixa Postal 73 e 261, Bauru, São Paulo

921 Faculdade de Odontologia, Universidade Catolica de Campinas, Rua Marechal Deodoro 1099, Campinas, São Paulo

922 Faculdade de Odontologia do Lins, Av. Tiradentes 375, Caixa Postal 118, Lins, São Paulo

923 Faculdade de Odontologia de Piracicaba, Universidade de Campinas, Rua Dom Pedro II, 627, Piracicaba, São Paulo

924 Faculdade de Odontologia de São Jose dos Campos, Rua Frederico Eyer 110, Bairro São Dimas, São Jose dos Campos, São Paulo

925 Faculdade de Farmacia e Odontologia de Ribeiro Preto, Rua Tibirica 714, Ribeiro Preto, São Paulo

926 Instituto Metodista de Ensino Superior, Faculdades Integradas, Rua do Sacramento 230, Caixa Postal 5002, 09720 Rudge Ramos, São Paulo

927 Faculdade de Odontologia, Universidade Federal de Sergipe, Rua Santo Amaro 285, Aracaju, Sergipe

Bulgaria

928 Faculty of Stomatology, Higher Institution of Medicine, Georgi Sofiiski 1, Sofia

Burma

929 College of Dental Medicine, Arts and Science University, Rangoon

Canada

930 Faculty of Dentistry, University of Alberta, Room 3032 Dent./Pharmacy Building, Edmonton, Alberta T6G 2NB

931 Faculty of Dentistry, University of British Columbia, 312–2194 Health Services Mall, Vancouver, British Columbia V6T 1W5

932 Faculty of Dentistry, University of Manitoba, 780 Bannatyne Avenue, Room D-113, Winnipeg, Manitoba R3E 0W3

933 Faculty of Dentistry, Dalhousie University, Halifax, Nova Scotia B3H 3J5

934 Faculty of Dentistry, University of Toronto, 124 Edward Street, Toronto, Ontario M5G 1G6

935 Faculty of Dentistry, University of Western Ontario, 1151 Richmond Street, London, Ontario N6A 5B7

936 Faculty of Dentistry, McGill University, Donner Building, Room 420, 740 Docteur Penfield, Montreal, Quebec H3A 1A4

937 Faculté de Médecine Dentaire, Université de Montréal, CP 6209, Succursale 'A', Montreal, Quebec H3C 3T9

938 Ecole de Médecine Dentaire, Université de Laval, Ste-Foy, Quebec G1K 7P4

939 University of Saskatchewan, College of Dentistry, Saskatoon, Saskatchewan S7N 0W0

Chile

940 Facultad de Odontología, Universidad de Concepción, Casilla No. 286, Concepción

941 Facultad de Odontología, Universidad de Chile, Avenida Santa Maria 571, Santiago

942 Carera de Odontología, Universidad de Valparaiso, Subida Carvallo s/n, Playa Ancha, Valparaiso

People's Republic of China

943 Faculty of Stomatology, Beijing Medical College, Beijing

Taiwan—China

944 School of Dentistry, College of Medicine of Kao-Haiung, Kao-Haiung

945 School of Dentistry, Chinese Medical College, Taichung

946 School of Dentistry, College of Medicine of Taichung, Taichung

947 Dental Department, National Defense Medical Centre, Taipei

948 School of Dentistry, College of Medicine, Taipei

949 School of Dentistry, National Yan-Ming Medical College, Taipei

Colombia

950 Faculdad de Odontología, Universidad Metropolitana, Apartado Aereo 50576, Barranquilla

951 Faculdad de Odontología, Universidad Nacional de Colombia, Ciudad Universitaria, Bogotá

952 Faculdad de Odontología, Fundación Universitaria 'San Martin', Calle 61A, 14–28, Bogotá

953 Faculdad de Odontología, Universidad Javeriana, Carrera 7a, 40–62, Bogotá

954 Faculdad de Odontología, Colegio Odontológico Colombiano, Apartado Aereo 34196, Bogotá

955 Faculdad de Odontología, Universidad de Santo Tomas, Carrera 18, 9–27, Bucaramanga

956 Depto. Estomatológia, Division de Salud, Universidad del Valle, Apartado Aereo 2188, Cali

957 Faculdad de Odontología, Universidad de Cartagena, Apartado Aereo 1610, Cartagena

958 Faculdad de Odontología, Fundación Autonoma Universitaria de Manizales, Manizales

959 Faculdad de Odontología, Universidad de Antoquia, Apartado Aereo 1226, Medellín

960 Faculdad de Odontología, Instituto de Ciencias de la Salud, Apartado Aereo 054591, Medellín

Costa Rica

961 Universidad de Costa Rica, Ciudad Universitaria 'Rodrigo Facio', Facultad de Odontología, Costa Rica

Cuba

962 Escuela de Estomatología, Ciencias Medicas, Universidad de la Habana, Carlos III y Ave. de los Presidentes, Havana

963 Escuela de Estomatología, Universidad de Oriente, Garzon y Ave. Martires del Moncada, Santiago de Cuba, Oriente

Czechoslovakia

964 The Dental Clinic, Bezrucova 5, Bratislava

965 Stomatologicka Klinika Lekarske Fakulty, University Komenskeko, Mickiewiczova c. 13, Bratislava

966 I. Stomatologicka Klinika Lekarske Faculty, J.E. Purkyně University, Silingrovo nam. c.2, Brno

967 II. Stomatologicka Klinika University, J.E. Purkyně University, Hybesova 43, Brno

968 Stomatologicka Klinika Lekarske Faculty, Karlovy University, Hradec Králové

969 Stomatologicka Klinika Lekarske Faculty, University v Kosicich, Rotislavova c. 41, Košice

970 Stomatologicka Klinika Lekarske Faculty, Palackého University, I.P. Pavlova c. 3, Olomouc

971 Stomatologicka Klinika Lekarske Fakulty, Karlovy University, Ul. 17. Listopadu c. 1, Plzen

972 I. Stomatologicka Klinika, Karlovy University, Katerinska ul. c. 32, 2 Praha

973 II. Stomatologicka Klinika, Karlovy University, Karlovo nam. c. 32, 2 Praha

Denmark

974 Århus Tandlaegehojskole, Vennelyst Boulevard, DK-8000 Århus C

975 Københavns Tandlaegehojskole, Universitetsparken 4, Købehavn

Dominican Republic

976 Faculdad de Ciencias Médicas, Escuela de Odontología, Universidad Autónoma de Santo Domingo, Ciudad Universitaria, Santo Domingo

977 Escuela Dental, Universidad Nacional Pedro Henríquez Ureña, Santo Domingo

Ecuador

978 Colegio Odontológico de Tungurahua, Centro Comercial Ambato, Bloque 1 – 40 Piso, Ambato

979 Colegio Odontológico del Canar, Ayacucho y Vintimilla, Azogues

980 Colegio Odontológico de los Rios, 5 de Junio 409 y 27 de Mayo, Babahoyo

981 Colegio Odontológico del Azuay, Manuel Vega 2–61, Casilla 479, Cuenca

982 Colegio Odontológico de Esmeraldas, Piedrahita 504 y Colon, Esmeraldas

983 Colegio Odontológico de Bolivar, Olmedo 221, Casilla 59, Guaranda

984 Colegio Odontológico del Guayas, Lorenzo de Garaicoa 7452, Casilla 4500, Guayaquil

985 Colegio Odontológico del Cotopaxi, Guayaquil 1442 Casilla 204, Latacunga

986 Colegio Odontológico de Loja, Av. 10 de Agosto 16–07, Loja

987 Colegio Odontológico de el Oro, Rocafuerte 620 Casilla 81, Machala

988 Colegio Odontológico de Manabi, Pedro Gual 515 y Olmedo, Portoviejo

989 Colegio Odontológico de Pichincha, Wilson 660 y Juan Leon Mera, Casilla 20–46, Quito

990 Colegio Odontológico del Chimborazo, Pinchincha 2117 y Guayaquil, Riobamba

991 Bolívar 12–12, Tulcán

Egypt

992 Faculty of Dentistry, University of Alexandria, Alexandria

993 Dental School, Faculty of Medicine, Alexandria University, Alexandria

994 Faculty of Dentistry, Asyût University, Asyût

995 Faculty of Dentistry, Al-Azhar University, Cairo

996 Faculty of Dentistry, Cairo University, El Manial, Cairo

997 Faculty of Oral and Dental Medicine, University of Cairo

998 Faculty of Dentistry, Mansoura University, Mansoura

999 Faculty of Dentistry, University of Tanta, Tanta

El Salvador

1000 Facultad de Odontología, Universidad de El Salvador, Ciudad Universitaria, San Salvador

Fiji

1001 Department of Dentistry, Fiji School of Medicine, Suva

Finland

1002 Institute of Dentistry, University of Helsinki, Fabiankatu 24, SF-00100 Helsinki 10

1003 Department of Dentistry, University of Kuopio, PL 138, SF-70101 Kuopio 10

1004 Department of Dentistry, University of Oulu, Kajaanintie 52A, SF-90230 Oulu 23

1005 Institute of Dentistry, University of Turku, Lemninkaisenkatu 2, SF-20520 Turku 52

France

1006 Faculté de Chirurgie Dentaire, 14–20 cours de la Marne, F-33082 Bordeaux Cedex

1007 Unité d'Enseignement et de Recherche, 4 rue Boussingault, F-29200 Brest

1008 Faculté de Chirurgie Dentaire, 11 boulevard Charles de Gaulle, BP 176, F-63005 Clermont Ferrand Cedex

1009 Faculté de Chirurgie Dentaire, Place de Verdun, F-59045 Lille Cedex

1010 Faculté de Chirurgie Dentaire, rue Guillaume Paradin, F-69372 Lyon Cedex 2

1011 Faculté de Chirurgie Dentaire, Centre Dentaire Gaston Berger, 17/19 rue Mireille Lauze, F-13010 Marseille

1012 Faculté de Chirurgie Dentaire, 219 rue Auguste Broussonnet, F-34000 Montpellier

1013 Faculté de Chirurgie Dentaire Paris V, 1 rue Maurice Arnoux, F-92120 Montrouge

1014 Faculté de Chirurgie Dentaire, rue du Docteur Heydenreich, F-54012 Nancy

1015 Faculté de Chirurgie Dentaire, Place Alexis Ricordeau, F-44000 Nantes

1016 Faculté de Chirurgie Dentaire, Chemin de Vallombrose, F-06000 Nice

1017 Faculté de Chirurgie Dentaire Paris VII, 5 rue Garancière, F-75006 Paris

1018 Faculté de Chirurgie Dentaire, 2 rue du Général Koenig, F-51100 Reims

1019 Faculté de Chirurgie Dentaire, 2 place Pasteur, F-35000 Rennes

1020 Faculté de Chirurgie Dentaire, 1 place de l'Hôpital, F-67000 Strasbourg

1021 Faculté de Chirurgie Dentaire, 3 chemin des Maraichers, F-31400 Toulouse

German Democratic Republic

1022 Humboldt-Universität Berlin, Medizinische Fakultät (Charité), Fachrichtung Stomatologie, Invalidenstrasse 87/89, X 104 Berlin

1023 Klinik und Poliklinik für Stomatologie an der Medizinischen Akademie 'Carl Gustav Carus', Friedlerstrasse 25, X 8019 Dresden

1024 Zahn- und Kieferklinik der Medizinischen Akademie Erfurt, X 50 Erfurt, Augustinerstrasse 38

1025 Klinik und Poliklinik für Stomatologie der Ernst-Moritz-Arndt-Universität Greifswald, Rotgerberstrasse 8, X 22 Greifswald

1026 Klinik und Poliklinik für Zahn-, Mund- und Kieferkrankheiten der Martin Luther Universität Halle, Gr. Steinstrasse 19, X Halle (Saale)

1027 Universitätsklinik und Poliklinik für Zahn-, Mund-, und Kieferkrankheiten, Bachstrasse 18, X 69 Jena

1028 Fachrichtung Stomatologie der Karl-Marx-Universität Leipzig, Nürnberger Strasse 57, X 701 Leipzig CI

1029 Klinik und Poliklinik für Stomatologie der Medizinischer Akademie Magdeburg, Leipzig Strasse 44, X 301 Magdeburg 1

1030 Klinik und Poliklinik für Zahn-, Mund- und Kieferkrankheiten der Universität Rostock, Strempelstrasse 13, X 25 Rostock

German Federal Republic

1031 Rheinisch-Westfälische Technische Hochschule Aachen, Goethestrasse 27/ 29, D-5100 Aachen

1032 Freie Universität Berlin, Poliklinik und Klinik für Zahn-, Mund- und Kieferkrankheiten, Assmannshauser Strasse 4–6, D-1000 Berlin 33

1033 Universitätsklinik und Poliklinik für Zahn-, Mund- und Kieferkrankheiten, Welschnonnenstrasse 17, D-5300 Bonn.

1034 Westdeutsche Kieferklinik, Poliklinik und Klinik für Zahn-, Mund- und Kieferkrankheiten, Moorenstrasse 5, D-4000 Düsseldorf 1.

1035 Westdeutsche Kieferklinik, Klinik für Kiefer- und Gesichtschirurgie, Moorenstrasse 5, D-4000 Düsseldorf 1

1036 Universitätsklinik und Poliklinik für Zahn-, Mund- und Kieferkranke, Glückstrasse 11, D-8520 Erlangen

1037 Klinikum Essen der Ruhr-Universität Bochum, Hufelandstrasse 55, D-4300 Essen 1

1038 Zahnärztliches Universitäts-Institut der Freiherr Carl von Rothschild'-schen Stiftung 'Carolinum', Theodor-Stern-Kai 7, D-6000 Frankfurt/Main

1039 Zahn- und Kieferklinik der Universität Freiburg i. Br., Hugstetter Strasse 55, D-7800 Freiburg

1040 Zahnärztliches Institut der Justus Liebig-Universität, Am Schlangenzahl 14, D-6300 Giessen

1041 Zahnärztliche Klinik und Poliklinik der Universität Göttingen, Robert-Koch-Strasse 40, D-3400 Göttingen

1042 Poliklinik für Zahn-, Mund- und Kieferkrankheiten, Karl-Wiechert-Allee 9, D-3000 Hannover 61

1043 Universitätsklinik und Poliklinik für Zahn-, Mund und Kieferkranke, Hospitalstrasse 1, D-6900 Heidelberg

1044 Universität des Saarlandes, Klinik für Zahn-, Mund- und Kieferkrankheiten der Medizinischen Facultät, D-6650 Homburg/Saar

1045 Universitätsklinik und Poliklinik für Zahn-, Mund und Kieferkrankheiten, Arnold-Heller-Strasse, D-2300 Kiel

1046 Universitäts-Zahn- und Kieferklinik, Kerpenerstrasse 32, D-5000 Köln 41

1047 Kliniken und Polikliniken für Zahn-, Mund- und Kieferheilkunde, Ratzeburger Allee 160, D-2400 Lübeck

1048 Klinik und Poliklinik für Zahn-, Mund- und Kieferkrankheiten an der Johannes-Gutenberg Universität Mainz, Augustusplatz 2, D-6500 Mainz

1049 Klinik und Poliklinik für Zahn-, Mund- und Kieferkrankheiten der Philipps Universität, Georg Voigt Strasse 3, D-3550 Marburg/Lahn

1050 Klinik für Zahn-, Mund- und Kieferkrankheiten der Universität München, Goethe Strasse 70, D-8000 München 2

1051 Poliklinik und Klinik für Zahn-, Mund- und Kieferkrankheiten, Waldeyes Strasse 30, D-4400 Münster

1052 Zahnärztliches Universitäts-Institut, Osianderstrasse 2–8, D-7400 Tübingen

1053 Universitätsklinik und Poliklinik für Zahn-, Mund- und Kieferkrankheiten, Pleicherwall 2, D-8700 Würzburg

Greece

1054 University of Athens, School of Dentistry, Thivon St 2, Goudi Athens 608

1055 University of Salonica (Aristotle's University), Vassileos Heracliou St. 28, Salonica

Guatemala

1056 Faculdad de Odontología, USAC, Ciudad Universitaria Zona 12, Guatemala City

Haiti

1057 Faculté d'Odontologie, Université d'Etat d'Haïti, rue Oswald Durand, Port-au-Prince

Honduras

1058 Faculdad de Odontología, Universidad Nacional Autónoma de Honduras, Carretera a Suyapa, Tegucigalpa

Hong Kong

1059 University of Hong Kong School of Dentistry, Prince Philip Dental Hospital, Hospital Road, Sai Ying Pun

Hungary

1060 Fogászati Fakultás, Orvos Tudományi Egyetem (Faculty of Dentistry, University of Medical Science), Ulloi út 26, H-1085 Budapest

1061 Stomatological Clinic, Faculty of Medicine, University of Debrecen, H-4012 Debrecen

1062 Stomatological Clinic, Faculty of Medicine, University of Pécs, H-7620 Pécs

1063 Fogászati Fakultás, Orvos Tudományi Egyetem (Faculty of Dentistry, University of Medical Science), Lenin körut 64, H-6721 Szeged

Iceland

1064 Tannlaeknadeild Háskóla Islands (Dental School, University of Iceland), Reykjavik

India

1065 Punjab Government Dental College and Hospital, Guru Nanak Dev University, Amritsar 143001

1066 Government Dental College, Bangalore University, Fort, Bangalore 560002

1067 Nair Hospital College, Bombay University, Dr. A. L. Nair Road, Byculla, Bombay 400008

1068 Dr R. Ahmed Dental College and Dental Hospital, Calcutta University, 114 Acharya J.C. Bose Road, Calcutta 700014

1069 Government Dental College and Hospital, Bombay University, P. Demello Road No. 1, Fort Bombay 400001

1070 Government Dental College and Principal Hospital, Osmania University, Afzalganj, Hyderabad 500012 (AP)

1071 Dental College Hospital, Lucknow University, Lucknow 220003

1072 Madras Dental College, Madras University, Opp. Fort Railway Station, Madras 600003

1073 Dental Wing, Government Medical College, Punjabi University, 147001 Patiala, Punjab State

1074 Dental Wing, Medical College, Kerala University, Trivandrum 895011, Kerala State

Indonesia

1075 Dental Faculty, State University Padjadjaran, Kompleks UNPAD, Sekeloa, Bandung

1076 Faculty of Dentistry, Trisakti University, Jalan Kyai Tapa – Grogol, Djakarta Barat

1077 Dental Faculty, University of Indonesia, Salemba Raya 4, Djakarta Pusat

1078 Faculty of Dentistry, Professor Moestopo University, Jalan Hanglekir 1/8, Kebayoran Baru, Djakarta Selatan

1079 Dental Faculty, Gadjah Mada University, Bulaksumur, Djojakarta

1080 Dental Faculty, University Sumatera Utara, Medan

1081 Faculty of Dentistry, Airlangga University, Jalan Dharmahusada 47, Surabaya

1082 Faculty of Dentistry, Hassanudin University, Jalan Satando 25, Ujung Pandang

Iran

1083 School of Dental Medicine, University of Isfahan, Isfahan

1084 School of Dental Medicine, Meshed University, Saad Abad, Meshed

1085 School of Dental Medicine, Shīrāz University, Shīrāz

1086 School of Dental Medicine, Tehran University, Enghelab Avenue, Tehran

1087 School of Dental Medicine, National University of Iran, Ewin, Tehran

Iraq

1088 College of Dentistry, University of Baghdad, Baghdad

Ireland

1089 Cork Dental School and Hospital, National University of Ireland, John Redmond Street, Cork

1090 School of Dental Science, Trinity College, Dublin 2

Israel

1091 Hadassah School of Dentistry, The Hebrew University, PO Box 1172, Jerusalem

Italy

1092 Clinica Odontoiatrica, Università di Bari, Bari

1093 Scuola di Specializzazione in Stomatologia (Malattia della Bocca e Protesi Dentaria), Università di Bologna, Bologna

1094 Clinica Odontoiatrica, Università di Cagliari, Cagliari

1095 Clinica Odontoiatrica, Università di Catania, Catania

1096 Clinica Odontoiatrica, Università di Ferrara, Ferrara

1097 Scuola di Specializzazione in Odontoiatrica e Protesi Dentaria della Clinica Odontoiatrica Università di Firenze, Via le Morgagni, Firenze

1098 Clinica Odontoiatrica, Università di Genova, Genova

1099 Clinica Odontoiatrica, Università di Messina, Messina

1100 Clinica Odontoiatrica, Università di Milano, Milano

1101 Cattedra di Chirurgia Maxillo-Facciale, Università di Milano, Milano

1102 Clinica Odontoiatrica, Università di Modena, Modena

1103 Clinica Odontoiatrica, Università di Napoli, Napoli

1104 Clinica Odontoiatrica, Università di Padova, Padova

1105 Clinica Odontoiatrica, Università di Palermo, Palermo

1106 Clinica Odontoiatrica, Università di Parma, Parma

1107 Scuola di Specializzazione in Odontoiatrica e Protesi Dentaria, Clinica Odontoiatrica, Università di Pavia, Pavia

1108 Clinica Odontoiatrica, Università di Perugia, Perugia

1109 Clinica Odontoiatrica, Università di Pisa, Pisa

1110 Clinica Odontoiatrica, Università di Roma, Via le Regina Elena 287/a, Roma

1111 Istituto di Clinica Odontoiatrica,Università Cattolica del Sacro Cuore, Via Pineta Sachetti 526, Roma

1112 Clinica Odontoiatrica, Università di Sassari, Sassari

1113 Clinica Odontoiatrica, Università di Siena, Siena

1114 Clinica Odontoiatrica, Università di Torino, Torino

1115 Clinica Odontoiatrica, Università di Trieste, Trieste

Japan

1116 Tokyo Dental College, 1–2–2 Masago, Chiba, Chiba

1117 Kyushu University, Faculty of Dentistry, 1–1, Maidashi, 3-chome, Higashi-ku, Fukuoka

1118 Fukuoka Dental College, 700 Ooaza Ta, Sawara-ku, Fukuoka

1119 Tohoku Dental University, 31–1, Misumido, Tomita-machi, Koriyama, Fukushima

1120 Gifu College of Dentistry, 1851–1, Hozumi, Hozumi-cho, Motosu-gun, Gifu

1121 Hiroshima University, School of Dentistry, 1–2–3, Kasumi, Minami-ku, Hiroshima

1122 Higashi Nippon Gakuen University, School of Dentistry, 1757, Kanazawa, Tobetsu-cho, Ishikari-gun, Hokkaido

1123 Kagoshima University Dental School, 1208–1, Usuki-cho, Kagoshima

1124 Kyushu Dental College, 6–1, Manazuru 2-chome, Kokurakita-ku, Kita-Kyūshū

1125 Nihon University School of Dentistry at Matsudo, 870–1, Sakae-cho Nishi, 2-chome, Matsudo

1126 Iwate Medical University, School of Dentistry, 3–27, Cho-dori 1-chome, Morioka

1127 Matsumoto Dental College, 1780 Gobara, Hirooka, Shiojiri, Nagano

1128 Nagasaki University, School of Dentistry, 7–1, Sakamoto-machi, Nagasaki

1129 Aichigakuin University, School of Dentistry, 2–11, Suemori-dori, Chikusa-ku, Nagoya

1130 Nippon Dental University, Niigata, 8, Hamaura-cho, 1-chome, Niigata

1131 Niigata University, School of Dentistry, 5274, 2 ban-cho, Gakkocho-dori, Niigata

1132 Okayama University Dental School, 5–1, Shikata-cho 2-chome, Okayama

1133 Osaka University, Faculty of Dentistry, 1–8, Yamadaoka, Suita, Osaka

1134 Osaka Dental University, 47, Kyobashi 1–chome, Higashi-ku, Osaka

1135 Josai Dental University, 1–1, Keyakidai, Sakado, Saitama

1136 Hokkaido University, School of Dentistry, Nishi 7–chome, Kita 13–jo, Kita-ku, Sapporo

1137 Tohoku University School of Dentistry, 4–1, Seiryo-machi, Sendai

1138 Tokushima University, School of Dentistry, 18–15, Kuramoto-cho 3-chome, Tokushima

1139 Tokyo Medical and Dental University, School of Dentistry, 5–45, Yushima 1-chome, Bunkyo-ku, Tokyo

1140 Nihon University, School of Dentistry, 8–13, Kanda-Surugadai 1-chome, Chiyoda-ku, Tokyo

1141 Showa University, School of Dentistry, 5–8, Hatanodai 1-chome, Shinagawa-ku, Tokyo

1142 Nippon Dental University, Tokyo, 9–20, Fujimi 1-chome, Chiyoda-ku, Tokyo

1143 Tsurumi University, School of Dental Medicine, 1–3, Tsurumi 2-chome, Tsurumi-ku, Yokahama

1144 Kanagawa Dental College, 82, Inaoka-cho, Yokusuka

Kenya

1145 Faculty of Medicine, Dental Surgery Chiromo, University of Nairobi, PO Box 30197, Nairobi

Korea

1146 College of Dentistry, Seoul National University, 28 Yunken-dong, Jongro-ku, Seoul

1147 College of Dentistry, Yonsei University, 15 San, Sinchon-dong, Seodaemoon-ku, Seoul

1148 Division of Dentistry, College of Medicine, Kyung Hee University, 4 San Heegi-dong, Dongdaemoon-ku, Seoul

Laos

1149 School of Dentistry, Mahosot Hospital, Vientiane

Lebanon

1150 Ecole Dentaire de la Faculté Française de Médecine et de Pharmacie, Université Saint-Joseph, rue de Damas, Beirut

Madagascar

1151 Ecole Supérieur de Chirurgie Dentaire, Mahajanga B.P. 652

Malaysia

1152 Faculty of Dentistry, University of Malaya, Pantai Valley, Kuala Lumpur

Malta

1153 Faculty of Dental Surgery, University of Malta Medical School, Gwardamanga

Mexico

1154 Facultad de Odontología, Universidad Autónoma de Guadalajara, Tolsa 238, Guadalajara, Jalisco

1155 Facultad de Odontología, Universidad de Guadalajara, Boulevard A. Tlaquepaque y Calle 40, Guadalajara, Jalisco

1156 Escuela de Odontología, Universidad de Yucatán, Calle 57 X 60, Merida, Yucatán

1157 Escuela Nacional de Odontología, Universidad Nacional Autónoma de México, Ciudad Universitaria, México DF

1158 Facultad de Odontología, Universidad de Nuevo Léon, Salvatierra y Silao, Col. Las Mitras Norte, Monterrey, Nuevo Léon

1159 Escuela de Odontología, Universidad Michoácana de San Nicolas de Hidalgo, Rayon No. 81, Morelia, Michoacán

1160 Escuela de Odontología, Universidad Autónoma de Puebla, Av. 3 Oriente N° 402, Puebla

1161 Escuela de Estomatología, Universidad Autónoma de San Luis Potosí, Jardín Guerrero N° 10, San Luis Potosí

1162 Escuela Dental de Tampico, Universidad de Tamaulipas, Tampico

1163 Escuela de Odontología, Universidad Autónoma del Estado de México, Ave. Constituyentes No. 100, Toluca, Edo. de México

1164 Escuela de Odontología, Universidad de Coahuila, Ave. Allende 1511 Pte., Torreon, Coahuila

1165 Facultad de Odontología, Universidad Veracruzana, 20 de Noviembre e Iturbide, Veracruz

1166 Escuela de Odontología, Universidad Autónoma de Zacatecas, Francisco Garcia Salinas, Ciudad Universitaria, Calz. López Velarde, Zacatecas

Netherlands

1167 Subfaculteit Tandheelkunde der Universiteit van Amsterdam, Louwesweg 1, NL-1066 EA Amsterdam

1168 Subfaculteit Tandheelkunde der Vrije Universiteit te Amsterdam, Provisorium De Boelelaan 1115, NL-1081 HV Amsterdam

1169 Subfaculteit Tandheelkunde der Rijksuniversiteit te Groningen, Ant. Deusinglaan 1, NL-9713 AV Groningen

1170 Subfaculteit Tandheelkunde der Katholieke Universiteit te Nijmegen, Philips van Leydenlaan 25, NL-6500 HB Nijmegen

1171 Tandheelkundig Institut der Rijksuniversiteit te Utrecht, De Uithof, NL-3584 CA Utrecht

New Zealand

1172 University of Otago Dental School, 318 Great King Street PO Box 647, Dunedin

Nicaragua

1173 Universidad Autónoma de Nicaragua, Facultad de Odontología, León

Nigeria

1174 School of Dentistry, University of Benin, Benin City

1175 School of Dentistry, University College Hospital, Ibadan

1176 Department of Dental and Oral Health, Faculty of Health Sciences, University of Ife, Ile-Ife

1177 School of Dental Sciences, College of Medicine, University of Lagos, PMB 12003, Lagos

Norway

1178 Odontologiske Fakultet, Universitetet i Bergen, Arstadveien 17, N-5000 Bergen

1179 Odontologiske Fakultet Universitetet i Oslo, Geitmyrsveien 71, Oslo 4

Pakistan

1180 Teaching Dental Section, Liaquat Medical College, Hyderabad

1181 De Montmorency College of Dentistry, Ravi Road, Lahore, Punjab

Panama

1182 Universidad de Panama, Facultad de Odontología, Estafeta Universitaria, Panama

Papua New Guinea

1183 Port Moresby Dental College, PO Box 1881, Boroko

Paraguay

1184 Faculdad de Odontología, Universidad Nacional de Asunción, Dr. Manuel Dominguez 208, Apartado Postal 517, Asunción

Peru

1185 Programa Académico de Odontología, Universidad Católica de Santa María, Apartado de Correo 135, Arequipa

1186 Programa Académico de Odontología, Universidad Nacional 'San Luis Gonzaga de Ica', Bolivar 236, Ica

1187 Programa Académico de Odontología, Universidad Nacional Mayor de San Marcos, Ciudad Universitaria, Apartado 454, Lima 1

1188 Programa Académico de Estomatología, Universidad Peruana 'Cayetano Heredia', Apartado 5045, Lima 1

1189 Programa Académico de Odontologia, Universidad Nacional 'Frederico Villarreal', San Marcos 385, Lima 21

Philippines

1190 College of Dentistry, Cebu Doctors' Hospital, Cebu City, Cebu

1191 College of Dentistry, Southwestern University, Cebu City, Cebu

1192 College of Dentistry, Davao Medical School, Circumferential Road, Bajada, Davao City

1193 College of Dentistry, Mindanao Medical Foundation, Mindanao Aeronautical and Technical School, Lapu-Lapu Extension, Agdao, Davao City

1194 College of Dentistry, Centro Escolar University, E. Mendiola Street, Sampaloc, Manila

1195 College of Dentistry, De Ocampo Memorial School, 2921 Nagtahan Street, Manila

1196 College of Dentistry, Manila Central University, Mayhaligue Street, Santa Cruz, Manila

1197 College of Dentistry, National University, Jhocson Street, Sampaloc, Manila

1198 College of Dentistry, University of the Philippines, Padre Faura Street, Ermita, Manila

1199 College of Dentistry, Virgen Milagrosa, San Carlos City, Pangasinan

1200 College of Dentistry, University of the East, Aurora Boulevard, Quezon City

Poland

1201 Oddzial Stomatologiczny, Wydzialu Lekarskiego, Akademii Medycznej, Ul. Curie-Skłodowskiej 3, Gdansk

1202 Oddzial Stomatologiczny, Wydzialu Lekarskiego, Akademii Medycznej, Ul. Poniatowskiego 15, Katowice

1203 Oddzial Stomatologiczny, Wydzialu Lekarskiego, Ul. Sw. Anny 12, Kraków

1204 Oddzial Stomatologiczny, Wydzialu Lekarskiego, Akademii Medycznej, Ul. Kosciuszki 4, Łódź

1205 Oddzial Stomatologiczny, Wydzialu Lekarskiego, Akademii Medycznej, Ul. Fedry 18, Poznań

1206 Oddzial Stomatologiczny, Wydzialu Lekarskiego, Akademii Medycznej, Ul. Postancow 72, Szczecin

1207 Oddzial Stomatologiczny, Wydzialu Lekarskiego, Akademii Medycznej, Ul. Filtrowa 30, Warszawa

1208 Oddzial Stomatologiczny, Wydzialu Lekarskiego, Akademii Medycznej, Ul. Curie Skłodowskiej 58, Wrocław

1209 Oddzial Stomatologiczny, Wydzialu Lekarskiego, Slaska Akademia Medyczna, Plac Dworcowy 3, Zabrze

Portugal

1210 Servicio do Estomatologia, Hospital de Aveiro, 3800 Aveiro

1211 Servicio de Estomatologia e Cirurgia Maxilo-Facial, Hospital da Universidade de Coimbra, Bloco de Celas, 3000 Coimbra

1212 Servicio de Estomatologia, Hospital de San Jose, Lisboa

1213 Servicio de Cirurgia Plastica e Estomatologia, Hospital de S. Maria, Lisboa

1214 Servicio de Estomatologia e Cirurgia Maxilo-Facial, Hospital Egas Moniz, Lisboa

1215 Escuela Superior de Medicina Dentaria de Lisboa, Cidade Universitaria, 1600 Lisboa

1216 Servicio de Estomatologia, Hospital de S. João, Porto

1217 Servicio de Estomatologia, Hospital General de S. Antonio, Porto

Romania

1218 Facultatea de Stomatologie, Calea Plevnei 19, Raion 16 Februarie, Bucureşti

1219 Institutul de Medicina si Farmacie, Biblioteca, Piata Liberyatii No. 10, Cluj

1220 Facultatea de Stomatologie, Institutul de Medicina si Farmacie, Str. Universitatii No. 16, Iasi

1221 Sectia de Stomatologie, Institutul de Medicina Timisoara, Piata 25 August No. 2, Timisoara

1222 Facultatea de Stomatologie Institutul de Medicina si Farmacie, Tg. Mures, Str. Universitatii No. 38, Tîrgu Mures

Senegal

1223 Ecole de Chirurgie Dentaire, Faculté mixte de Médecine et de Pharmacie, Université de Dakar, Dakar

Singapore

1224 Faculty of Dentistry, University of Singapore, General Hospital, Sepoy Lines 3

South Africa

1225 Dept. of Dentistry, University of Durban—Westville, Private Bag X3, Dormerton 4015

1226 Hospital vir Tand- en Mondheelkunde, Universiteit van Pretoria, Beatrix-straat, Pretoria

1227 Faculty of Dentistry, Medical University of Southern Africa, P.O. Medunsa

1228 Faculty of Dentistry, University of Stellenbosch, Private Bag X1, Tyge-burg, 7505

1229 Dental Faculty, University of the Western Cape, Private Bag X17, Bellville 7530

1230 Oral and Dental Hospital, University of the Witwatersrand, Milner Park, Johannesburg

Spain

1231 Escuela de Estomatología, Casanova, 143, Barcelona – 36

1232 Escuela de Estomatología, Facultad de Medicina, Lejona (Vizcaya)

1233 Escuela de Estomatología, Facultad de Medicina, Ciudad Universitaria, Madrid

1234 Escuela de Estomatología, Facultad de Medicina, Oviedo

1235 Escuela de Estomatología, Departamento de Microbiología y Medicina Preventiva, Facultad de Medicina, Sevilla

1236 Escuela de Estomatología, Avenida Blasco Ibañez, 16, Valencia – 10

Sri Lanka

1237 Department of Dental Surgery, University of Ceylon, Augusta Road, Paradeniya, Kandy

Sweden

1238 University of Göteborg, Faculty of Odontology, Fack, S-500 33 Göteborg 33

1239 University of Lund, School of Dentistry, S-214 21 Malmö

1240 Karolinska Institutet, School of Dentistry, Box 3207, S-103 64 Stockholm

1241 University of Umea School of Dentistry, S-901 87 Umeä

Switzerland

1242 Zahnärztliches Institut der Universität Basel, Peterplatz 14, CH-4051 Basel

1243 Zahnmedizinische Kliniken der Universität Bern, Freiburgstrasse 7, CH-3030 Berne

1244 Institut de Médecine Dentaire, Université de Genève, 19 rue Barthelémy-Menn, CH-1205 Genève

1245 Zahnärztliches Institut, Universität Zürich, Plattenstrasse 11, CH-8028 Zürich

Syria

1246 Faculty of Medicine, University of Damascus, Damascus

Thailand

1247 Faculty of Dentistry, Chulalongkorn University, Henri Dunant Road, Bangkok

1248 Faculty of Dentistry, Mahidol University, Yotee Street, Bangkok

1249 Faculty of Dentistry, Chiang Mai University, Chiang Mai

1250 Faculty of Dentistry, Khon Kaen University, Khon Kaen

Turkey

1251 School of Dentistry, Hacettepe Faculty of Medicine and Health Sciences, University of Ankara, Ankara

1252 Faculty of Dentistry, Istanbul University, Istanbul

1253 School of Dentistry, Büyükciftlik sok. No. 6, Güselbahce-Nisantasi, Istanbul

Union of Soviet Socialist Republics

1254 Faculty of Stomatology, Erevan Medical Institute, Ul. Kirova 2, Erevan, Armenian SSR

1255 Faculty of Stomatology, Azerbaijan Medical Institute, Ul. Karaganova 13, Baku, Azerbaijan SSR

1256 Faculty of Stomatology, Minsk Medical Institute, Bazarnaja ul. 10, Minsk, Byelorussian SSR

1257 Faculty of Stomatology, University of Tartu, Tartu, Estonian SSR

1258 Faculty of Stomatology, Kalinin Medical Institute, Sovetskaja ul. 4, Kalinin, SFSR

1259 Faculty of Stomatology, Kazań Medical Institute, Universitetskaja ul. 13, Kazań, SFSR

1260 Faculty of Stomatology, Kemerovo Medical Institute, Volgogradskaja ul. 1, Kemerovo, SFSR

1261 Faculty of Stomatology, Kubarskov Medical Institute, Ul. Krasnaja 4, Krasnodar, SFSR

1262 Faculty of Stomatology, Leningrad Medical Institute, Ul. Lva Tolstogo 6/8, Leningrad, SFSR

1263 Moscow Medical Stomatological Institute, Kalzaevskaja ul. 18, Moscow, SFSR

1264 Faculty of Stomatology, Omsk Medical Institute, Ul. Lenina 9, Omsk, SFSR

1265 Faculty of Stomatology, Perm' Medical Institute, Kommunisticeskaja ul. 26, Perm', SFSR

1266 Faculty of Stomatology, Smolensk Medical Institute, Ul. Proletarskaja 3, Smolensk, SFSR

1267 Faculty of Stomatology, Stavropol' Medical Institute, Morozova ul. 8, Stavropol, SFSR

1268 Faculty of Stomatology, Volgograd Medical Institute, Leninskaja ul. 21, Volgograd, SFSR

1269 Faculty of Stomatology, Voronezh Medical Institute, Studenceskaja ul. 10, Voronezh, SFSR

1270 Faculty of Stomatology, Tadzhik Medical Institute, Ul. Kirova 68/87, Dushanbe, Tadzhik SSR

1271 Faculty of Stomatology, Dnepropetrovsk Medical Institute, Ul. Dzerzinskogo 9, Dnepropetrovsk, Ukrainian SSR

1272 Faculty of Stomatology, Donetsk Medical Institute, Ul. Artema 57, Donetsk, Ukrainian SSR

1273 Harkov Medical Stomatological Institute, Ul. Luskina 53, Harkov, Ukrainian SSR

1274 Faculty of Stomatology, Kiev Medical Institute, Ul. Sevcenko 15, Kiev, Ukrainian SSR

1275 Faculty of Stomatology, L'vov Medical Institute, Pekarskaja ul. 69, L'vov, Ukrainian SSR

1276 Faculty of Stomatology, Odessa Medical Institute, Medicinskij per. 2, Odessa, Ukrainian SSR

1277 Faculty of Stomatology, Tashkent Medical Institute, Ul. Karla Marksa 25, Tashkent, Uzbekistan SSR

United Kingdom—England

1278 Dental School, University of Birmingham, St Chad's, Queensway, Birmingham B4 6NN

1279 Dental School, University of Bristol, Lower Maudlin Street, Bristol BS1 2LY

1280 School of Dentistry, University of Leeds, Clarendon Way, Leeds LS2 9LU

1281 School of Dental Surgery, University of Liverpool, Pembroke Place, Liverpool L3 5PS

1282 United Medical and Dental Schools of Guy's and St. Thomas's Hospitals, St. Thomas's Street, London Bridge, London SE1 9RT

1283 Kings College Hospital Medical School, School of Dental Surgery, Denmark Hill, London SE5 8RX

1284 London Hospital Medical College, Dental School, Turner Street, London E1 2AD

1285 University College Hospital Dental School, Mortimer Market, Tottenham Court Road, London WC1E 6JD

1286 Institute of Dental Surgery, Eastman Dental Hospital, Gray's Inn Road, London WC1X 8LD

1287 Turner Dental School, University of Manchester, Bridgeford Street, Manchester M15 6FH

1288 Dental School, University of Newcastle upon Tyne, Framlington Place, Newcastle upon Tyne NE2 4BW

1289 School of Clinical Dentistry, University of Sheffield, Charles Clifford Dental Hospital, Wellesley Road, Sheffield S10 2SZ

United Kingdom—Northern Ireland

1290 Queen's University of Belfast, Grosvenor Road, Belfast BT7 1NN

United Kingdom—Scotland

1291 Dental School, University of Dundee, Park Place, Dundee DD1 4HR

1292 School of Dental Surgery, University of Edinburgh, Chambers Street, Edinburgh EH1 1JA

1293 University of Glasgow, Glasgow Dental School, 378 Sauchiehall Street, Glasgow G2 3JZ

United Kingdom—Wales

1294 Welsh National School of Medicine, Dental School, Heath Park, Cardiff CF4 4XY

USA

1295 School of Dentistry, University of Alabama, 1919 Seventh Avenue S, Birmingham, Alabama 35294

1296 School of Dentistry, Loma Linda University, Loma Linda, California 92345

1297 School of Dentistry, University of California at Los Angeles, Center for the Health Sciences, Los Angeles, California 90024

1298 School of Dentistry, University of Southern California, 925 West 34th Street, Los Angeles, California 90007

1299 School of Dentistry, University of California, San Francisco, California 94143

1300 School of Dentistry, University of the Pacific, 2155 Webster Street, San Francisco, California 94115

1301 School of Dentistry, University of Colorado Medical Center, 4200 East Ninth Avenue, Denver, Colorado 80262

1302 School of Dental Medicine, The University of Connecticut Health Center, 263 Farmington Avenue, Farmington, Connecticut 06032

1303 School of Dentistry, Georgetown University, 3900 Reservoir Road, NW, Washington, DC 20007

1304 College of Dentistry, Howard University, 600 'W' Street, NW, Washington, DC 20059

1305 College of Dentistry, University of Florida, J. Hillis Miller Health Center, Gainesville, Florida 32610

1306 School of Dentistry, Emory University, Atlanta, Georgia 30322

1307 School of Dentistry, Medical College of Georgia, Augusta, Georgia 30902

1308 College of Dentistry, University of Illinois, 801 South Paulina Street, Chicago, Illinois 60612

1309 Northwestern University Dental School, 311 East Chicago Avenue, Chicago, Illinois 60611

1310 School of Dentistry, Loyola University of Chicago, 2160 South First Avenue, Maywood, Illinois 60153

1311 School of Dental Medicine, Southern Illinois University, Edwardsville, Illinois 62025

1312 School of Dentistry, Indiana University, 1121 West Michigan Street, Indianapolis, Indiana 46202

1313 College of Dentistry, The University of Iowa, Dental Building, Iowa City, Iowa 52242

1314 College of Dentistry, University of Kentucky Medical Center, Lexington, Kentucky 40506

1315 School of Dentistry, University of Louisville, Health Sciences Building, Box 35260, Louisville, Kentucky 40232

1316 School of Dentistry, Louisiana State University, Medical Center, 1100 Florida Avenue, Building 101, New Orleans, Louisiana 70119

1317 Baltimore College of Dental Surgery, University of Maryland, 666 West Baltimore Street, Baltimore, Maryland 21201

1318 Harvard School of Dental Medicine, 188 Longwood Avenue, Boston, Massachusetts 02115

1319 School of Dental Medicine, Tufts University, 1 Kneeland Street, Boston, Massachusetts 12111

1320 Goldman School of Graduate Dentistry, Boston University, 100 East Newton Street, Boston, Massachusetts 02118

1321 School of Dentistry, University of Michigan, Ann Arbor, Michigan 48109

1322 School of Dentistry, University of Detroit, 2985 East Jefferson Avenue, Detroit, Michigan 48207

1323 School of Dentistry, University of Minnesota, 515 SE Delaware Street, Minneapolis, Minnesota 55455

1324 University of Mississippi, School of Dentistry, Medical Center, 2500 North State Street, Jackson, Mississippi 39216

1325 School of Dentistry, University of Missouri at Kansas City, 650 East 25th Street, Kansas City, Missouri 54108

1326 School of Dental Medicine, Washington University, 4559 Scott Avenue, St. Louis, Missouri 63110

1327 College of Dentistry, University of Nebraska, 40th and Holdrege Street, Lincoln, Nebraska 68583

1328 Boyne School of Dental Science, Creighton University, 2500 California Street, Omaha, Nebraska 68178

1329 College of Medicine and Dentistry of New Jersey, New Jersey Dental School, 100 Bergen Street, Newark, New Jersey 07103

1330 School of Dentistry, Fairleigh Dickinson University, 110 Fuller Place, Hackensack, New Jersey 07601

1331 School of Dentistry, State University of New York at Buffalo, Farber Hall, 3435 Main Street, Buffalo, New York 14214

1332 School of Dental Medicine, State University of New York at Stony Brook, Health Sciences Center, Stony Brook, New York 11794

1333 School of Dental and Oral Surgery, Columbia University, 630 West 168th Street, New York, New York 10032

1334 College of Dentistry, New York University, 421 First Avenue, New York NY 10010

1335 School of Dentistry, University of North Carolina, PO Box 750, Chapel Hill 27514, North Carolina

1336 School of Dentistry, Ohio State University, 305 West 12th Avenue, Columbus, Ohio 43210

1337 College of Dentistry, University of Oklahoma, Health Science Center, PO Box 26901, Oklahoma City, Oklahoma 73190

1338 Oral Roberts University School of Dentistry, 7777 South Lewis Avenue, Tulsa, Oklahoma 74136

1339 School of Dentistry, University of Oregon, Health Science Center, 611 SW Campus Drive, Sam Jackson Park, Portland, Oregon 97201

1340 School of Dental Medicine, University of Pennsylvania, 4001 West Spruce Street, Philadelphia, Pennsylvania 19104

1341 School of Dentistry, Temple University, 3223 North Broad Street, Philadelphia, Pennsylvania 19140

1342 School of Dental Medicine, University of Pittsburgh, 3501 Terrace Street, Pittsburgh, Pennsylvania 15261

1343 School of Dentistry, University of Puerto Rico, San Juan, Puerto Rico 00905

1344 College of Dental Medicine, Medical University of South Carolina, 171 Ashley Avenue, Charleston, South Carolina 29403

1345 College of Dentistry, University of Tennessee, 875 Union Avenue, Memphis, Tennessee 38163

1346 School of Dentistry, Meharry Medical College, 1005 18th Avenue N, Nashville, Tennessee 37208

1347 Baylor College of Dentistry, 3302 Gasston Avenue, Dallas, Texas 75246

1348 University of Texas, Health Sciences Center at Houston, Dental Branch, 6516 John Freeman Avenue, Houston, Texas 77025

1349 University of Texas, Health Sciences Center at San Antonio, Dental School, 7703 Floyd Curl Drive, San Antonio, Texas 78229

1350 School of Dentistry, Virginia Commonwealth University, Medical College of Virginia, Box 637 MCV Station, Richmond, Virginia 23298

1351 School of Dentistry, University of Washington, Health Sciences Building SC 62, Seattle, Washington 98195

1352 School of Dentistry, West Virginia University, Medical Center, Morgantown, West Virginia 26506

1353 School of Dentistry, Marquette University, 604 North 16th Street, Milwaukee, Wisconsin 53233

Uruguay

1354 Facultad de Odontología, Universidad de la República Oriental del Uruguay, General Las Heras 1925, Montevideo

Venezuela

1355 Facultad de Odontología, Universidad Central de Venezuela, Apartado del Este No. 5351, Caracas

1356 Facultad de Odontología, Universidad de Los Andes, Mérida

1357 Facultad de Odontología, Universidad del Zulia, Calle 65 Esq. Avenida 19, Maracaibo, Zulia

Vietnam

1358 Faculty of Dentistry, University of Saigon, Ho Chi Minh City

Yugoslavia

1359 Stomatoloski Fakultet, Univerzitet u Beogradu, Rankeová 4, 11000 Beograd

1360 Medicinska Fakulteta, Odsek za Stomatologijo, Univerzitet Edvarda Kardelja u Ljubljani, Vrazov trg 2, 61000 Ljubljana

1361 Stomatoloski Odsek Med. Fak., Univerzitet u Nisu, Bracé Tascovica b.b., 1800 Nisu

1362 Stomatoloski Odsek Med. Fak. Univerzitet u Novom Sadu, Hajduk Velkova 12, 21000 Novi Sad

1363 Stomatoloski Odsek Med. Fak. 38000 Priština

1364 Stomatoloski Odsek Med. Fak., Borisa Kidrica 40, 51000 Rijeka

1365 Stomatoloski Fakultet, Univerzitet u Sarajevu, Mose Pijada 4a, 71000 Sarajevo

1366 Stomatoloski Fakultet, Univerzitet vu Skopje, Vodnjanska 17, 91000 Skopje

1367 Stomatoloski Fakultet, Sveucilista u Zagrebu, Gunduliceva 5, 41000 Zagreb

Publishers

1368 Academic Press, 24–28 Oval Road, London NW1 7DX, England

1369 Ballinger Publishers, 54 Church Street, Cambridge, Massachusetts 02138, USA

1370 Johann Ambrosius Barth, DDR 7010 Leipzig, Salomonstrasse 18B, Postfach 109, German Democratic Republic

1371 Blackwell Scientific Publications, Osney Mead, Oxford OX2 0EL, England

1372 Bowker Ltd, 1180 Avenue of the Americas, New York, New York 10036, USA

1373 British Library Lending Division, Boston Spa, Wetherby, West Yorkshire LS23 7BQ, England

1374 Butterworth & Co., Borough Green, Sevenoaks, Kent TN15 8PH, England

1375 Cadmos (Gruppo Editoriale Cadmos), Via L. da Viagana 9, I-20122 Milan, Italy

1376 Editions de Chabassol, 30 rue de Gramont, F-75002 Paris, France

1377 Chadwyck-Healey Ltd, 20 Newmarket Road, Cambridge CB5 8DT, England

1378 Churchill Livingstone, Robert Stevenson House, 1–3 Baxters Place, Leith Walk, Edinburgh EH1 3AF, Scotland

1379 Council for Postgraduate Medical Education, 7 Marylebone Road, London NW1 5HH, England

1380 Chroma Inc., 5323 Brainerd Road, Chattanooga, Tennessee 37411, USA

1381 CRC Press Inc., 2000 Corporate Boulevard NW, Boca Raton, Florida 33431, USA

1382 Datapharm Publications, 12 Whitehall, London SW1A 2DY, England

1383 Marcel Dekker Inc., 270 Madison Avenue, New York, NY 10016, USA

1384 Demeter Verlag, D-8032 Grafeling, German Federal Republic

1385 Department of Health and Social Security, Leaflets, PO Box 21, Stanmore, Middlesex HA7 1AY, England

1386 Deutsche Arzte Verlag, Postfach 40 04 40, D-5000 Cologne 40, German Federal Republic

1387 Dumont Buchverlag, Apostelnkloster 21–25, D-5000 Cologne 1, German Federal Republic

1388 Editoriale Scientifica, Via Chiamone 60B, I-80121 Naples, Italy

1389 Elsevier Science Publishers, PO Box 211, NL-1000 AE Amsterdam, Netherlands

1390 Faber & Faber, 3 Queen Square, London WC1N 3AU, England

1391 Greenwood Press, 88 Post Road West, Westport, Connecticut 06881, USA

1392 G. K. Hall, 70 Lincoln Street, Boston, Massachusetts 02111, USA

1393 Carl Hanser Verlag, Kolbergerstrasse 22, Postfach 86 04 20, D-8000 Munich 80, German Federal Republic

1394 Heinemann Medical Books, 22 Bedford Square, London WC1B 3HH, England

1395 HMSO (Her Majesty's Stationery Office), Atlantic House, Holborn Viaduct, London EC1P 1BN, England

1396 Hobsons Press (Cambridge), Bateman Street, Cambridge CB2 1LZ, England

1397 Huthig Esco, 1405 North Main Street, San Antonio, Texas, USA

1398 A. Huthig Verlag, Postfach 10 28 69, D-6900 Heidelberg 1, German Federal Republic

1399 Institute for Scientific Information, 3501 Market Street, University City Science Center, Philadelphia, Pennsylvania 19104,USA

1400 Interamericana Ltda, Rua Coronel Cabrita 8, San Cristovao, CP 21176, 20920 Rio de Janeiro, Brazil

1401 Ishiyaku Publishers, 7–10 Honkomagome-1, Bunkyo-Ku, Tokyo, Japan

1402 S. Karger, PO Box, CH-4009 Basle, Switzerland.

1403 King Edward's Hospital Fund for London (King's Fund), 126 Albert Street, London NW1 7NF, England

1404 Lea & Febiger, 600 South Washington Square, Philadelphia, Pennsylvania 19106, USA

1405 J. Libbey & Co., 80–84 Bondway, London SW8 1SF, England

1406 J. B. Lippincott, PO Box 1430, East Washington Square, Philadelphia, Pennsylvania 19105, USA

1407 Maloine SA, 27 rue de l'Ecole de Médecine, F-75006 Paris, France

1408 Masson SA, 120 Boulevard St. Germain, F-75280 Paris, France

1409 Masson Italia Editori, Via G. Pascoli 55, I-20133 Milan, Italy

1410 Masson Italia Periodici, Via Pinturicchio 1, I-20133 Milan, Italy

1411 Medica Verlag, Reutlingerstrasse 13, Stuttgart Degerloch, German Federal Republic

1412 MEDSI (Médecine et Sciences Internationales), 31 rue Falguiere, F-75015 Paris, France

1413 Microinfo, PO Box 3, Alton, Hampshire GU34 2PG, England

1414 Minerva Medica, Corso Bramante 83, I-10126 Torino, Italy

1415 A. E. Morgan, Stanley House, 9 West Street, Epsom, Ewell, Surrey KT18 7RL, England

1416 C. V. Mosby Co., 11830 Westline Industrial Drive, St. Louis, Missouri 63141, USA

1417 Munksgaard International Publishers, 35 Norre Sogade, DK-1370 Copenhagen K, Denmark

1418 Noyes Data Corporation, Mill Road, Grand Avenue, Park Ridge, New Jersey 07656, USA

1419 Nueva Editorial Interamericana, Cedro 512, Apartado 26370, Mexico 4DF, Mexico

1420 Oxford University Press, Walton Street, Oxford OX2 6DP, England

1421 Pennwell Books, PO Box 1260, Tulsa, Oklahoma 74101, USA

1422 Pergamon Press, Headington Hill Hall, Oxford OX3 0BW, England

1423 Piccin Editore, Via Brunnacci 12, I-35100 Padua, Italy

1424 Praeger Publishers, 521 5th Avenue, New York, NY 10175, USA

1425 Julien Prelat, 17 rue du Petit Pont, F-75005 Paris, France

1426 Quintessence Publishing Co., Suite 2301, 8 South Michigan Avenue, Chicago, Illinois 60603, USA

1427 Quintessenz Verlag, 2–4 Ifenpfad, D-1000 Berlin 42, German Federal Republic

1428 Raven Press, 1140 Avenue of the Americas, New York, NY 10036, USA

1429 W. B. Saunders Co., W. Washington Square, Philadelphia, Pennsylvania 19105, USA

1430 Saccardin, Via Franceschini 3, I-40128 Bologna, Italy

1431 Scienza e Technica Dentistica, Via Capecelatro 75, I-20148 Milan, Italy

1432 SEU (Società Editricé Universo), Via Morgagni 1, I-00161 Rome, Italy

1433 Shorin Co., Sankyo Building, 11–5 Tidabashi, 3 Chome, Chiyoda-ku, Tokyo, Japan

1434 Société d'Edition de l'Information Dentaire, 42 rue Vignon, F-75009 Paris, France

1435 G. Thieme Verlag, Rudigerstrasse 14, Postfach 732, D-7000 Stuttgart 1, German Federal Republic

1436 C. C. Thomas, 2600 South First Street, Springfield, Illinois 62717, USA

1437 University Microfilms International, 300 North Zeeb Road, Ann Arbor, Michigan 48105, USA

1438 Urban & Schwarzenberg, Pettenkoferstrasse 18, D-8000 Munich 2, German Federal Republic

1439 Verduci, Via Gregorio VIII 132, I-00165 Rome, Italy

1440 Volk und Gesundheit, Neuer Grunstrasse 18, Postfach 53, 1020 Berlin, German Democratic Republic

1441 Westview Press, 5500 Central Avenue, Boulder, Colorado 80301, USA

1442 John Wiley & Sons, 605 3rd Avenue, New York, NY 10158, USA

1443 Williams & Wilkins, 428 East Preston Street, Baltimore, Maryland 21202, USA

1444 John Wright & Sons, 823–825 Bath Road, Bristol BS4 5NU, England

1445 Verlag Zahnärztlich-medizinisches Schrifttum, Insterburgerstrasse 2, Postfach 81 05 09, D-8000 Munich 81, German Federal Republic

Index

Numbers in square brackets refer to items in Parts II and III. Numbers without brackets refer to pages in Part I.